# Ion and Molecule Transport in Lysosomes

# Methods in Signal Transduction

*Series Editors*
*Joseph Eichberg, Jr. and Michael X. Zhu*

The overall theme of this series continues to be the presentation of the wealth of up to date research methods applied to the many facets of signal transduction. Each volume is assembled by one or more editors who are pre-eminent in their specialty. In turn, the guiding principle for editors is to recruit chapter authors who will describe procedures and protocols with which they are intimately familiar in a reader-friendly format. The intent is to assure that each volume will be of maximum practical value to a broad audience, including students and researchers just entering an area, as well as seasoned investigators.

**Signaling by Toll-Like Receptors**
*Gregory W. Konat*

**Lipid-Mediated Signaling**
*Eric J. Murphy and Thad A. Rosenberger*

**TRP Channels**
*Michael Xi Zhu*

**Cyclic Nucleotide Signaling**
*Xiaodong Cheng*

**Gap Junction Channels and Hemichannels**
*Donglin Bai and Juan C. Sáez*

**Signaling Mechanisms Regulating T Cell Diversity and Function**
*Jonathan Soboloff and Dietmar J. Kappes*

**Lipid-Mediated Signaling Transduction, Second Edition**
*Eric Murphy, Thad Rosenberger, and Mikhail Golovko*

**Calcium Entry Channels in Non-Excitable Cells**
*Juliusz Ashot Kozak and James W. Putney, Jr.*

**Autophagy and Signaling**
*Esther Wong*

**Signal Transduction and Smooth Muscle**
*Mohamed Trebak and Scott Earley*

**Polycystic Kidney Disease**
*Jinghua Hu and Yong Yu*

**New Techniques for Studying Biomembranes**
*Qiu-Xing Jiang*

**Ion and Molecule Transport in Lysosomes**
*Bruno Gasnier and Michael X. Zhu*

# Ion and Molecule
# Transport in Lysosomes

Edited by
## Bruno Gasnier and Michael X. Zhu

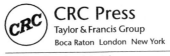

CRC Press
Taylor & Francis Group
Boca Raton  London  New York

CRC Press is an imprint of the
Taylor & Francis Group, an **informa** business

First edition published 2020
by CRC Press
6000 Broken Sound Parkway NW, Suite 300, Boca Raton, FL 33487-2742

and by CRC Press
2 Park Square, Milton Park, Abingdon, Oxon, OX14 4RN

First issued in paperback 2021

Typeset in Times
by Deanta Global Publishing Services, Chennai, India

ISBN 13: 978-1-138-56039-0 (hbk)
ISBN 13: 978-1-03-224115-9 (pbk)

DOI: 10.1201/b22460

Publisher's Note
The publisher has gone to great lengths to ensure the quality of this reprint but points out that some imperfections in the original copies may be apparent.

# Contents

# Editors

**Bruno Gasnier** is a senior scientist at the French National Center for Scientific Research (CNRS) and a group leader at the Saints-Pères Paris Institute for the Neurosciences (SPPIN), Université de Paris, France. He studied at the École Normale Supérieure in Paris from 1980 to 1985 and received his M.S. and Ph.D. degrees in molecular pharmacology from Pierre and Marie Curie University (now Sorbonne University), Paris, France, in 1982 and 1985, respectively. After a postdoctoral training in yeast biochemistry at the Instituto Gulbenkian de Ciência, Oeiras, Portugal, he joined the Institut de Biologie Physico-Chimique in Paris as a CNRS scientist in 1988. He started there his independent research work in 1994 and earned a senior scientist position in 2002. In 2011, he moved his lab to its current place at the University of Paris, Campus Saint-Germain-des-Prés. Dr. Gasnier's research interests cover the compartmentalization of eukaryotic cells and the dynamics of membrane-bound organelles, including the filling of synaptic vesicles with neurotransmitters and the export of metabolites from lysosomes. His studies have identified and/or characterized several organellar transporters, including their participation in human diseases. He served as a director of CNRS research units (alike departments) in 2005–2008 and 2014–2018. He has chaired or co-chaired several international conferences, including the 3rd Gordon Research Conference on Organellar Channels and Transporters, Vermont, 2019.

**Michael Xi Zhu** is a professor in the Department of Integrative Biology and Pharmacology, McGovern Medical School, The University of Texas Health Science Center at Houston, Houston, Texas. He received his B.S. degree in Biology from Fudan University, Shanghai, China, in 1984, and his M.S. and Ph.D. degrees from University of Houston, Houston, Texas, in 1988 and 1991, respectively. He had his postdoctoral training in Cellular and Molecular Biology from 1991–1994 at Baylor College of Medicine, Houston, Texas. He then worked as an Assistant Researcher in the Department of Anesthesiology, UCLA, California, from 1994 to 1997. In autumn of 1997, he went to the Ohio State University to build his own lab and moved from the rank of assistant professor to full professor in the Department of Neuroscience there. In 2010, he moved to his current position at the University of Texas-Houston. Dr. Zhu's research interests include several aspects of cell signaling, especially those that involve heterotrimeric G proteins and ion channels that affect $Ca^{2+}$ signaling. He has published more than 150 research papers, reviews, and monographs on these topics and delivered lectures at many international conferences and symposia. His main contributions include identification and characterization of multiple TRPC channels in mammalian species and determination of the molecular identity of endolysosomal $Ca^{2+}$ release channels activated by the $Ca^{2+}$ mobilizing messenger, NAADP. He currently serves on editorial boards of *Journal of Cellular Physiology*, *Pflügers Archiv*, *Biophysics Reports*, *Cells*, and *Molecular Pharmacology*. He also serves as a series editor of the CRC Methods in Signal Transduction book series. He has chaired or co-chaired several international conferences, including the 17th

International Symposium on $Ca^{2+}$-Binding Proteins and $Ca^{2+}$ Function in Health and Disease, Beijing, 2011, and the 2nd Gordon Research Conference on Organellar Channels and Transporters, Vermont, 2017. He served as a regular member of the US NIH Molecular and Integrative Signal Transduction study section from 2010–2014.

# Contributors

**Matthias R. Baumgartner**
University Children's Hospital
Zurich, Switzerland

**Martin Biel**
Ludwig-Maximilians-Universität
  München
Munich, Germany

**Anja Blessing**
Leibniz-Forschungsinstitut für
  Molekulare Pharmakologie (FMP)
and
Max Delbrück Centrum für Molekulare
  Medizin (MDC),
Berlin, Germany

**Cheng-Chang Chen**
Ludwig-Maximilians-Universität
  München
Munich, Germany

**Guangwei Du**
University of Texas Health Sciences
  Center at Houston
Houston, Texas

**Anne-Marie Ellegaard**
Danish Cancer Society Research Center
Copenhagen, Denmark

**Sean Froese**
University Children's Hospital
Zurich, Switzerland

**Bruno Gasnier**
Université de Paris, SPPIN – Saints-
  Pères Paris Institute for the
  Neurosciences
Paris, France

**Christian Grimm**
Ludwig-Maximilians-Universität
  München
Munich, Germany

**Line Groth-Pedersen**
Danish Cancer Society Research Center
Copenhagen, Denmark

**Mingxue Gu**
University of Michigan
Ann Arbor, Michigan

**Salwa Y. Hafez**
Brown University
Providence, Rhode Island

**Jingquan He**
University of Texas Health Sciences
  Center at Houston
Houston, Texas

**Meiqin Hu**
University of Michigan
Ann Arbor, Michigan
and
Zhejiang University of Technology
Hangzhou, China

**Marja Jäättelä**
Danish Cancer Society Research Center
Copenhagen, Denmark

**Thomas J. Jentsch**
Leibniz-Forschungsinstitut für
  Molekulare Pharmakologie (FMP)
and
Max Delbrück Centrum für Molekulare
  Medizin (MDC)
Berlin, Germany

**Nicholas E. Karagas**
University of Texas Health Sciences
  Center at Houston
Houston, Texas

**Jeffrey J. Kelu**
Hong Kong University of Science and
  Technology
Hong Kong, China

**Donald C. Koroma**
Brown University
Providence, Rhode Island

**Xavier Leray**
Université d'Angers
Angers, France

**Andrew L. Miller**
Hong Kong University of Science and
  Technology
Hong Kong, China

**Elena Oancea**
Brown University
Providence, Rhode Island

**Morgan A. Rousseau**
University of Texas Health Sciences
  Center at Houston
Houston, Texas

**Corinne Sagné**
Université de Paris, SPPIN – Saints-
  Pères Paris Institute for the
  Neurosciences
Paris, France

**Sonali Saha**
Leibniz-Forschungsinstitut für
  Molekulare Pharmakologie (FMP)
and
Max Delbrück Centrum für Molekulare
  Medizin (MDC)
Berlin, Germany

**Kartik Venkatachalam**
University of Texas Health Sciences
  Center at Houston
Houston, Texas

**Christian Wahl-Schott**
Ludwig-Maximilians-Universität
  München
Munich, Germany

**Sarah E. Webb**
Hong Kong University of Science and
  Technology
Hong Kong, China

**Jian Xiong**
University of Texas Health Sciences
  Center at Houston
Houston, Texas

**Haoxing Xu**
University of Michigan
Ann Arbor, Michigan

**Yexin Yang**
University of Michigan
Ann Arbor, Michigan

**Xiaoli Zhang**
University of Michigan
Ann Arbor, Michigan

**Michael X. Zhu**
University of Texas Health Sciences
  Center at Houston
Houston, Texas

# 1 Endosomal and Lysosomal Electrophysiology

*Xiaoli Zhang, Mingxue Gu, Meiqin Hu,*
*Yexin Yang, and Haoxing Xu*

## CONTENTS

## 1.1 INTRODUCTION

Lysosomes, acidic organelles containing more than 60 types of hydrolytic enzymes in the lumen, were traditionally viewed as the "digestion centre" of the cell "passively" involved in the digestion and recycling of cellular macromolecules (Kolter and Sandhoff, 2005; Perera and Zoncu, 2016). A more "active" signal transduction role of lysosomes has recently been discovered, and lysosomes are now known to regulate biomaterial recycling, membrane trafficking, catabolite export, nutrient sensing, and energy homeostasis (Perera and Zoncu, 2016; Xu and Ren, 2015). The mechanistic target of rapamycin (mTOR), the primary nutrient sensor in the cell, is found to be localized on the lysosomal membrane to regulate various lysosomal functions (Zoncu et al., 2011). The ionic composition of the lysosome lumen plays an essential role in both "digestive" and "signalling" functions of the lysosome (Xiong and Zhu, 2016; Xu and Ren, 2015). For instance, the 1,000–5,000 fold concentration gradients for $H^+$ and $Ca^{2+}$ in the lumen vs. cytosol are required for both degradation and nutrient-dependent signal transduction of lysosomes (Xu and Ren, 2015). Lysosomal ion homeostasis is established and maintained by lysosomal ion channels and transporters that mediate ionic flux across the lysosomal membranes in response to various cellular cues that are derived from either the cytoplasm or the lysosome lumen (Perera and Zoncu, 2016; Xu and Ren, 2015). Dysregulation of lysosomal ion flux leads to a lysosome storage phenotype with the characteristic accumulation of enlarged vacuoles, cellular wastes, and lipofuscin in the cell (Ferreira and Gahl, 2017; Kolter and Sandhoff, 2005; Xu and Ren, 2015).

Unlike their plasma membrane counterparts, ion channels and transporters localized on the intracellular membranes have been inaccessible for conventional electrophysiology, e.g., the patch-clamp method, in studying their ionic selectivity and gating/modulation mechanisms (Xu et al., 2015). The primary challenge is that the size of lysosomes, typically 100–500 nm in diameter, is sub-optimal for patch clamping (Xu et al., 2015). Early studies of lysosomal channels relied on liposome reconstitution or cell surface re-routing that allows examination of intracellular channels using the whole-cell patch-clamp technique (Arai et al., 1993; Sawada et al., 2008). However, the non-native membrane environment (e.g., the lack of lysosome-specific phospholipids and interacting proteins) has limited the physiological studies of lysosomal membranes and channels (Xu et al., 2015). In contrast, the development of the whole-endolysosome patch-clamp technique on artificially enlarged endolysosomes has allowed direct studies of lysosomal channels in a more "native" environment under more "physiological" conditions (Dong et al., 2008; Schieder et al., 2010; Xiong and Zhu, 2016; Xu and Ren, 2015). Hence, a new avenue has been opened for lysosomal channel research, which provides a promising platform for the discovery of new lysosomal channels and their cellular modulators (Dong et al., 2008; Schieder et al., 2010; Xiong and Zhu, 2016; Xu and Ren, 2015). In this chapter, we describe detailed protocols of endosomal and lysosomal electrophysiology and discuss several examples of lysosomal channels that have been characterized using this method.

## 1.2 LYSOSOMAL IONIC COMPOSITION

The lysosome lumen contains $H^+$, $Na^+$, $K^+$, $Ca^{2+}$, and $Cl^-$ (Mindell, 2012; Morgan et al., 2011; Xu and Ren, 2015). With the exceptions of $H^+$ and $Ca^{2+}$, luminal concentrations of other ions have not been accurately determined (Xu and Ren, 2015). Indeed, it remains controversial whether lysosomes are $Na^+$ or $K^+$ enriched compartments (Steinberg et al., 2010; Wang et al., 2012). Given that lysosomes constantly undergo membrane fusion or fission with other intracellular membrane compartments, the ionic compositions are likely heterogeneous for individual lysosomes. For example, peripheral lysosomes are less acidic than the perinuclear lysosomes (Johnson et al., 2016), suggesting that lysosomal positioning may affect the luminal ionic composition. Likewise, the primary and terminal lysosomes are likely $Na^+$-dominant, whereas secondary lysosomes (e.g., the newly formed autolysosomes) may have a much lower luminal $Na^+$ concentration due to the prior fusion with the cytosol-generated $K^+$-dominant autophagosomes (Xu and Ren, 2015). Furthermore, due to the small volume of individual lysosomes, ion flux mediated by transient openings of organellar channels may be sufficient to cause drastic changes in the luminal ionic composition (Xu et al., 2015; Xu and Ren, 2015).

$H^+$: A hallmark feature of the lysosome is its acidic pH (pH 4.6) in the lumen, which is required for the activity of most lysosome hydrolases (Kolter and Sandhoff, 2005; Mindell, 2012). During endosome maturation, the V-ATPase is responsible for decreasing luminal pH from 6.5 in early endosomes to 4.6 in late endosomes and lysosomes (LELs) (Huotari and Helenius, 2011). Disruption of lysosomal pH gradient using V-ATPase inhibitors (e.g., bafilomycin-A1) or protonophores results in accumulation of the endocytic and autophagic cargos (Kawai et al., 2007; Padman et al., 2013). In addition, lysosomal pH or V-ATPase regulates other lysosomal functions, including autophagosome-lysosome fusion (Kawai et al., 2007; Mauvezin and Neufeld, 2015) and nutrient sensing (Zoncu et al., 2011).

$Na^+/K^+$: The lysosome lumen was thought to be high in $K^+$, but low in $Na^+$, suggesting that like endoplasmic reticulum (ER), there are no significant concentration gradients of $Na^+$ or $K^+$ across lysosomal membranes (Morgan et al., 2011; Steinberg et al., 2010; Xu and Ren, 2015). This view has been challenged by several recent lysosomal physiological studies. First, whole-endolysosome recordings have revealed the presence of multiple $Na^+$-selective and $K^+$-selective channels in the lysosome (Cang et al., 2015; Cao et al., 2015b; Wang et al., 2017; Wang et al., 2012). Second, isolated lysosomes, like the extracellular space, may contain high concentrations of $Na^+$ (i.e., >100 mM) (Wang et al., 2012). The ion transporters that are required to establish the $Na^+$ gradient are not known. Importantly, activation of $Na^+$ and $K^+$-selective channels may rapidly change lysosome membrane potential ($\Delta\psi$, defined as $\Delta\psi = \psi_{cytosol} - \psi_{lumen}$), which may be required for various lysosomal functions, such as catabolite export (Cang et al., 2013) and $Ca^{2+}$ import (Wang et al., 2017).

$Ca^{2+}$: $[Ca^{2+}]_{lumen}$ (~0.5 mM) is about 5,000 times higher than $[Ca^{2+}]_{cyto}$ (100 nM). Hence, like ER, lysosomes are recognized as important intracellular $Ca^{2+}$ stores (Yang et al., 2018). The uptake/import mechanisms that maintain such high $Ca^{2+}$ gradient across lysosomal membranes are not clear (Yang et al., 2018). Many lysosomal functions, including lysosomal membrane trafficking and lysosome biogenesis, are reportedly regulated by lysosomal $Ca^{2+}$ through various downstream $Ca^{2+}$ effectors, such as synaptotagmin VII, ALG-2, calcineurin, and calmodulin (Chu et al., 2015; Li et al., 2016a; Li et al., 2016b; Medina et al., 2015). $Ca^{2+}$-permeable channels in the lysosome mediate lysosomal $Ca^{2+}$ release in response to changes in nutrient availability, redox status, and lipid abundance (Cao et al., 2015a; Dong et al., 2010; Shen et al., 2012; Xiong and Zhu, 2016; Xu and Ren, 2015; Zhang et al., 2016).

$Cl^-$: Lysosomes also store high concentrations of $[Cl^-]_{lumen}$ (Chakraborty et al., 2017), which are connected with the luminal pH, presumably through the $Cl^-$ and $H^+$-dependent transporter CLC7 (Graves et al., 2008; Jentsch, 2007; Neagoe et al., 2010).

## 1.3 LYSOSOMAL ION CHANNELS

Lysosomal ion channels (LICs) include those that reside primarily on LELs, e.g., TRPML1–TRPML3, TPC1–TPC2, and TMEM175, the so-called "committed" lysosomal channels, as well as plasma membrane channels that are also localized in the lysosomes, i.e., the large conductance $Ca^{2+}$- and voltage-activated $K^+$ (BK) channels and P2X4 puringergic receptors/channels, referred to as "non-committed" lysosomal channels (Figure 1.1) (Cang et al., 2015; Cang et al., 2013; Cao et al., 2015a; Cao et al., 2015b; Cheng et al., 2010; Wang et al., 2017; Wang et al., 2012; Xiong and Zhu, 2016). Lysosome-targeting trafficking motifs, e.g., double leucine (LL) motifs, are required for the highly specific expression of LICs in the lysosome (Bonifacino and Traub, 2003; Xu and Ren, 2015). Both "committed" and "non-committed" LICs, regardless of their primary locations in the cell, display significant endogenous currents in the lysosome (Xiong and Zhu, 2016). Importantly, genetic or pharmacological inhibition of the known lysosomal channels impairs lysosome function to cause lysosome storage disease (LSD)-like phenotypes in the cell (Wang et al., 2017; Xiong and Zhu, 2016; Xu and Ren, 2015).

### 1.3.1 LYSOSOMAL CA²⁺ CHANNELS

Transient receptor potential mucolipins (TRPML1–TRPML3) are principal $Ca^{2+}$ release channels in the lysosome (Cheng et al., 2010; Xu and Ren, 2015). Whereas TRPML2 and TRPML3 are also present in early and recycling endosomes; all three TRPMLs are highly expressed in LELs (Cheng et al., 2010; Grimm et al., 2017). TRPML1 is most extensively studied, as loss-of-function mutations of TRPML1 cause type IV mucolipidosis (ML-IV) in humans, an autosomal recessive LSD that shows neurodegeneration, motor impairment, and retinal defects (Cheng et al., 2010; Grimm et al., 2017). Since potent TRPML1 agonists trigger lysosomal $Ca^{2+}$ release and promote the clearance of cellular waste, TRPML1 has become a potential therapeutic target for many lysosomal diseases, including Niemann–Pick disease type C (Shen et al., 2012; Wang et al., 2015; Xu and Ren, 2015).

TRPML1 was the first lysosomal channel studied using whole-endolysosome recordings, the use of which quickly led to the discovery of phosphatidylinositol 3,5-bisphosphate ($PI(3,5)P_2$) as the endogenous agonist for TRPMLs (Dong et al., 2010) and $PI(4,5)P_2$ and sphingomyelin as the endogenous inhibitors of TRPML1 (Shen et al., 2012; Zhang et al., 2012) (Figure 1.1). TRPML1 currents are also potentiated by acidic pH (Dong et al., 2008), likely through three aspartate residues in the luminal pore region (Li et al., 2017). Hence, the channel activity of TRPML1 is potentiated by lysosome-specific cellular cues, conferring lysosome-specific cell biological functions of TRPML1 (Xu and Ren, 2015).

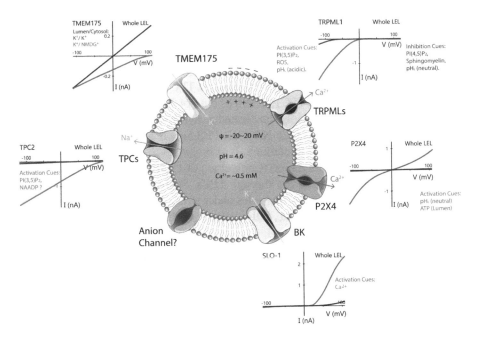

**FIGURE 1.1** Lysosomal ion channels (LICs): ionic selectivity and gating by cellular cues. Lysosomal $Ca^{2+}$-permeable channels include TRPMLs and $P2X_4$. TRPML1 is activated by lysosomal membrane $PI(3,5)P_2$ and cellular ROS, and $P2X_4$ is regulated by luminal ATP and pH. Two major $K^+$-selective LICs are TMEM175 and BK. TPCs are lysosomal $Na^+$-selective channels that are activated by $PI(3,5)P_2$, and possibly NAADP.

TRPML1 is also a lysosomal sensor of reactive oxygen species (ROS) that is required for lysosomal adaptation (i.e., changes in lysosome function) to oxidative stress (Zhang et al., 2016). TRPML1 itself is a substrate of the transcriptional factor EB (TFEB), a master regulator of autophagosome and lysosome biogenesis (Settembre et al., 2011; Settembre et al., 2013). Activation of TFEB (dephosphorylated and translocated from the cytosol to the nucleus) under stress conditions, such as nutrient-deprivation and oxidative stress, may increase the expression levels of TRPML1 (Wang et al., 2015; Zhang et al., 2016). On the other hand, TRPML1-mediated lysosomal $Ca^{2+}$ release may activate TFEB through the $Ca^{2+}$-calcineurin pathway (Medina et al., 2015; Zhang et al., 2016). Thus, TRPML1 and TFEB may form a positive feedback loop that is activated by various cellular stresses for the purpose of lysosomal adaptation (Medina et al., 2015; Wang et al., 2015; Xu and Ren, 2015).

### 1.3.2 Lysosomal Na⁺ Channels

Mammalian two-pore channels (TPC1, 2), constituted by two 12 transmembrane subunits (She et al., 2018), are predominantly localized on early endosomes and LELs (Calcraft et al., 2009). TPC2 is believed by many investigators to mediate the NAADP-induced lysosomal $Ca^{2+}$ release, based on $Ca^{2+}$ imaging studies (Calcraft et al., 2009; Grimm et al., 2017; Ruas et al., 2015). However, later whole-endolysosome studies

#### 1.4.1.4   Limitations of Current Lysosomal Patch-Clamp Methods

Although whole-endolysosome recordings provide a direct analysis of lysosomal membranes, one should be aware that the recording conditions are quite simplified compared to intact cells. First, genetically or chemically enlarged vacuoles may contain membranes from non-lysosomal intracellular organelles (Wang et al., 2017). Second, the endolysosome enlargement process may result in changes of membrane lipid composition. Third, the lysosome isolation process may also cause a loss of interaction proteins and cytosolic factors. Fourth, the ionic environments are determined by pipette and bath solutions, but the real ionic compositions of lysosomes have not been accurately determined (Wang et al., 2012). Hence, complementary approaches are necessary to validate the conclusions that are drawn based on the whole-endolysosome patch-clamp method.

#### 1.4.2   Optical Imaging of Lysosomal Physiology

The transport of many ions, such as $Ca^{2+}$, $Na^+$, $K^+$, $H^+$, and $Cl^-$, across lysosomal membranes can also be analyzed using ion-sensitive dyes or genetically engineered ionic indicators (Chakraborty et al., 2017; Xu et al., 2015). In addition, voltage-sensitive dyes and protein sensors can be developed to study lysosomal $\Delta\psi$ regulation (Koivusalo et al., 2011).

#### 1.4.2.1   Chemical Ion Indicators

Ion-sensitive fluorescent dyes are often utilized to measure cytosolic or luminal concentrations of ions, with $Ca^{2+}$ dyes being the most well developed (Morgan et al., 2015). The emission intensity ratio (F340/F380) of the Fura-2 dye can be used to detect the synchronized $Ca^{2+}$ release from lysosomes (Morgan et al., 2015). Fluorescence dyes for $Na^+$, $K^+$, and $Cl^-$ have also been developed, but accurate calibrations of these dyes have proven to be difficult (Christensen et al., 2002; Garrity et al., 2016; Morgan et al., 2011). Whereas an increase in cytosolic $Ca^{2+}$ upon lysosome stimulation is suggestive of lysosomal $Ca^{2+}$ release, a more direct way is to measure the lysosomal luminal $Ca^{2+}$ content using luminal $Ca^{2+}$ dyes, such as Oregon Green Dextran 488 BAPTA (Morgan et al., 2015; Wang et al., 2017). Dextran is a large molecule that will be endocytosed and transported into lysosomes over time. A common challenge for luminal $Ca^{2+}$ measurement is that most ion-sensitive dyes are also pH sensitive (Garrity et al., 2016). As a result, a large portion of the presumed-to-be $Ca^{2+}$ signal might be contaminated by changes in luminal pH (Garrity et al., 2016; Wang et al., 2017).

#### 1.4.2.2   Genetically Encoded Ion Indicators

Compared to $Ca^{2+}$ dyes, genetically encoded $Ca^{2+}$ indicators (GECIs) have the advantage of precise organelle-targeting (Garrity et al., 2016). GECIs usually consist of a calcium-binding domain (e.g., calmodulin), fused to one or two fluorescent proteins. By linking GECIs, such as GCaMPs and GECOs, onto the N-terminal (facing cytosol) of the lysosomal $Ca^{2+}$-release channel TRPML1, real-time observation of $Ca^{2+}$ efflux from lysosomes through TRPML1 has been achieved (Shen et al., 2012; Yang et al., 2018). GCaMP3-TRPML1 has proven to be helpful in confirming the agonists identified in the lysosomal electrophysiology (Shen et al., 2012; Wang et al., 2015). Tissue-specific GCaMP3-TPRML1 knock-in mice have been generated and utilized to investigate the *in vivo* roles of TRPML1 (Sahoo et al., 2017). A caveat of GCaMP3 is its high affinity. Hence, GCaMP3-TPRML1 may also detect $Ca^{2+}$ release from other compartments (Shen et al., 2012). It is possible that low-affinity cytosolic GECIs may allow a more specific detection of lysosomal $Ca^{2+}$ release. However, in the intact cells, $Ca^{2+}$ release from the lysosomes is likely to be very small (Yang et al., 2018), so a low-affinity probe may not be efficient in detecting lysosomal $Ca^{2+}$ release. Another potential pitfall for lysosome-targeted GECIs is that they are also pH sensitive (Garrity et al., 2016; Wang et al., 2017), and many cellular cues are known to induce both $Ca^{2+}$ release and $H^+$ release from the lysosomes (Morgan et al., 2015).

## 1.5  PROTOCOL OF ENDOLYSOSOMAL PATCH CLAMP

### 1.5.1  RECORDING SOLUTIONS

For most whole-endolysosome recordings, the bath (internal or cytosolic) solution contains (in mM): 145 K-gluconate, 4 NaCl, 2 $MgCl_2$, 20 HEPES, 1 EGTA, 0.39 $CaCl_2$ (free $Ca^{2+}$ is estimated to be ~100 nM with MaxChelator), pH adjusted to 7.2 with KOH, and the osmolality adjusted to 290 mOsm. When necessary, 2 mM ATP and 0.3 mM GTP are added into the solution. Pipette (luminal) solution contains (in mM): 145 NaCl, 5 KCl, 2 $CaCl_2$, 1 $MgCl_2$, 10 glucose, 10 MES, 10 HEPES, and pH adjusted to 4.6 with HCl (osmolality = 300 mOsm).

### 1.5.2  EQUIPMENT

Conventional electrophysiological setups are used, which include a micropipette puller, a microforge, an air table, an inverted microscope, a patch-clamp amplifier, a digitizer, a multi micromanipulator, and a solution-exchange perfusion system. Data are acquired with an Axopatch 200B patch-clamp amplifier and a Digidata 1440 digitizer, which are controlled by the pClamp 10.0 software (Axon Instruments).

### 1.5.3  WHOLE-ENDOLYSOSOMAL RECORDING PROCEDURES

Whole-endolysosomal recordings are performed on vacuolin-1 enlarged LELs that are mechanically isolated (Dong et al., 2008; Wang et al., 2012). Below is the step-by-step protocol for lysosomal recordings on Cos-1 cells that are transfected with EGFP-TRPML1.

**Step 1: Transfection**
  A. Cos-1 cells are cultured with high glucose DMEM medium supplemented with 10% fetal bovine serum at 37°C under 5% $CO_2$.
  B. Cells are split into a 35-mm dish the day before transfection in a density that will reach 60–70% confluence on the transfection day.
  C. EGFP-TRPML1 plasmid (in pEGFP vector) is transfected with a Lipofectamine™ 2000 (Thermo Fisher) system. Briefly, 1.5–2 µg plasmid

of EGFP-TRPML1 is mixed with 200 μl of Opti-MEM™ (solution A) and 5 μl of Lipofectamine™ 2000 reagent is mixed with another 200 μl of Opti-MEM™ (solution B). After standing for 5 min, solution A is mixed with solution B, and 20 min later, the transfection mixture is transferred into the 35-mm culture dish prepared in step B, containing 1.6 ml of fresh culture medium (final volume = 2 ml).

**D.** 12 h after transfection, Cos-1 cells are re-plated onto poly-L-lysine coated coverslips.

## Step 2: Enlargement of LELs

At 24–36 h after transfection, 1 μM vacuolin-1 (Cerny et al., 2004) is added to the transfected Cos-1 cells for 1–12 h. The enlarged LELs of 1–5 μm in diameter are subject to recording. Note that the concentration and treatment time of vacuolin-1 need to be optimized for each individual cell types.

## Step 3: Preparation of Glass Electrodes

Glass electrodes are made from glass capillaries (World Precision Instruments, 1B150F-4) in a micropipette puller (Sutter Instrument Co., P97). The pulling protocol is optimized to obtain electrodes with a tip diameter of 0.5–0.9 μm and a resistance of 9–11 MΩ. Glass electrodes are slightly polished before recording.

## Step 4: Whole-Endolysosomal Patch Clamp

**A.** On the day of the experiment, coverslips are transferred into a recording chamber and bathed with the internal solution. EGFP-positive vacuoles are monitored under a fluorescent microscope. Once an enlarged vacuole with bright green fluorescence is selected, a glass electrode is used to tear the cell membrane apart to release the vacuole for recording (Wang et al., 2012).

**B.** The electrode is filled with the pipette solution and applied with a positive pressure (~5cm $H_2O$) before entering the bath solution in the recording chamber.

**C.** The voltage offset of the pipette is adjusted to 0 mV after being immersed into the bath solution. The resistance is monitored with a 5 mV step pulse (Figure 1.2).

**D.** The electrode is pushed against the isolated vacuole under the control of a micromanipulator until it slightly touches the vacuole membrane. A negative pressure is applied in order to form a gigaseal (5–20 GΩ). The pipette resistance and capacitance are compensated.

**E.** A voltage protocol is used to break-in the vacuole membrane (Figure 1.2). Briefly, three voltage pulses are sequentially applied with 2 ms intervals. The first pulse is used for break-in, and its voltage and duration are tailored for each individual vacuole. In general, it starts with a pulse of 400 mV of 1 ms, then the voltage and duration are gradually increased until break-in. The second and the third pulses are for the membrane test: 150 mV for 2 ms and 100 mV for 4 ms, respectively.

**F.** After break-in, the whole-endolysosome configuration is verified by the reappearance of capacitance transients (Figure 1.2). A membrane resistance at GΩ levels usually indicates a good membrane seal. The "inside-out patch" configuration is then set for the whole-endolysosome recording.

G. For voltage-clamp recordings, the holding voltage is set at 0 mV. TRPML1 currents are elicited and recorded with repeated voltage ramps (–140 to +140 mV; 400 ms) every 4 s in interval. All recordings are analyzed in pCLAMP10 (Axon Instruments).

## Step 5: Recordings from Excised Endolysosome Membranes

A. Cytosolic side-out (C/O) patch clamp: after break-in, the glass electrode is slowly pulled away from the vacuole to achieve the C/O patch configuration.

B. Luminal side-out (L/O) patch clamp: the L/O patch configuration is achieved by pulling the pipette from the vacuole after the gigaseal is established. This configuration can be used to study channel modulators in the luminal side. Note that the aforementioned internal solution and luminal solution are used as the pipette and bath solution, respectively.

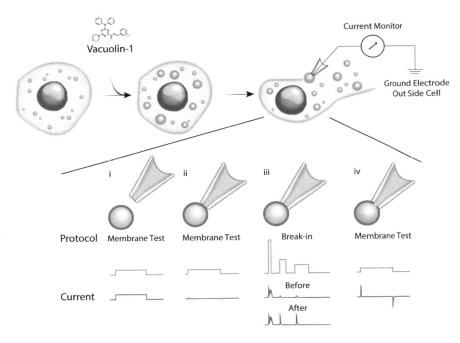

**FIGURE 1.2** Illustration of whole-endolysosome patch-clamp recording. Late endosomes and lysosomes are enlarged by vacuolin-1 and related compounds. After the cell is cut open, a glass electrode is pushed against the targeted isolated vacuole. After a gigaseal is formed, break-in is achieved with a strong voltage pulse. There are four different steps: (i) approach, (ii) seal, (iii) break-in, and (iv) record/verify, each with a voltage protocol (blue lines). The ideal corresponding current responses are shown below (red traces). The membrane test voltage protocol for the approach, seal, and record (verify) steps is composed of test pulses at 5 mV with a 5 ms duration; break-in voltage protocol includes three pulses at 400 mV, 150 mV, and 100 mV, with 1, 2, and 4 ms durations, respectively, at an intra-pulse interval of 2 ms.

## 1.6   ELECTROPHYSIOLOGICAL STUDIES OF LYSOSOME FUNCTION

The cell biological functions of lysosomal ion channels are determined by two basic features of ion channels: selectivity and gating. The $Na^+$- and $K^+$- selectivity of TPC and BK/TMEM175 channels, respectively, suggest that the cellular cues that activate these channels may regulate lysosomal $\Delta\psi$ (Xiong and Zhu, 2016; Xu and Ren, 2015). While activation of TPCs increases lysosomal $\Delta\psi$, opening of BK channels reduces $\Delta\psi$ (Xiong and Zhu, 2016; Xu and Ren, 2015). The changes in lysosomal $\Delta\psi$ may in turn alter the driving forces for the flux of other ions. On the other hand, activation of $Ca^{2+}$-permeable channels in the lysosome may mediate $Ca^{2+}$-dependent functions of lysosomes, e.g., membrane trafficking (Morgan et al., 2011).

Cellular cues that are known to activate lysosomal channels include lysosomal pH, $Ca^{2+}$, lipids, and oxidants (Figure 1.1). Lysosome-localized $PI(3,5)P_2$ activates TRPMLs and TPCs (Dong et al., 2010; Wang et al., 2012), suggesting that $PI(3,5)P_2$ plays an essential role in regulating lysosomal $Ca^{2+}$ signalling and $\Delta\psi$ regulation. Likewise, TPC2 is negatively regulated by mTOR, suggesting that nutrients may regulate lysosomal $\Delta\psi$ through TPC2 (Cang et al., 2013). In addition, ROS may regulate lysosome function by direct activation of TRPML1. Finally, synthetic channel modulators of lysosomal channels may directly regulate lysosome function (Shen et al., 2012; Xu and Ren, 2015). For example, TRPML1 agonists promote autophagy through the $Ca^{2+}$-TFEB pathway, providing new opportunities to treat LSDs (Grimm et al., 2017; Xiong and Zhu, 2016; Xu and Ren, 2015).

## 1.7   PERSPECTIVES AND FUTURE DIRECTIONS

Lysosome membrane proteomics reveals the presence of more than 70 lysosome-enriched ion channel/transporter-like proteins (Chapel et al., 2013; Wyant et al., 2018). Only a subset of them have been characterized using endolysosomal electrophysiology. In the future, we may witness the discovery of many new lysosomal channel and transporters, including the $Ca^{2+}$ import channels/transporters in the lysosome (Garrity et al., 2016). Because artificial ionic conditions are used in the current lysosomal recordings, how $\Delta\psi$ is regulated in the native settings for individual lysosomes is unknown. Genetically encoded voltage sensors are proven to be helpful in monitoring action potentials in neurons. A lysosomal voltage sensor that should be developed to study lysosomal $\Delta\psi$ regulation would need to satisfy at least the three following criteria: excellent lysosome localization, appropriate voltage spectrum with a $V_{1/2}$ at around 0 mV, and a high voltage sensitivity.

Lysosomal channels represent promising therapeutic targets for lysosomal diseases. Activation of TRPML1 has been shown to promote the clearance of accumulated cholesterol in cells from patients with Niemann–Pick disease type C (Wang et al., 2015) and neuronal $A\beta$ in the mouse model of Alzheimer's disease (Bae et al., 2014). Likewise, TPC2 inhibitors have been reported to prevent the infection of Ebola virus (Sakurai et al., 2015). Hence designing or screening lysosomal channel modulators is of great basic research and clinical interests. The recent sprout up of atomic structures of lysosomal ion channels (Chen et al., 2017b; Guo et al., 2016;

Hirschi et al., 2017; Schmiege et al., 2017; She et al., 2018) may help the structure-guided drug discovery.

## ACKNOWLEDGEMENT

We apologize to colleagues whose works are not cited due to space limitations. The research in the authors' laboratory is supported by NIH grants (NS062792, AR060837, and DK115471).

## REFERENCES

Abu-Remaileh, M., Wyant, G.A., Kim, C., Laqtom, N.N., Abbasi, M., Chan, S.H., Freinkman, E., and Sabatini, D.M. (2017). Lysosomal metabolomics reveals V-ATPase and mTOR-dependent regulation of amino acid efflux from lysosomes. *Science 358*(6364), 807–813.

Arai, K., Shimaya, A., Hiratani, N., and Ohkuma, S. (1993). Purification and characterization of lysosomal H(+)-ATPase: An anion-sensitive v-type H(+)-ATPase from rat liver lysosomes. *The Journal of Biological Chemistry 268*(8), 5649–5660.

Bae, M., Patel, N., Xu, H., Lee, M., Tominaga-Yamanaka, K., Nath, A., Geiger, J., Gorospe, M., Mattson, M.P., and Haughey, N.J. (2014). Activation of TRPML1 clears intraneuronal Abeta in preclinical models of HIV infection. *The Journal of Neuroscience : The Official Journal of the Society for Neuroscience 34*(34), 11485–11503.

Bonifacino, J.S., and Traub, L.M. (2003). Signals for sorting of transmembrane proteins to endosomes and lysosomes. *Annual Review of Biochemistry 72*, 395–447.

Calcraft, P.J., Ruas, M., Pan, Z., Cheng, X., Arredouani, A., Hao, X., Tang, J., Rietdorf, K., Teboul, L., Chuang, K.-T., et al. (2009). NAADP mobilizes calcium from acidic organelles through two-pore channels. *Nature 459*(7246), 596.

Cang, C., Aranda, K., Seo, Y.-j., Gasnier, B., and Ren, D. (2015). TMEM175 is an organelle K+ channel regulating lysosomal function. *Cell 162*(5), 1101–1112.

Cang, C., Bekele, B., and Ren, D. (2014). The voltage-gated sodium channel TPC1 confers endolysosomal excitability. *Nature Chemical Biology 10*(6), 463.

Cang, C., Zhou, Y., Navarro, B., Seo, Y.J., Aranda, K., Shi, L., Battaglia-Hsu, S., Nissim, I., Clapham, D.E., and Ren, D. (2013). mTOR regulates lysosomal ATP-sensitive two-pore Na(+) channels to adapt to metabolic state. *Cell 152*(4), 778–790.

Cao, Q., Zhong, X.Z., Zou, Y., Murrell-Lagnado, R., Zhu, M.X., and Dong, X.P. (2015a). Calcium release through P2X4 activates calmodulin to promote endolysosomal membrane fusion. *The Journal of Cell Biology 209*(6), 879–894.

Cao, Q., Zhong, X.Z., Zou, Y., Zhang, Z., Toro, L., and Dong, X.-P. (2015b). BK channels alleviate lysosomal storage diseases by providing positive feedback regulation of lysosomal Ca2+ release. *Developmental Cell 33*(4), 427–441.

Cerny, J., Feng, Y., Yu, A., Miyake, K., Borgonovo, B., Klumperman, J., Meldolesi, J., McNeil, P.L., and Kirchhausen, T. (2004). The small chemical vacuolin-1 inhibits Ca(2+)-dependent lysosomal exocytosis but not cell resealing. *EMBO Reports 5*(9), 883–888.

Chakraborty, K., Leung, K., and Krishnan, Y. (2017). High lumenal chloride in the lysosome is critical for lysosome function. *eLife 6*, e28862.

Chang, D., Nalls, M.A., Hallgrimsdottir, I.B., Hunkapiller, J., van der Brug, M., Cai, F., International Parkinson's Disease Genomics, C., and Me Research, T., Kerchner, G.A., Ayalon, G., et al. (2017). A meta-analysis of genome-wide association studies identifies 17 new Parkinson's disease risk loci. *Nature Genetics 49*(10), 1511-1516.

Perera, R.M., and Zoncu, R. (2016). The lysosome as a regulatory hub. *Annual Review of Cell and Developmental Biology 32*, 223–253.

Ruas, M., Davis, L.C., Chen, C.C., Morgan, A.J., Chuang, K.T., Walseth, T.F., Grimm, C., Garnham, C., Powell, T., Platt, N., et al. (2015). Expression of Ca2+ permeable two-pore channels rescues NAADP signalling in TPC-deficient cells. *The EMBO Journal 34*(13), 1743–1758.

Sahoo, N., Gu, M., Zhang, X., Raval, N., Yang, J., Bekier, M., Calvo, R., Patnaik, S., Wang, W., King, G., et al. (2017). Gastric acid secretion from parietal cells is mediated by a Ca2+ efflux channel in the tubulovesicle. *Developmental Cell 41*(3), 262–273, e266.

Saito, M., Hanson, P.I., and Schlesinger, P. (2007). Luminal chloride-dependent activation of endosome calcium channels: Patch clamp study of enlarged endosomes. *The Journal of Biological Chemistry 282*(37), 27327–27333.

Sakurai, Y., Kolokoltsov, A.A., Chen, C.C., Tidwell, M.W., Bauta, W.E., Klugbauer, N., Grimm, C., Wahl-Schott, C., Biel, M., and Davey, R.A. (2015). Ebola virus. Two-pore channels control Ebola virus host cell entry and are drug targets for disease treatment. *Science 347*(6225), 995–998.

Sawada, K., Echigo, N., Juge, N., Miyaji, T., Otsuka, M., Omote, H., Yamamoto, A., and Moriyama, Y. (2008). Identification of a vesicular nucleotide transporter. *Proceedings of the National Academy of Sciences of the United States of America 105*(15), 5683–5686.

Schieder, M., Rötzer, K., Brüggemann, A., Biel, M., and Wahl-Schott, C. (2010). Planar patch clamp approach to characterize ionic currents from intact lysosomes. *Science Signaling 3*(151), pl3–pl3.

Schmiege, P., Fine, M., Blobel, G., and Li, X. (2017). Human TRPML1 channel structures in open and closed conformations. *Nature 550*(7676), 366–370.

Settembre, C., Di Malta, C., Polito, V.A., Garcia Arencibia, M., Vetrini, F., Erdin, S., Erdin, S.U., Huynh, T., Medina, D., Colella, P., et al. (2011). TFEB links autophagy to lysosomal biogenesis. *Science 332*(6036), 1429–1433.

Settembre, C., Fraldi, A., Medina, D.L., and Ballabio, A. (2013). Signals from the lysosome: A control centre for cellular clearance and energy metabolism. *Nature Reviews Molecular Cell Biology 14*(5), 283–296.

She, J., Guo, J., Chen, Q., Zeng, W., Jiang, Y., and Bai, X.C. (2018). Structural insights into the voltage and phospholipid activation of the mammalian TPC1 channel. *Nature 556*(7699), 130–134.

Shen, D., Wang, X., Li, X., Zhang, X., Yao, Z., Dibble, S., Dong, X.P., Yu, T., Lieberman, A.P., Showalter, H.D., and Xu, H. (2012). Lipid storage disorders block lysosomal trafficking by inhibiting a TRP channel and lysosomal calcium release. *Nature Communications 3*, 731.

Steinberg, B.E., Huynh, K.K., Brodovitch, A., Jabs, S., Stauber, T., Jentsch, T.J., and Grinstein, S. (2010). A cation counterflux supports lysosomal acidification. *The Journal of Cell Biology 189*(7), 1171–1186.

Stenmark, H., Parton, R.G., Steele-Mortimer, O., Lutcke, A., Gruenberg, J., and Zerial, M. (1994). Inhibition of rab5 GTPase activity stimulates membrane fusion in endocytosis. *The EMBO Journal 13*(6), 1287–1296.

Wang, W., Gao, Q., Yang, M., Zhang, X., Yu, L., Lawas, M., Li, X., Bryant-Genevier, M., Southall, N.T., Marugan, J., et al. (2015). Up-regulation of lysosomal TRPML1 channels is essential for lysosomal adaptation to nutrient starvation. *Proceedings of the National Academy of Sciences of the United States of America 112*(11), E1373–E1381.

Wang, W., Zhang, X., Gao, Q., Lawas, M., Yu, L., Cheng, X., Gu, M., Sahoo, N., Li, X., Li, P., et al. (2017). A voltage-dependent K+ channel in the lysosome is required for refilling lysosomal Ca2+ stores. *The Journal of Cell Biology 216*(6), 1715–1730.

Wang, X., Zhang, X., Dong, X.P., Samie, M., Li, X., Cheng, X., Goschka, A., Shen, D., Zhou, Y., Harlow, J., et al. (2012). TPC proteins are phosphoinositide- activated sodium-selective ion channels in endosomes and lysosomes. *Cell 151*(2), 372–383.

Wyant, G.A., Abu-Remaileh, M., Frenkel, E.M., Laqtom, N.N., Dharamdasani, V., Lewis, C.A., Chan, S.H., Heinze, I., Ori, A., and Sabatini, D.M. (2018). NUFIP1 is a ribosome receptor for starvation-induced ribophagy. *Science 360*(6390), 751–758.

Xiong, J., and Zhu, M.X. (2016). Regulation of lysosomal ion homeostasis by channels and transporters. *Science in China (Life Sciences) 59*(8), 777–791.

Xu, H., Martinoia, E., and Szabo, I. (2015). Organellar channels and transporters. *Cell Calcium 58*(1), 1–10.

Xu, H., and Ren, D. (2015). Lysosomal physiology. *Annual Review of Physiology 77*, 57–80.

Yang, J., Zhao, Z., Gu, M., Feng, X., and Xu, H. (2018). Release and uptake mechanisms of vesicular Ca(2+) stores. *Protein and Cell 10*(1), 8–19.

Zhang, X., Cheng, X., Yu, L., Yang, J., Calvo, R., Patnaik, S., Hu, X., Gao, Q., Yang, M., Lawas, M., et al. (2016). MCOLN1 is a ROS sensor in lysosomes that regulates autophagy. *Nature Communications 7*, 12109.

Zhang, X., Li, X., and Xu, H. (2012). Phosphoinositide isoforms determine compartment-specific ion channel activity. *Proceedings of the National Academy of Sciences of the United States of America 109*(28), 11384–11389.

Zoncu, R., Bar-Peled, L., Efeyan, A., Wang, S., Sancak, Y., and Sabatini, D.M. (2011). mTORC1 senses lysosomal amino acids through an inside-out mechanism that requires the vacuolar H(+)-ATPase. *Science 334*(6056), 678–683.

# 2 Chloride Transport across the Lysosomal Membrane

*Sonali Saha, Anja Blessing, and Thomas J. Jentsch*

## CONTENTS

## 2.1 INTRODUCTION

Lysosomes mediate a range of biological processes, such as the degradation of macromolecules, plasma membrane repair, regulation of cellular metabolism and immune response (Appelqvist et al., 2013; Ballabio, 2016; Settembre et al., 2013). For its normal function, the lysosome needs to generate and maintain an acidic luminal pH, a process which requires several ion-transporting proteins embedded in its limiting membrane (Scott and Gruenberg, 2011). Acidification of the lysosomal lumen is directly mediated by a V-type proton ATPase, which needs, however, parallel anion or cation conductive pathways to allow bulk proton transport by compensating the electric charge transported by the ATPase (Grabe and Oster, 2001).

In endosomes, electrogenic transport of chloride into the lumen was shown to be essential for acidification (Günther et al., 2003; Hara-Chikuma et al., 2005; Novarino et al., 2010; Van Dyke, 1993). Similarly, chloride flux across lysosomal membranes was proposed to enable luminal acidification of isolated lysosomes (Dell'Antone, 1979; Ohkuma et al., 1982). Since $Cl^-/H^+$-antiporters of the CLC family of $Cl^-$-channels and $Cl^-$-transporters (Jentsch, 2015; Jentsch and Pusch, 2018), in particular ClC-5 (Günther et al., 2003; Novarino et al., 2010; Piwon et al., 2000) and ClC-3 (Hara-Chikuma et al., 2005), facilitated endosomal acidification, the lysosome-residing member of this family ClC-7, together with its ß-subunit Ostm1 (Kasper et al., 2005; Kornak et al., 2001; Lange et al., 2006), was supposed to mediate the same process in lysosomes (Kornak et al., 2001). However, using ratiometric fluorescence measurements, we did not detect differences in lysosomal pH between cells derived from WT and ClC-7 knockout mice (Kasper et al., 2005; Lange et al., 2006; Steinberg et al., 2010; Weinert et al., 2010).

In contrast, Graves et al. (2008), using technically less convincing non-ratiometric LysoTracker fluorescence integrated over entire cells, reported an increase in lysosomal pH upon siRNA-mediated partial knockdown of ClC-7. Another report suggested an involvement of ClC-7 in lysosomal acidification of activated microglia (Majumdar et al., 2011). Such measurements can only report stationary lysosomal pH and do not exclude the possibility that the kinetics of lysosomal acidification during the formation from late endosomes is influenced by ClC-7. It is important to stress that lysosomes also express various cation channels (Cang et al., 2015; Cao et al., 2015; Grimm et al., 2017; Grimm et al., 2012), which could serve as shunt pathway by releasing e.g. $Na^+$ from lysosomes. Indeed, there is convincing evidence for the role of cations in lysosomal acidification (Steinberg et al., 2010; Weinert et al., 2010).

Despite unchanged lysosomal pH (Kasper et al., 2005; Lange et al., 2006; Steinberg et al., 2010; Weinert et al., 2014; Weinert et al., 2010), disruption of lysosomal ClC-7 (Kasper et al., 2005; Kornak et al., 2001) or loss-of-function mutations of its ancillary β-subunit Ostm1 (Lange et al., 2006) lead to osteopetrosis, lysosomal storage and neurodegeneration in mice and humans. Qualitative similar pathologies were also observed in a knock-in mouse model, in which a point mutation disrupted the ion transport of ClC-7/Ostm1, but not its expression and localization (Weinert et al., 2014), excluding that these symptoms are caused by the loss of interactions of ClC-7 with other proteins. Furthermore, converting the $2Cl^-/H^+$-exchanger ClC-7 into a pure $Cl^-$ conductance by a single point mutation also resulted in osteopetrosis and neurodegeneration (Weinert et al., 2010). These experiments point to an important physiological role of lysosomal $Cl^-$ which, driven by the large inside-out lysosomal $H^+$-gradient, is transported into lysosomes by the $2Cl^-/H^+$ exchange activity of ClC-7/Ostm1.

Cystic fibrosis transmembrane conductance regulator (CFTR)-mediated $Cl^-$ currents were also claimed to foster the acidification of lysosome-like organelles (Barasch and al-Awqati, 1993; Barasch et al., 1991; Di et al., 2006). Electron microscopical studies employing immunogold labelling suggested that CFTR is expressed on vesicles of the recycling pathway and on autophagosomes (Di et al., 2006; Puchelle et al., 1992; Webster et al., 1994). However, loss-of-function mutations of CFTR did not affect the steady-state pH of endocytic organelles in all cell types (Haggie and Verkman, 2009; Lukacs et al., 1992; Steinberg et al., 2010). Furthermore, several studies reporting an effect of CFTR on lysosomal and autolysosomal pH (Deriy et al., 2009; Di et al., 2006) used sensors that are not suitable to report the low lysosomal pH because their fluorescence already saturates at endosomal pH values (pH 5–6). This casts a shadow of doubt on the suggested importance of CFTR for lysosomal acidification.

Any ion conductance shunting $H^+$-ATPase currents during vesicular acidification will change the luminal concentration of the respective ion – an increase of anions or a decrease of cations for currents carried by anions and cations, respectively. Although both $Cl^-$-channels and $2Cl^-/H^+$-exchangers will raise the luminal $Cl^-$ concentration during lysosomal acidification, $Cl^-$ accumulation by $2Cl^-/H^+$-exchangers will be more pronounced, owing to the coupling to the pH gradient (Weinert et al., 2010). Somewhat counterintuitively, model calculations predict that $2Cl^-/H^+$-exchangers will lead to a more pronounced luminal acidification than $Cl^-$-channels when operating in parallel to an $H^+$-ATPase (Ishida et al., 2013; Weinert et al., 2010). This is owed to an effect on lysosomal potential, which is calculated to be more negative-inside with an exchanger (Ishida et al., 2013; Weinert et al., 2010). It should also be borne in mind that an altered concentration of one ionic species will most likely affect the luminal abundance of other ions because of boundary conditions for electroneutrality and osmolarity.

The mechanisms by which changes in lysosomal $Cl^-$ concentration entail pathology remain presently unclear. The elucidation of underlying processes requires reliable quantitative information on the lysosomal chloride concentration and currents (or fluxes) under both normal and pathological conditions. Electrophysiological techniques are the conventional method to study ionic currents across biological membranes. However, the small size of lysosomes has made the study of ion transport across lysosomal membranes and its regulators technically challenging. Patch-clamp analysis of artificially enlarged lysosomes is feasible (Chen et al., 2017), but to the best of our knowledge, no patch-clamp analysis of lysosomal $Cl^-$ currents has been published to date. The difficulties to obtain pure lysosomal preparations also limit the study of ion fluxes with isolated lysosomes. Moreover, both approaches remove lysosomes from their cellular context and change their composition. Therefore, lysosomal [$Cl^-$] should be quantified in native lysosomes within cells. Imaging techniques based on ratiometric fluorescent probes specifically targeted to lysosomes enable measurements of steady-state luminal [$Cl^-$] within lysosomes in intact cells, and might also be useful to assess lysosomal $Cl^-$ transport in cells using selective permeabilization of the plasma membrane to control the ionic composition of the cytosol, as reported in a study using lysosomal pH measurements as read-out (Steinberg et al., 2010). Considering the low lysosomal pH and its variations, pH-sensitive $Cl^-$-sensors cannot be used without measuring lysosomal pH in parallel. Therefore, one needs a fluorescent $Cl^-$-sensor that operates over the entire physiological range of [$Cl^-$] and is pH-independent.

In this chapter, we describe different methods to study lysosomal $Cl^-$ concentration and permeability, highlighting their principles of operation, advantages and disadvantages. Finally, we discuss how these measurements have advanced our understanding about the role of lysosomal $Cl^-$.

## 2.2   METHODS TO SENSE LYSOSOMAL CHLORIDE

### 2.2.1   Assays with Isolated Lysosomes

Assays using isolated lysosomes are suited to measure ionic fluxes across lysosomal membranes, but cannot be used to determine native steady-state ion concentrations because these are likely to change during the purification procedure. Reports on lysosomal ion concentrations determined by ICP-MS with lysosomal preparations (Wang et al., 2012) have to be viewed extremely critically. After several hours of centrifugation in non-physiological media, the obtained values are unlikely to reflect the native luminal ion composition.

However, measurements of changes of external or luminal ion concentrations of vesicle preparations in response to imposed ion gradients can yield important insights into ion transport pathways. Since the bulk flux of ions through channels or electrogenic transporters generates electrical currents that will soon change the voltage across vesicular membranes, the addition of ionophores for other ions (such as valinomycin in the presence of potassium) may strongly enhance net transport and show that the respective transport process is electrogenic. Chloride fluxes can be measured directly using radioactive isotopes (unfortunately, $^{36}$Cl is extremely long-lived, and thus displays low specific activity). Changes in luminal [Cl$^-$] can be also detected by using fluorescent dyes, whereas Cl$^-$-specific electrodes are able to record alterations in [Cl$^-$] in the external solution. Another more indirect approach to monitor Cl$^-$ fluxes is the detection of changes in other ions whose transport is coupled to that of Cl$^-$ (e.g. measuring changes in pH with the 2Cl$^-$/H$^+$-exchanger ClC-7/Ostm1).

Cl$^-$ permeability properties of lysosomal membranes can be studied by isotope flux assays with purified lysosomes in a rather simple and sensitive fashion. However, they do not necessarily reflect native kinetics because regulatory factors may have been lost during the isolation procedure. Such an approach was taken by Graves et al. (2008) to examine properties of lysosomal Cl$^-$/H$^+$-exchange. Subcellular fractions enriched for lysosomal marker proteins were prepared from tissues using differential sedimentation. The vesicles were then loaded with a high concentration of KCl by freeze/thawing followed by sonication. Shortly before the assay, the external Cl$^-$ was replaced by a relatively impermeant anion, such as gluconate, using Sephadex G-50 columns equilibrated in external buffer. Their experiments confirmed that lysosomes possess an electrogenic transport pathway for Cl$^-$. As a consequence of the Cl$^-$ gradient and a lysosomal Cl$^-$-conductive pathway, a lumen-positive electrical diffusion potential was set up that drove the uptake of externally added $^{36}$Cl (Figure 2.1a) and was inversed by the addition of the K$^+$-ionophore valinomycin (because of the large outward K$^+$ gradient) (Figure 2.1a). Uptake was stimulated by luminal acidic pH, which is either compatible with the modulatory role of pH on transport rates, or with Cl$^-$/H$^+$-exchange. To test for the latter possibility, $^{36}$Cl$^-$ uptake was driven by a pH gradient across the lysosomal membrane in the presence of valinomycin that abolished the electrical gradient. Collapse of the pH gradient with the protonophore FCCP abolished the H$^+$-driven Cl$^-$ accumulation (Figure 2.1b). Graves and colleagues further measured the reversal potential of H$^+$ and for Cl$^-$ transport, using the pH indicator BCECF (2',7'-Bis-(2-Carboxyethyl)-5-(and-6)-Carboxyfluorescein) and the Cl$^-$-sensitive dye SPQ (6-methoxy-N-(3-sulphopropyl)quinolinium) trapped

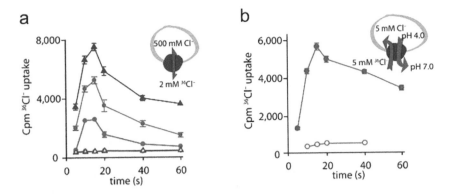

**FIGURE 2.1** Measurement of radioactive chloride fluxes across the lysosomal membrane in isolated lysosomes. (a) In order to assess Cl⁻ transport pathways of lysosomes, isolated lysosomes were preloaded with 500 mM KCl and transferred to Cl⁻-free medium, leading to an inside-positive potential. The presence of a lysosomal Cl⁻ conductance would drive the uptake of Cl⁻. Addition of $^{36}$Cl⁻ (with a final Cl⁻ concentration of 2 mM) to the external medium led to an uptake of $^{36}$Cl⁻ into the lysosomal lumen, which was measured by rapidly washing the vesicle suspension at the indicated time points and determining the trapped radioactivity. This uptake process was enhanced by lowering the luminal pH from pH 7 (red) to pH 5.5 (green), and to pH 4 (blue), by previously loading with respective solutions. After 15 s, the luminal $^{36}$Cl⁻ concentrations decreased again because of progressive equilibration of luminal and external solutions. The addition of 1 mM of the potassium ionophore valinomycin, which will create a lumen-negative potential owed to the large inside-out K⁺ gradient, prevented the uptake of radioactive Cl⁻ into the lysosomal lumen (open symbols). (b) To explore whether the pH-dependent accumulation of luminal Cl⁻ was due to a coupled H⁺/Cl⁻ transport, isolated lysosomes were kept in symmetrical [Cl⁻] while a pH gradient was set up. The luminal pH of the isolated lysosomes was kept at pH 4, whereas the external solution had a pH of 7. The proton-motive force enabled the luminal accumulation of externally added $^{36}$Cl⁻, which was abolished when the protonophore FCCP was added to the isolated lysosomes (open symbols). Adapted from Graves et al. (2008).

into vesicles, respectively, with the membrane voltage set by defined K⁺ gradients in the presence of valinomycin. This suggested a 2Cl⁻/1H⁺ stoichiometry for ClC-7, the predominant CLC on lysosomes (Kasper et al., 2005; Kornak et al., 2001), like previously determined for bacterial EcClC-1 (Accardi and Miller, 2004) and later confirmed for plasma membrane-targeted ClC-7/Ostm1 (Leisle et al., 2011).

Whereas Graves et al. (2008) used poorly controlled siRNA knockdown of ClC-7 to suggest that ClC-7 mediated the measured transport activity, Weinert et al. (2010) compared the transport activity of lysosomes isolated from wildtype, *Clcn7⁻/⁻* and *Clcn7unc/unc* mice using luminal pH measurements under different conditions. The results, which were compared to model calculations, showed that ClC-7 indeed mediated lysosomal Cl⁻/H⁺-exchange, and like EcClC-1 (Accardi and Miller, 2004), ClC-4 and ClC-5 (Picollo and Pusch, 2005; Scheel et al., 2005), ClC-7 is converted into an uncoupled Cl⁻ conductor by the *unc* point mutation of the 'gating' glutamate residue in the pore. Furthermore, the study showed that ClC-7 supports ATP-dependent lysosomal acidification *in vitro* (Weinert et al., 2010).

Although measurements with isolated lysosomes can provide valuable insight into lysosomal ion transport, the method is associated with several pitfalls. First, lysosomal preparations, depending on the particular protocol for their isolation, may be rather impure. This problem can be largely circumvented by loading membrane-impermeable ion indicators by endocytosis and subsequent chase into lysosomes of living cells before their preparation (Weinert et al., 2010), or potentially by using genetically encoded ion sensors specifically targeted to lysosomes. Second, the transport properties of isolated lysosomes may not correspond exactly to those in their native environment as, e.g. cytosolic factors that only transiently interact with the channels or transporters might be lost during the purification (Waller-Evans and Lloyd-Evans, 2015). In addition, relatively large quantities of lysosomes are needed. Finally, as a consequence of the small volume of vesicles, the uptake and efflux will saturate within a short time. This requires, e.g. short uptake times and rapid washing of vesicle preparations to remove external radioisotopes with flux measurements. Small differences in manual handling might therefore have large impacts on the final result.

## 2.2.2 Fluorescent Chloride-Sensitive Dyes

Ion-sensitive fluorescent dyes have substantially advanced our knowledge of the biological importance of $H^+$ and $Ca^{2+}$. These fluorescent dyes sense $H^+$ and $Ca^{2+}$ by binding to these ions. In contrast, fluorescent small molecule $Cl^-$-indicators detect $Cl^-$ by collisional fluorescence quenching and, unlike some $Ca^{2+}$-sensors, are therefore unlikely to change the biologically important ion concentrations – a concern that also seems remote because the biological concentrations of $Cl^-$ are orders of magnitude higher than cytosolic $Ca^{2+}$ or $H^+$ concentrations.

Based on the finding that quinine fluorescence is quenched by $Cl^-$, a variety of quinolone-based dyes with quaternary nitrogens have been developed as $Cl^-$-indicators (Geddes, 2001). In spite of their sensitivity to many halides ($I^- > Br^- > Cl^- > F^-$), these small molecules are mainly considered as $Cl^-$-sensors because of the much higher concentration of $Cl^-$ compared to other halides in cells (Geddes, 2001). These probes have been used to image intracellular $Cl^-$ in many cell types, including neurons (Dallwig et al., 1999; Frech et al., 1999; Inglefield and Schwartz-Bloom, 1997; Marandi et al., 2002; Schwartz and Yu, 1995), glia (Bevensee et al., 1997), epithelial cells (Krapf et al., 1988; Lau et al., 1994), fibroblasts (Chao et al., 1989; Munkonge et al., 2004; Wöll et al., 1996), human gastric cancer cells (Miyazaki et al., 2008) and pancreatic beta-cells (Eberhardson et al., 2000). However, these probes are mostly excited at ultraviolet wavelengths and are therefore problematic for prolonged live cell imaging because of associated phototoxicity (Biwersi et al., 1994). This problem could be solved by the development of long-wavelength fluorescent $Cl^-$-indicators that are based on acridinium compounds (Biwersi et al., 1994).

All $Cl^-$-sensitive small molecules display fast response to changes in the $Cl^-$ concentration which usually occurs in less than a millisecond (Verkman, 1990). Importantly, they are also insensitive to pH in the physiological pH range, including the acidic environment of lysosomes (Geddes, 2001).

The Cl⁻-dependent fluorescence of these sensors must be normalized to their concentrations within the respective compartment, and/or must be calibrated in those compartments, to obtain quantitative results. For pH- and Ca²⁺-sensors, normalization is possible with ratiometric dyes that display both ion-sensitive and ion-insensitive fluorescence at different wavelengths. However, all fluorescent Cl⁻-indicators lack a Cl⁻-dependent spectral shift (Poenie, 1992). To overcome this problem, Cl⁻-insensitive fluorophores were linked to Cl⁻-sensitive probes via various spacer groups, resulting in a dual wavelength ratiometric chloride indicator (Jayaraman et al., 1999; Li et al., 2014). As a caveat, bleaching may affect the used fluorophores differentially, thereby leading to shifts in fluorescence ratios over time that may be wrongly interpreted as reflecting changes in ion concentration. Li et al. (2014) designed a new fluorescence ratiometric probe consisting of two fluorophores with identical excitation wavelengths: a Cl⁻-sensitive 6-methoxyquinolinium (MQ) group and a Cl⁻-insensitive dansyl (DS) group (Figure 2.2a). Importantly, the emission profiles of the two fluorophores differed when simultaneously excited at the same wavelength (Figure 2.2b). The dimethylamino group of the dansyl fluorophore enabled the targeting to acidic intracellular organelles. Although this strategy does not allow the specific staining of lysosomes, it enables chloride measurements in compartments with low luminal pH. Without the 'acidity trapping strategy', the Cl⁻-indicators would remain homogeneously distributed throughout the cytoplasm.

There is a need to develop strategies to measure Cl⁻ in defined subcellular compartments. For the endosomal-lysosomal pathway, this could be achieved by synthesizing dextran-conjugatable long-wavelength indicators, for example 10,10'-Bis [3-carboxypropyl]-9,9'-biacridiniumdinitrate (BAC), for chloride (Biwersi et al.,

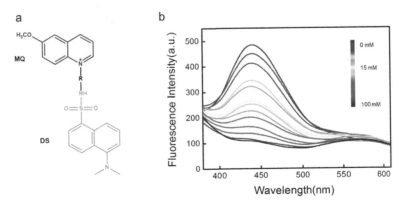

**FIGURE 2.2** MQ-DS as ratiometric Cl⁻-sensor for intracellular acidic organelles. (a) Structure of MQ-DS with the Cl⁻-sensitive moiety 6-methoxyquinolinium (MQ) coupled to a Cl⁻-insensitive dansyl group (DS) via a benzyl linker. By protonation of the dimethylamino group of DS, the ratiometric dye concentrates inside acidic organelles. (b) Cl⁻-dependent fluorescence changes of MQ-DS (12 µM) in 5.0 mM phosphate/citric acid buffer (pH 4.5) upon excitation at $\lambda = 330$ nm. [Cl⁻] ranged from 0 mM (purple line) to 100 mM (brown line). Fluorescence decreased with increasing [Cl⁻] and saturated at 80–100 mM. Adapted from Li et al. (2014).

1992; Sonawane et al., 2002) (Figure 2.3a). Dextran conjugation facilitates endo-lysosomal delivery of the Cl⁻-indicator via fluid-phase endocytosis and prevents its escape from vesicular lumina to the cytosol. Unfortunately, the chemical conjugation of Cl⁻-indicators to dextran or other macromolecules often leads to fluorescence quenching and/or highly variable sensor characteristics between batches because the location and degree of functionalization on the polymer cannot be properly controlled (Biwersi et al., 1994; Geddes, 2001; Sonawane et al., 2002; Sonawane and Verkman, 2003).

BAC is currently the best-suited Cl⁻-sensitive small sensor module for organellar Cl⁻ measurements (Figure 2.3b) (Sonawane et al., 2002). (i) It is bioconjugatable and hence can be targeted to specific intracellular locations, (ii) it can be excited in the visible range and (iii) it can sense chloride over a wide range of concentrations (0–200 mM). Verkman and coworkers pioneered quantitative ratiometric imaging methods for measuring endosomal chloride concentrations by using dextrans that had been coupled to both BAC and the chloride-insensitive

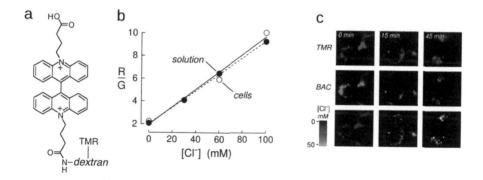

**FIGURE 2.3** Fluorescence-based ratiometric Cl⁻ imaging with BAC-TMR-dextran. (a) Schematic presentation of BAC-TMR-dextran. The dye was synthesized by covalently linking the Cl⁻-sensitive fluorophore BAC and the Cl⁻-insensitive chromophore TMR to 40 kDa amino dextran. (b) Intensity ratio of TMR (R) and BAC (G) in response to increasing [Cl⁻] in solution (filled circles) and in living cells (open circles). For *in vitro* calibration, 10 µM BAC-TMR-dextran was diluted in 5 mM phosphate buffer with pH 7.4 while microliter amounts of NaCl were added to the solution to increase [Cl⁻]. *In vivo* calibration profiles required the loading of cells with 18 mg/ml BAC-TMR-dextran while different [Cl⁻] were clamped by the addition of 10 µM nigericin, 10 µM valinomycin, 5 µM CCCP, 10 µM monensin and 200 nM bafilomycin for 1 h. Addition of the K⁺/H⁺-exchanger, potassium ionophore, protonophore, Na⁺/H⁺-exchanger and V-ATPase blocker should allow the passive equilibration of [Cl⁻] between the external solution and the lumen of BAC-TMR-dextran containing organelles. Both *in vitro* and *in vivo* calibrations showed a linear decrease in BAC fluorescence between 0 mM and 100 mM Cl⁻. (c) To determine [Cl⁻] in the endosomal pathway, J774 cells were loaded with 18 mg/ml BAC-TMR-dextran for 2 min and chased for 0 min, 15 min and 45 min at 37°C to allow the trafficking of the sensor to different organelles along the endo-lysosomal pathway. Pictures display the fluorescence intensity for TMR, BAC and the ratio of both channels converted to the absolute Cl⁻ concentration. Longer chase times were accompanied by an increase in luminal [Cl⁻]. Adapted from Sonawane et al. (2002).

fluorophore tetramethylrhodamine (TMR) (BAC-TMR-dextran) (Sonawane et al., 2002). Their measurements show that endosomal Cl⁻ concentration progressively increases from 20–30 mM in newly formed endosomes to 50–70 mM in late endosomes (Sonawane et al., 2002) (Figure 2.3c). However, lysosomal [Cl⁻] was not reported (Sonawane et al., 2002).

The saturation of fluorescence changes with higher chloride concentrations has hampered measurements of lysosomal Cl⁻ concentrations (which exceed 100 mM) (Weinert et al., 2010). Jentsch and coworkers (Weinert et al., 2010) attempted to measure lysosomal Cl⁻ concentration by using a ratiometric dye (MEQ (6-methoxy-N-ethylquinolinium) and TMR (tetramethylrhodamine) coupled to dextran). However, the Cl⁻-sensitivity of MEQ saturates beyond ~60–80 mM, much lower than the expected lysosomal [Cl⁻]. Therefore, Weinert et al. performed experiments under non-physiological conditions where lysosomal [Cl⁻] was shifted to a measurable range by pre-incubating cells in a low chloride-containing medium (see protocol I). These measurements suggested lower lysosomal [Cl⁻] in $Clcn7^{-/-}$ and $Clcn7^{unc/unc}$ fibroblasts compared to wildtype cells and thus indicate a role for ClC-7-mediated Cl⁻/H⁺-exchange in lysosomal Cl⁻ accumulation (Weinert et al., 2014; Weinert et al., 2010).

## 2.2.3 Genetically Encoded Chloride Indicators

YFP (yellow fluorescent protein) fluorescence is sensitive to anions with relative potencies $I^- > NO_3^- > Cl^- > Br^-$~formate > acetate (Jayaraman et al., 2000). YFP's sensitivity to these small anions results from their binding near the chromophore as revealed by the crystal structure (Wachter et al., 2000). This binding alters the chromophore ionization constant and hence its fluorescence (Arosio et al., 2007; Wachter and Remington, 1999; Wachter et al., 2000). Unfortunately, pH- and Cl⁻-sensitivity of YFP are highly interrelated. The anion binding constant for YFP is influenced by the amount of proton binding, and *vice versa*, with positive cooperativity. YFP-based genetically encoded sensors have been extensively used to monitor cytoplasmic changes in [Cl⁻] at near neutral pH in pharmacological and genetic screens (Galietta et al., 2001; Ma et al., 2002; Metzger et al., 2002; Muanprasat et al., 2007; Muanprasat et al., 2004; Voss et al., 2014; Yang et al., 2003). Mutagenesis of YFP resulted in brightly fluorescent YFP-H148G with higher Cl⁻-sensitivity, but stronger pH-dependence (Wachter et al., 1998). However, the Cl⁻ affinity of both YFP and YFP-H148G is too high for the whole range of [Cl⁻] along the endo-lysosomal pathway (Wachter et al., 1998), seriously limiting the use of these probes in lysosomes.

Four different ratiometric YFP-based Cl⁻-sensors were developed, namely Clomeleon (Kuner and Augustine, 2000), SuperClomeleon (Grimley et al., 2013), 'Cl⁻ Sensor' (Markova et al., 2008) and ClopHensor (Arosio et al., 2010). Clomeleon consists of two fluorescent proteins, Cl⁻-insensitive CFP and a variant of YFP named topaz fluorescent protein (TFP), connected with a 24-mer polypeptide linker. Binding of Cl⁻ to anion-sensitive TFP reduces its emission, whereas CFP fluorescence remains constant, thereby allowing a ratiometric, FRET-based measurement of Cl⁻. Clomeleon could be successfully applied for long-term imaging in mice (Berglund et al., 2008). A major disadvantage of Clomeleon is its rather low sensitivity to Cl⁻ at physiological pH. To address this problem, the Cl⁻-sensitivity of Clomeleon was improved by inserting two point mutations in YFP, yielding in SuperClomeleon with a better signal to noise ratio in the physiologically relevant Cl⁻ concentration range (Boffi et al., 2018; Grimley et al., 2013). Likewise, another genetically encoded sensor, 'Cl⁻ Sensor', was developed with fivefold higher Cl⁻-sensitivity at physiological concentrations than Clomeleon (Markova et al., 2008). This construct contains YFP coupled to CFP via a polypeptide linker. The higher Cl⁻-sensitivity of 'Cl⁻ Sensor' was achieved by incorporating three point mutations in YFP that enhance the sensitivity and accelerate its binding kinetics. However, the sensor still shows a relatively large pH-dependence (Markova et al., 2008) that introduces errors by pH variations of up to 50% when Cl⁻ approaches higher concentrations. Given that the Cl⁻ affinity of all YFP-derived sensors is strongly pH-dependent, the concomitant assessment of pH is required for [Cl⁻] measurements. To achieve simultaneous measurement of pH and Cl⁻, ClopHensor was developed (Arosio et al., 2010). Ratiometric ClopHensor is constructed by fusion of an $E^2GFP$ variant, which contains a specific chloride-binding site, to a chloride- and pH-insensitive DsRed-monomer (Figure 2.4a). Even though the fusion protein overcomes the limitations of previous genetically encoded Cl⁻-sensors, quantification of [Cl⁻] using ClopHensor requires complicated data analysis involving the following steps: (i) estimate $pH_i$ in a region of interest; (ii) calculate the corresponding $K_d^{Cl}$ (pH); (iii) use this value to estimate $[Cl^-]_i$ in the selected region of interest (Figure 2.4b–d). As a proof of principle, Arosio et al. (2010) quantified [Cl⁻] in large dense-core vesicles (LDCVs) of PC12 cells. Targeting to these granules was achieved by fusing an N-terminal signal sequence of neuropeptide Y to the Cl⁻-sensor. ClopHensor fluorescence indicated a high [Cl⁻] (~110 mM) within LDCVs at an average pH of ~5.2. However, the measurements showed a large variability in both WSS-1 and PC12 cells that seemed to be related to the need for assessing both [Cl⁻] and pH, since measurement errors sum up in this approach (Figure 2.4e,f).

On the other hand, genetically encoded Cl⁻-sensors have many advantages over small organic dyes. They can be targeted to specific cell types or subcellular compartments in a rather straight-forward manner. Yet, YFP-based Cl⁻-sensors are not suitable for lysosomal [Cl⁻] measurement as the acidic environment of lysosomes considerably quenches their basal fluorescence and decreases the signal to noise ratio. Moreover, poor proteolytic stability of genetically encoded Cl⁻-indicators inside lysosomes may increase the variability of the measurements or may bias results towards late endosomes which display less proteolytic activity.

## 2.2.4  DNA Scaffold-Based pH-Independent Chloride Indicator

The first quantitative measurement of physiological lysosomal [Cl⁻] was achieved with a DNA scaffold-based pH-independent ratiometric sensor named *Clensor* (Saha et al., 2015). Nucleic acids provide an excellent scaffold for designing quantitative sensors with high specificity and sensitivity (Bhatia et al., 2011a; Krishnan and Bathe, 2012; Krishnan and Simmel, 2011; Modi et al., 2010). Inside living cells and

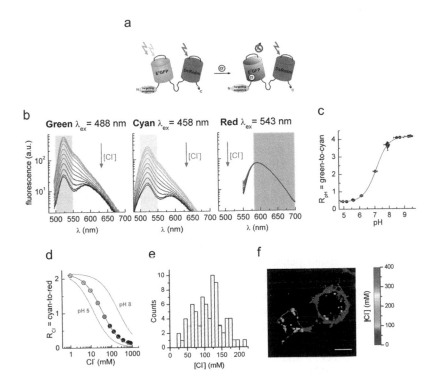

**FIGURE 2.4** Genetically encoded Cl⁻-sensor ClopHensor and its application to measure luminal [Cl⁻] in large dense-core vesicles (LDCVs). (a) Scheme of the genetically encoded Cl⁻-sensor, ClopHensor. The sensor consists of an E²GFP, which shows a decrease in fluorescence upon Cl⁻ binding and a Cl⁻-insensitive DsRed-monomer. The two fluorophores are coupled by a flexible 20-amino-acid linker. (b) The purified sensor was used to determine the change in fluorescence emission upon the binding of Cl⁻ to E²GFP *in vitro* at pH 6.9. [Cl⁻] was changed from 0 mM (lightest colour line) to 1 M (darkest colour line). The Cl⁻-dependent decrease in emission could be seen for both excitation maxima at 488 nm and 458 nm. The fluorescence emission of DsRed was not changed after the addition of increasing amounts of Cl⁻ to the solution. The shaded areas represent the emission parameters used for *in vivo* studies. (c) To monitor the pH-dependent change in E²GFP emission, the purified protein was excited at 488 nm (pH-dependent component) and at 458 nm (pH-independent signal) under conditions with varying pH values from 4.5 to 9.5. The ratio of emission signals obtained by exciting ClopHensor at 488 nm and 458 nm showed a sigmoidal curve in response to increasing pH. (d) Cyan-to-red ratio values of the purified construct at various [Cl⁻] values. Light and dark blue spots represent experimental data obtained from measurements in (b). Light grey lines represent the theoretical calculated pH-dependent change of ClopHensor in the presence of increasing [Cl⁻]. Lower pH values led to a stronger decrease in E²GFP emission upon Cl⁻ binding. (e) Distribution of the measured luminal [Cl⁻] in large dense-core vesicles (LDCVs) in PC12 cells. Differentiated PC12 cells were transfected with ClopHensor fused to the N-terminal signal sequence of neuropeptide Y (NPY) for targeting ClopHensor into LDCVs. Chloride clamping was achieved by incubating cells in solutions with different Cl⁻ concentrations, containing nigericin, valinomycin, CCCP and tributyltinchloride (TBT-Cl). The applied ionophores allowed the passive flow of sodium, potassium, protons and chloride across all membranes. (f) Cl⁻ concentration heat map of WSS-1 cells expressing ClopHensor in LDCVs and at the plasma membrane. The Cl⁻ calibration in WSS-1 cells was performed as mentioned for PC12 cells in (e). The measurement clearly showed higher [Cl⁻] in LDCVs compared to the low levels of Cl⁻ in the cytosol surrounding the plasma membrane. Adapted from Arosio et al. (2010).

multicellular organisms, synthetic nucleic acid-based sensors have been employed to detect ions (Bhatia et al., 2011a; Modi et al., 2009; Modi et al., 2013; Surana et al., 2011), small molecules (Kellenberger et al., 2013; Paige et al., 2012) and nucleic acids themselves (Tyagi, 2009; Volpi and Bridger, 2008). Quantitative stability assays in *Caenorhabditis elegans* revealed that such DNA scaffold-based sensors have a half-life of 8 h *in vivo* in the absence of illumination (Surana et al., 2011). Since most experiments can be performed within a few hours, these sensors are suitable for intracellular ion measurements.

DNA-based sensors are not genetically encoded, limiting somewhat their targeting to specific compartments. However, they can be coupled to targeting moieties, which allow, for instance, their targeting to compartments along the endo-lysosomal pathway and to the Golgi (Modi et al., 2013). The combination of such targeting strategies and the modular nature of nucleic acid-based nanosensors enable a wide spectrum of quantitative measurements of biologically important chemicals at their site of action.

The DNA-based pH-independent fluorescent ratiometric Cl$^-$-sensor *Clensor* (Saha et al., 2015) integrates a sensing module (P), a normalizing module (D2) and a targeting module (D1) on a single structure by nucleic acid hybridization. The sensing module (P) is a 12-mer peptide nucleic acid (PNA) sequence conjugated to the Cl$^-$-sensitive dye, BAC. The normalizing module (D2) is a 38 nt DNA sequence carrying an Alexa 647 fluorescent label that is Cl$^-$-insensitive. The targeting module (D1) is a 26-mer DNA sequence. P and D1 are hybridized to adjacent sites on D2 as shown in Figure 2.5a. The dsDNA domain on *Clensor*, comprising D1 and D2, functions as a negatively charged ligand for trafficking along the endo-lysosomal pathway mediated by anionic ligand binding receptors (ALBRs) (Bhatia et al., 2011b; Modi et al., 2009; Surana et al., 2011). Alternatively, *Clensor* can be targeted to the endocytic pathway by integrating an aptamer module binding to the transferrin receptor (Saha et al., 2015). In contrast to the conjugation of BAC-TMR to dextran (Sonawane et al., 2002), the stoichiometry of dye conjugation can be strictly controlled by DNA hybridization, which eliminates batch-to-batch variations. The fluorescent read-out of *Clensor* is based on the collisional quenching of BAC by Cl$^-$, leading to a linear decrease in fluorescence intensity with increasing [Cl$^-$] (Sonawane et al., 2002), whereas the fluorescence intensity of Alexa 647 remains constant. This results in different ratios of the emission intensities (R/G) for A647 (R) and BAC (G) over physiological [Cl$^-$] (Figure 2.5b,c).

*Clensor* is capable of reliably mapping [Cl$^-$] during endo-lysosomal maturation (see protocol II) (Figure 2.5d) and was used to measure lysosomal [Cl$^-$] in *Drosophila* hemocytes (Saha et al., 2015). Quantification of the mean R/G values obtained from a population of lysosomes revealed a mean lysosomal [Cl$^-$] of 108.5 ± 1.4 mM that is consistent with the model calculation for lysosomal [Cl$^-$] (Saha et al., 2015; Weinert et al., 2010). More recently, Krishnan and coworkers have used *Clensor* to measure lysosomal [Cl$^-$] in *Caenorhabditis elegans* and in mammalian cell culture models of lysosomal storage diseases (Chakraborty et al., 2017). Their measurements suggested that reduced lysosomal [Cl$^-$] leads to inefficient Ca$^{2+}$ release from lysosomes and is correlated with a loss in their degradative function, bolstering the notion that luminal Cl$^-$ is crucial for proper lysosomal function.

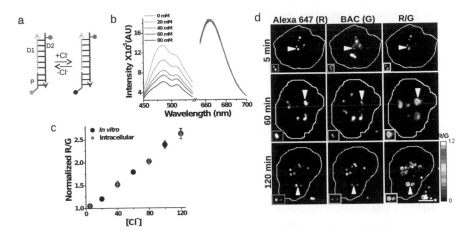

**FIGURE 2.5** Determination of vesicular [Cl⁻] using *Clensor*. (a) Schematic drawing of *Clensor*. The pink line shows the sensing module (P) carrying a Cl⁻-sensitive fluorophore, BAC (green filled circle). The brown line depicts the normalizing module (D2) containing a Cl⁻-insensitive fluorophore, Alexa 647 (red filled circle). The orange line represents the targeting module D1. In the presence of Cl⁻, the fluorescence intensity of BAC experiences collisional quenching, whereas the fluorescence of Alexa 647 is chloride-independent and serves as reference fluorophore. (b) Graph showing the fluorescence emission spectra of BAC and Alexa 647 at the indicated values of [Cl⁻] obtained using $\lambda_{Ex}$ BAC = 435 nm (green) and $\lambda_{Ex}$ Alexa 647 = 650 nm (red). (c) *In vitro* (black) and vesicular (red) Cl⁻ calibration profile of *Clensor*. The calibration curves were generated by plotting normalized R/G intensity (Alexa 647/BAC) ratios as a function of [Cl⁻]. Under both conditions, the DNA-based sensor responded in a linear fashion to changes in Cl⁻ ranging from 0–120 mM. For vesicular calibration, cells were loaded with 2 µM *Clensor* by endocytosis and fixed for 2 min with 2.5% paraformaldehyde to allow the permeabilization of the plasma membrane. Clamping solutions with varying Cl⁻ concentrations were applied together with the ionophores nigericin, valinomycin and tributyltinchloride (TBT-Cl). (d) Pseudo-colour R/G map of hemocytes labelled with 2 µM *Clensor* by endocytosis showed spatiotemporal change of [Cl⁻] along the endo-lysosomal pathway. Maturation of early endosomes to late endosomes and lysosomes was accompanied by a successive increase in luminal [Cl⁻]. Adapted from Saha et al. (2015).

## 2.3   PROTOCOLS FOR DETERMINING LYSOSOMAL [CL⁻]

To date, there are only two published protocols for *in vivo* measurements of 'resting' luminal [Cl⁻] of the lysosome. In the following section we will describe the detailed protocol to perform lysosomal Cl⁻ measurements in adherent cells with a dextran-coupled fluorophore MEQ-TMR-dextran (Weinert et al., 2014; Weinert et al., 2010) and the DNA-based fluorescent dye *Clensor* (Saha et al., 2015).

### 2.3.1   PROTOCOL I: LYSOSOMAL CL⁻ MEASUREMENT
####           WITH DEXTRAN-COUPLED CL⁻-SENSOR

The detailed protocol for the synthesis of MEQ-TMR-dextran by chemically conjugating MEQ (N-(7-carboxyhexyl)-6-methoxy-quinolinium bromide) and TMR

(N,N,N′,N′-tetramethylrhodamine) to 10 kDa dextran via amide linkage is described elsewhere (Weinert et al., 2010).

### 2.3.1.1 *In Vitro* Characterization

(i) Dissolve lyophilized powder of MEQ-TMR-dextran in DMSO to obtain a stock solution. A concentration of 20 mg/ml should be suitable for all applications.

(ii) Dilute the stock solution to 20 μg/ml MEQ-TMR-dextran in 10 mM HEPES pH 7.4.

(iii) To characterize the $Cl^-$-dependent change of the fluorescence ratio of MEQ-TMR-dextran, adjust $[Cl^-]$ to 0–100 mM in the solution in suitable increments (e.g. 20 mM) by adding aliquots of NaCl solution to MEQ-TMR-dextran dissolved in 10 mM HEPES pH 7.4. Make sure that the solution is mixed well after the addition of NaCl. (After mixing, an additional incubation step up to 30 min might help to ensure complete equilibration of the solution.) Record the emission spectra for MEQ at the excitation wavelength $(\lambda_{ex})$ of 360 nm and for TMR at the $\lambda_{ex} = 524$ nm. Measurements can be performed with a spectrofluorometer, e.g. a Safire II plate reader (Tecan).

(iv) Record the same spectra with the 0 mM $Cl^-$ buffer containing only the solvent (DMSO) that was used to dissolve the MEQ-TMR-dextran, because it might additionally emit a fluorescence signal at the used wavelengths. These measurements do not need to be performed with different $[Cl^-]$.

(v) Subtract the fluorescence intensity obtained with the buffer sample (in step iv) from the ones obtained with MEQ-TMR-dextran (in step iii). Then, calculate the fluorescence ratio of MEQ and TMR at the respective wavelength of peak emission.

### 2.3.1.2 Labelling Cells with MEQ-TMR-dextran

(i) Seed cells on a glass-bottom culture dish (e.g. MatTek P35G-0-10-C) and allow the cells to adhere/settle by incubation overnight at 37°C (in a $CO_2$ incubator if the medium contains bicarbonate). Make sure that the cell layer is not too dense to allow proper spreading of the cells. This helps to obtain images with well separated lysosomes.

(ii) Wash cells ≥3 times with 1× phosphate-buffered saline (PBS).

(iii) Prior to cell loading, dilute MEQ-TMR-dextran in growth medium to a concentration of 2 mg/ml.

(iv) Load cells by incubating them with the working solution from step (iii) for 1 h at 37°C in an incubator (with 5% $CO_2$ if the medium contains bicarbonate). Cells take up MEQ-TMR-dextran via fluid-phase endocytosis (this step is referred to as pulse). We recommend testing different pulse times, which may have to be adjusted to the cell type used.

*Note*: Using live cell imaging dishes from MatTek (P35G-0-10-C) with a small glass cavity in the middle reduces the amount of solution (and hence precious sensor) that needs to be added to the cells (typically 50 μl).

(v) Wash cells ≥3 times with 1× PBS while gently shaking the dish.

(vi) In order to chase MEQ-TMR-dextran to lysosomes, incubate cells for 2 h in a 37°C incubator with 5% $CO_2$ in low $Cl^-$ IMDM (Iscove's Modified Dulbecco's Medium; PAN-Biotech) with remaining 7 mM $Cl^-$. Depending on the cell type used, the trafficking from early endosomes to lysosomes takes up to 2 h.

*Note*: As the $Cl^-$-sensitivity of MEQ saturates at ~60–80 mM, Weinert et al. (2010) incubated cells in media with 7 mM $[Cl^-]$ during the entire chase and measurement period to restrict the lysosomal $[Cl^-]$ within the sensitive range of MEQ.

(vii) After chasing MEQ-TMR-dextran into lysosomes, wash cells ≥3 times with 1x PBS.

(viii) Add imaging buffer (in mM: 135 Na-gluconate, 5 KCl, 1 $CaCl_2$, 1 $MgCl_2$, 10 HEPES, 10 glucose, pH 7.4) and immediately take the dish for live cell imaging.

*Note*: To avoid an increase in lysosomal $[Cl^-]$ during the measurement, an imaging buffer with low $[Cl^-]$ was used.

### 2.3.1.3 Fluorescence Microscope Setup

Different fluorescence microscope setups can be used for intracellular $Cl^-$ imaging. It is important to have a sensitive camera such as a CCD (charge-coupled device) camera. For imaging lysosomes, one should use an objective with high magnification (e.g. 63x or 100x) that is suited for fluorescence microscopy. Depending on the fluorophores, adequate filter sets must be selected. For MEQ, the set should allow excitation at 344 nm and enable fluorescence detection at 442 nm. TMR is excited at 550 nm while the emission peak is at 580 nm.

(In Weinert et al. (2010), images were taken with an inverted microscope (Axiovert 200, Zeiss) equipped with a $100 \times 1.30$ NA oil immersion objective. The dye was excited with a Polychrom II monochromator (TILL photonics) while using a 440 ± 20 nm emission filter for MEQ and a 580 ± 20 nm emission filter for TMR. An emission filter wheel Lambda 10-2 (Sutter instruments) allowed for the rapid switch between the two channels during image acquisition. The setup was connected with a Sensicam CCD (PCO).)

### 2.3.1.4 Image Analysis

(i) For image analysis choose at least 10 lysosomes per cell as regions of interest (ROI) with ImageJ.

(ii) Calculate mean fluorescence intensity from MEQ and TMR for each ROI followed by appropriate background subtraction for each channel. Background subtraction is optimally done by measuring the mean fluorescence intensity (for each wavelength) that surrounds the ROI. For this purpose, three regions can be selected that surround the ROI.

(iii) Then calculate the mean background-corrected fluorescence intensity ratio between MEQ and TMR.

(iv) To obtain a reliable result, the experiment should be repeated at least three times on different days, because small changes in the experimental setup, e.g. intensity of the light source, might influence the result. When using permanently transfected cells or, e.g. cells generated by CRISPR-Cas9 gene editing, we recommend performing the experiments with three different cell lines to avoid potential effects of clonal selection. The same holds true for primary cell lines.

## 2.3.2  PROTOCOL II: LYSOSOMAL CL⁻ MEASUREMENT USING A DNA SCAFFOLD-BASED RATIOMETRIC SENSOR

The description for the synthesis of *Clensor* is not part of the following section, but can be found in detail in Saha et al. (2015).

### 2.3.2.1  Characterization of *Clensor In Vitro*

  (i) Dilute 10 µM stock of *Clensor* to a final concentration of 200 nM using 10 mM sodium phosphate buffer pH 7.2.
 (ii) Acquire emission spectra of BAC (495–550 nm) and Alexa 647 (650–700 nm) by exciting the sample at 435 nm ($_{\lambda Ex}^{BAC}$) and 650 nm ($_{\lambda Ex}^{Alexa\ 647}$), respectively. Record emission spectra of 10 mM sodium phosphate buffer pH 7.2 for blank subtraction.
(iii) In order to study the Cl⁻-sensitivity of *Clensor*, adjust final [Cl⁻] to values between 5 mM and 200 mM in 20 mM increments by addition of microliter aliquots of 1 M stock of NaCl to the sample and mix well by pipetting. (Even though the Cl⁻-induced quenching of BAC occurs within milliseconds, a 30-min incubation step is recommended as a precaution to allow proper mixing of the added NaCl.)
 (iv) Calculate the ratio (R/G) of emission intensity of Alexa 647 at 670 nm (R) and BAC at 505 nm (G). Plot R/G vs. [Cl⁻] to obtain the *in vitro* calibration profile of *Clensor*.

To investigate Cl⁻-sensitivity of *Clensor* at low pH, dilute the stock solution of *Clensor* to a final concentration of 200 nM using the following buffer (in mM: 150 $KNO_3$, 5 $NaNO_3$, 1 $Ca(NO_3)_2$, 1 $Mg(NO_3)_2$, 20 MES, pH 5). [Cl⁻] can be adjusted from 5 mM to 200 mM in 20 mM increments by addition of appropriate amounts of 1 M NaCl.

### 2.3.2.2  Labelling Cells with *Clensor*

  (i) Wash cells ≥3 times with standard imaging solution (in mM: 150 NaCl, 5 KCl, 1 $CaCl_2$, 1 $MgCl_2$, 20 HEPES, pH 7.4).
 (ii) Prior to labelling, dilute 10 µM *Clensor* stock to a final concentration of 2 µM with imaging solution and add the dye-containing solution to cells. Depending on the cell type used for the experiment, the concentration of *Clensor* may need to be adjusted in pilot experiments.

  *Note*: As mentioned in Section 3.1.2, you may wish to employ small amounts of the sensor, by using, e.g. live cells imaging dishes from MatTek.
(iii) Incubate cells with *Clensor* for 5–10 min to allow receptor-mediated endocytosis of the Cl⁻-sensor. The uptake is mediated by the interaction of the negatively charged backbone of the sensor with the anionic ligand binding

receptor (ALBR) (LaPlante et al., 2002). Since not all cell types express ALBRs, *Clensor* can be fused to an aptamer that enables, for example, the internalization via the transferrin receptor, allowing measurements along the endo-lysosomal pathway. (Binding of *Clensor* to the transferrin receptor is disrupted by the acidic pH of endosomes. The transferrin receptor is recycled to the plasma membrane, whereas the sensor is trafficked to late endosomes and finally to lysosomes.)

(iv) Wash cells ≥3 times with imaging solution and incubate the cells additionally for 5–120 min to label different compartments along the endo-lyso-somal pathway. This step is referred to as 'chase'. For a chase longer than 5 min, replace the imaging solution by complete growth media and transfer the cells to an incubator (with 5% $CO_2$ if the medium contains bicarbonate). The time required for the Cl⁻-sensor to reach different compartments needs to be established by using different chase times while staining the endo-lysosomal organelles with different marker proteins.

(v) Prior to imaging, wash cells ≥3 times with imaging solution and keep the cells in the same buffer during live cell imaging.

### 2.3.2.3  Vesicular Calibration of *Clensor*

In order to convert the obtained fluorescence ratios of BAC and Alexa 647 into Cl⁻ concentrations, calibration of *Clensor* needs to be performed *in situ*, using iono-phores to set the intracellular and intra-compartmental [Cl⁻]. Due to the fast maturation of endosomes and the slow equilibration with Cl⁻-clamping buffer (which takes 1 h), the calibration of *Clensor* cannot be performed in early endosomal compartments (after 1 h the majority of the sensor will be trafficked to late endosomal and lysosomal compartments). Vesicular calibrations should be performed after every experiment on the same day, since experimental settings, e.g. the intensity of the light source, might differ from day to day. Due to the fast bleaching of the Cl⁻-sensitive fluorophore BAC, the calibration on the same cells that were used for intra-cellular Cl⁻ imaging is problematic. Therefore, additional glass-bottom dishes with *Clensor*-loaded cells should be prepared for calibration exactly like those used for the experiment.

(i) Load cells with *Clensor* as mentioned above.

(ii) Incubate cells for 1 h at room temperature with an externally added Cl⁻-clamping buffer containing the desired [Cl⁻], supplemented with a mixture of ionophores such as nigericin (10 µM), valinomycin (10 µM), monensin (10 µM) and TBT-Cl (10 µM). (Tributyltin chloride (TBT-Cl) exchanges Cl⁻ for OH⁻. To collapse pH and voltage gradients the K⁺/H⁺-exchanger nigericin, the Na⁺/H⁺-exchanger monensin and the K⁺-ionophore valinomy-cin are added.) Chloride calibration buffers containing different chloride concentrations are prepared by appropriately mixing Cl⁻ containing buffer (in mM: 120 KCl, 40 NaCl, 1 $CaCl_2$, 1 $MgCl_2$, 20 K-acetate buffer, pH 4.5) with Cl⁻-free buffer (in mM: 120 $KNO_3$, 40 $NaNO_3$, 1 $Ca(NO_3)_2$, 1 $Mg(NO_3)_2$, 20 K-acetate buffer, pH 4.5) in different ratios, supplemented with the above-mentioned ionophores. After 1 h, cells are then imaged in the different clamping buffers, but each dish can only be used for one Cl⁻ concentration due to the high toxicity of TBT-Cl. Replacement of the solution would lead to the loss of many cells. Five different [Cl⁻]'s ranging from 5 mM to 160 mM are sufficient for calibration (e.g. 0 mM, 40 mM, 80 mM, 120 mM and 160 mM). We recommend comparing the obtained values with the *in vitro* calibration curve. If the two calibration profiles differ by more than a standard deviation, the obtained vesicular Cl⁻ concentrations should be discarded, because there is likely an experimental problem.

*Note*: TBT-Cl is highly toxic for cells. If 1-h incubation with TBT-Cl induces cell death, the incubation time can be reduced to 30–45 min, but this may lead to an incomplete equilibration of the intra-compartmental [Cl⁻].

(iii) For direct comparison, it is crucial to keep all acquisition settings (e.g. light intensity, detector sensitivity, image resolution and channel configuration) identical during imaging for all cell treatments and calibration.

*Note*: Krishnan and coworkers additionally introduced a fixation step in their calibration protocol (Saha et al., 2015) (i) to partially permeabilize the cells to allow the passive diffusion of chloride across the membrane, (ii) to maintain the integrity of the primary cells like *Drosophila* hemocytes that would de-adhere due to the prolonged exposure to the calibration solution and (iii) to antagonize the action of ion forces while the cells are being clamped.

### 2.3.2.4 Fluorescence Microscope Set-Up

Imaging of *Clensor* requires the use of an inverted microscope coupled to an adequate light source, such as a polychromator or a HBO lamp. To resolve single lysosomes within cells, objectives with a high magnification (63x or 100x) suitable for fluorescence microscopy are recommended. Fluorescence signals can be captured with sensitive CCD cameras. Specific illumination of BAC can be achieved by using a 480/20 band pass excitation filter, 535/40 band pass emission filter and 86023bs-FITC/Cy5 as dichroic filter. Image acquisition of Alexa 647 requires the use of 640/30 band pass excitation filter, 690/50 band pass emission filter and an HQ665lp-665 long pass dichroic filter.

(For example, in Saha et al. (2015) live cell imaging was performed with an inverted Olympus IX81 microscope connected to a mercury halide lamp. Images were taken with an iXon^EM CCD camera from Andor. All excitation, emission and dichroic filters used in this study were purchased from Chroma technology corp. USA.)

### 2.3.2.5 Image Analysis

Due to the rapid photobleaching of BAC (Sonawane et al., 2002) and the resulting low signal to noise ratio of the Cl⁻-sensitive fluorophore, image analysis needs careful background subtraction.

(i) Identify regions of cells containing well-demarcated punctate structures in each Alexa 647 (R) image and mark as 'regions of interest' (ROI) using image analysis software such as ImageJ.

(ii) For background determination, mark three nearby regions surrounding each punctate structure that was chosen as ROI.

(iii) Calculate the average mean background intensity from the three selected regions for each ROI.

(iv) Determine the mean intensity (R) for each ROI followed by background subtraction.

(v) Identify the same regions in the BAC (G) image by recalling the selected ROIs and follow the same steps to measure the mean background-subtracted intensity from BAC (G) in the images.

(vi) Calculate the mean intensity ratio of R to G (R/G) for each selected ROI.

## 2.4 OUTLOOK

The discovery of critical roles of CLC proteins in a number of physiological processes (Jentsch, 2015; Jentsch and Pusch, 2018) has put the role of chloride, which had previously been largely neglected, into the limelight. In particular, mouse models and human diseases owed to mutations in endosomal and lysosomal CLCs suggested important roles of luminal Cl$^-$ in the endosomal-lysosomal pathway (Jentsch, 2007).

Especially, the work on ClC-7 knockout mice changed the concepts of lysosomal ion homeostasis, including pH. The importance of lysosomal Cl$^-$/H$^+$ exchange becomes obvious when considering the pathologies of $Clcn7^{-/-}$ mice. The loss of this transporter or its beta subunit Ostm1 in neurons leads to the accumulation of lysosomal storage material, resembling a special type of lysosomal storage disease, neuronal ceroid lipofuscinosis (Kasper et al., 2005; Wartosch et al., 2009). Newer studies from cells and kidneys allow the conclusion that a reduced lysosomal enzymatic activity and hence an impaired substrate degradation are at least in part causative for the accumulation of storage material (Chakraborty et al., 2017; Wartosch et al., 2009). So far, luminal pH was considered to be the major regulator of lysosomal enzyme activity (López-Otín and Bond, 2008; Turk et al., 2012), however, in various cell types derived from ClC-7 knockout mice, no pH defect was observed (Kasper et al., 2005; Steinberg et al., 2010; Weinert et al., 2014; Weinert et al., 2010), leading to the hypothesis that changed lysosomal [Cl$^-$] plays a major role in these pathologies (Jentsch, 2007; Smith and Schwappach, 2010). This conclusion was significantly bolstered by the analysis of $Clcn5^{unc/unc}$ (Novarino et al., 2010) and $Clcn7^{unc/unc}$ (Weinert et al., 2010) mice, in which point mutations converted the endosomal ClC-5 and lysosomal ClC-7 2Cl$^-$/H$^+$-exchangers into pure Cl$^-$ conductors. Although these should provide the countercurrent for vesicular acidification, as directly shown for ClC-5$^{unc}$ (Novarino et al., 2010), these mice displayed almost the same pathologies as the respective KOs. The severe underdevelopment of the acid-secreting ruffled border of $Clcn7^{-/-}$ osteoclasts (Kornak et al., 2001; Weinert et al., 2014), which is built up by lysosomal exocytosis, points to the role of ClC-7 in vesicular trafficking, as does the role of ClC-5 in renal endocytosis (Novarino et al., 2010).

How these effects may be related to the observed decrease in lysosomal Cl$^-$ concentration, however, remains unclear. It is unlikely that the impaired protein degradation of $Clcn7^{-/-}$ cells can be entirely explained by a reduced activity of Cl$^-$-sensitive cathepsin C (Cigić and Pain, 1999). The effects of luminal Cl⁻ might be indirect. For instance, other transporters in the lysosomal membrane, many of which are not yet identified, may need Cl⁻ for co- or counter-transport, or luminal Cl⁻ may affect signalling molecules on the cytosolic face of the membrane. One should neither exclude the possibility that the loss of ClC-7 may impinge on the transmembrane voltage of lysosomes, as suggested by model calculations (Weinert et al., 2010). Furthermore, the observed drastic change in lysosomal [Cl⁻] will certainly change concentrations of other anions in the lysosomal lumen for reasons of electroneutrality and osmotic pressure, and may also somehow affect cations including $Ca^{2+}$ (Chakraborty et al., 2017). Addressing these important questions will not only require reliable measurements of lysosomal [Cl⁻], but also of other lysosomal anions and cations as well as the lysosomal membrane potential under different conditions and in cells lacking lysosomal transporters. This information must then be integrated into the increasingly complex picture of lysosomes, which are far from being only 'cellular dustbins', but are, for instance, also intimately involved in cellular metabolism. We are only beginning to understand the complex regulation of lysosomal ion homeostasis and function.

## REFERENCES

Accardi, A., and Miller, C. (2004). Secondary active transport mediated by a prokaryotic homologue of ClC Cl⁻ channels. *Nature 427*(6977), 803–807.

Appelqvist, H., Waster, P., Kagedal, K., and Ollinger, K. (2013). The lysosome: From waste bag to potential therapeutic target. *J Mol Cell Biol 5*(4), 214–226.

Arosio, D., Garau, G., Ricci, F., Marchetti, L., Bizzarri, R., Nifosi, R., and Beltram, F. (2007). Spectroscopic and structural study of proton and halide ion cooperative binding to gfp. *Biophys J 93*(1), 232–244.

Arosio, D., Ricci, F., Marchetti, L., Gualdani, R., Albertazzi, L., and Beltram, F. (2010). Simultaneous intracellular chloride and pH measurements using a GFP-based sensor. *Nat Methods 7*(7), 516–518.

Ballabio, A. (2016). The awesome lysosome. *EMBO Mol Med 8*(2), 73–76.

Barasch, J., and al-Awqati, Q. (1993). Defective acidification of the biosynthetic pathway in cystic fibrosis. *J Cell Sci Suppl 17*, 229–233.

Barasch, J., Kiss, B., Prince, A., Saiman, L., Gruenert, D., and al-Awqati, Q. (1991). Defective acidification of intracellular organelles in cystic fibrosis. *Nature 352*(6330), 70–73.

Berglund, K., Schleich, W., Wang, H., Feng, G., Hall, W.C., Kuner, T., and Augustine, G.J. (2008). Imaging synaptic inhibition throughout the brain via genetically targeted Clomeleon. *Brain Cell Biol 36*(1–4), 101–118.

Bevensee, M.O., Apkon, M., and Boron, W.F. (1997). Intracellular pH regulation in cultured astrocytes from rat hippocampus. II. Electrogenic Na/HCO₃ cotransport. *J Gen Physiol 110*(4), 467–483.

Bhatia, D., Sharma, S., and Krishnan, Y. (2011a). Synthetic, biofunctional nucleic acid-based molecular devices. *Curr Opin Biotechnol 22*(4), 475–484.

Bhatia, D., Surana, S., Chakraborty, S., Koushika, S.P., and Krishnan, Y. (2011b). A synthetic icosahedral DNA-based host-cargo complex for functional in vivo imaging. *Nat Commun 2*, 339.

Biwersi, J., Farah, N., Wang, Y.X., Ketcham, R., and Verkman, A.S. (1992). Synthesis of cell-impermeable Cl⁻-sensitive fluorescent indicators with improved sensitivity and optical properties. *Am J Physiol 262*(1), C242–C250.

Biwersi, J., Tulk, B., and Verkman, A.S. (1994). Long-wavelength chloride-sensitive fluorescent indicators. *Anal Biochem 219*(1), 139–143.

Boffi, J.C., Knabbe, J., Kaiser, M., and Kuner, T. (2018). KCC2-dependent steady-state intracellular chloride concentration and pH in cortical Layer 2/3 neurons of anesthetized and awake mice. *Front Cell Neurosci 12*, 7.

Cang, C., Aranda, K., Seo, Y.J., Gasnier, B., and Ren, D. (2015). TMEM175 is an organelle $K^+$ channel regulating lysosomal function. *Cell 162*(5), 1101–1112.

Cao, Q., Zhong, X.Z., Zou, Y., Zhang, Z., Toro, L., and Dong, X.P. (2015). BK channels alleviate lysosomal storage diseases by providing positive feedback regulation of lysosomal $Ca^{2+}$ release. *Dev Cell 33*(4), 427–441.

Chakraborty, K., Leung, K., and Krishnan, Y. (2017). High lumenal chloride in the lysosome is critical for lysosome function. *eLife 6:e28862*.

Chao, A.C., Dix, J.A., Sellers, M.C., and Verkman, A.S. (1989). Fluorescence measurement of chloride transport in monolayer cultured cells: Mechanisms of chloride transport in fibroblasts. *Biophys J 56*(6), 1071–1081.

Chen, C.C., Butz, E.S., Chao, Y.K., Grishchuk, Y., Becker, L., Heller, S., Slaugenhaupt, S.A., Biel, M., Wahl-Schott, C., and Grimm, C. (2017). Small molecules for early endosome-specific patch clamping. *Cell Chem Biol 24*(7), 907–916, e904.

Cigić, B., and Pain, R.H. (1999). Location of the binding site for chloride ion activation of cathepsin C. *Eur J Biochem 264*(3), 944–951.

Dallwig, R., Deitmer, J.W., and Backus, K.H. (1999). On the mechanism of GABA-induced currents in cultured rat cortical neurons. *Pflügers Arch 437*(2), 289–297.

Dell'Antone, P. (1979). Evidence for an ATP-driven "proton pump" in rat liver lysosomes by basic dyes uptake. *Biochem Biophys Res Commun 86*(1), 180–189.

Deriy, L.V., Gomez, E.A., Zhang, G., Beacham, D.W., Hopson, J.A., Gallan, A.J., Shevchenko, P.D., Bindokas, V.P., and Nelson, D.J. (2009). Disease-causing mutations in the cystic fibrosis transmembrane conductance regulator determine the functional responses of alveolar macrophages. *J Biol Chem 284*(51), 35926–35938.

Di, A., Brown, M.E., Deriy, L.V., Li, C., Szeto, F.L., Chen, Y., Huang, P., Tong, J., Naren, A.P., Bindokas, V., et al. (2006). CFTR regulates phagosome acidification in macrophages and alters bactericidal activity. *Nat Cell Biol 8*(9), 933–944.

Eberhardson, M., Patterson, S., and Grapengiesser, E. (2000). Microfluorometric analysis of $Cl^-$ permeability and its relation to oscillatory $Ca^{2+}$ signalling in glucose-stimulated pancreatic beta-cells. *Cell Signal 12*(11–12), 781–786.

Frech, M.J., Deitmer, J.W., and Backus, K.H. (1999). Intracellular chloride and calcium transients evoked by gamma-aminobutyric acid and glycine in neurons of the rat inferior colliculus. *J Neurobiol 40*(3), 386–396.

Galietta, L.J., Springsteel, M.F., Eda, M., Niedzinski, E.J., By, K., Haddadin, M.J., Kurth, M.J., Nantz, M.H., and Verkman, A.S. (2001). Novel CFTR chloride channel activators identified by screening of combinatorial libraries based on flavone and benzoquinolizinium lead compounds. *J Biol Chem 276*(23), 19723–19728.

Geddes, C.D. (2001). Optical halide sensing using fluorescence quenching: Theory, simulations, and applications - A review. *Meas Sci Technol 12*(9), R53–R88.

Grabe, M., and Oster, G. (2001). Regulation of organelle acidity. *J Gen Physiol 117*(4), 329–344.

Graves, A.R., Curran, P.K., Smith, C.L., and Mindell, J.A. (2008). The $Cl^-/H^+$ antiporter ClC-7 is the primary chloride permeation pathway in lysosomes. *Nature 453*(7196), 788–792.

Grimley, J.S., Li, L., Wang, W., Wen, L., Beese, L.S., Hellinga, H.W., and Augustine, G.J. (2013). Visualization of synaptic inhibition with an optogenetic sensor developed by cell-free protein engineering automation. *J Neurosci 33*(41), 16297–16309.

Grimm, C., Chen, C.C., Wahl-Schott, C., and Biel, M. (2017). Two-pore channels: Catalyzers of endolysosomal transport and function. *Front Pharmacol 8*, 45.

Grimm, C., Hassan, S., Wahl-Schott, C., and Biel, M. (2012). Role of TRPML and two-pore channels in endolysosomal cation homeostasis. *J Pharmacol Exp Ther 342*(2), 236–244.

Günther, W., Piwon, N., and Jentsch, T.J. (2003). The ClC-5 chloride channel knock-out mouse - An animal model for Dent's disease. *Pflügers Arch 445*(4), 456–462.

Haggie, P.M., and Verkman, A.S. (2009). Unimpaired lysosomal acidification in respiratory epithelial cells in cystic fibrosis. *J Biol Chem 284*(12), 7681–7686.

Hara-Chikuma, M., Yang, B., Sonawane, N.D., Sasaki, S., Uchida, S., and Verkman, A.S. (2005). ClC-3 chloride channels facilitate endosomal acidification and chloride accumulation. *J Biol Chem 280*(2), 1241–1247.

Inglefield, J.R., and Schwartz-Bloom, R.D. (1997). Confocal imaging of intracellular chloride in living brain slices: Measurement of GABA$_A$ receptor activity. *J Neurosci Methods 75*(2), 127–135.

Ishida, Y., Nayak, S., Mindell, J.A., and Grabe, M. (2013). A model of lysosomal pH regulation. *J Gen Physiol 141*(6), 705–720.

Jayaraman, S., Biwersi, J., and Verkman, A.S. (1999). Synthesis and characterization of dual-wavelength Cl⁻-sensitive fluorescent indicators for ratio imaging. *Am J Physiol 276*(3), C747–C757.

Jayaraman, S., Haggie, P., Wachter, R.M., Remington, S.J., and Verkman, A.S. (2000). Mechanism and cellular applications of a green fluorescent protein-based halide sensor. *J Biol Chem 275*(9), 6047–6050.

Jentsch, T.J. (2007). Chloride and the endosomal-lysosomal pathway: Emerging roles of CLC chloride transporters. *J Physiol 578*(3), 633–640.

Jentsch, T.J. (2015). Discovery of CLC transport proteins: Cloning, structure, function and pathophysiology. *J Physiol 593*(18), 4091–4109.

Jentsch, T.J., and Pusch, M. (2018). CLC chloride channels and transporters: Structure, function, physiology, and disease. *Physiol Rev 98*(3), 1493–1590.

Kasper, D., Planells-Cases, R., Fuhrmann, J.C., Scheel, O., Zeitz, O., Ruether, K., Schmitt, A., Poët, M., Steinfeld, R., Schweizer, M., et al. (2005). Loss of the chloride channel ClC-7 leads to lysosomal storage disease and neurodegeneration. *EMBO J 24*(5), 1079–1091.

Kellenberger, C.A., Wilson, S.C., Sales-Lee, J., and Hammond, M.C. (2013). RNA-based fluorescent biosensors for live cell imaging of second messengers cyclic di-GMP and cyclic AMP-GMP. *J Am Chem Soc 135*(13), 4906–4909.

Kornak, U., Kasper, D., Bösl, M.R., Kaiser, E., Schweizer, M., Schulz, A., Friedrich, W., Delling, G., and Jentsch, T.J. (2001). Loss of the ClC-7 chloride channel leads to osteopetrosis in mice and man. *Cell 104*(2), 205–215.

Krapf, R., Illsley, N.P., Tseng, H.C., and Verkman, A.S. (1988). Structure-activity relationships of chloride-sensitive fluorescent indicators for biological application. *Anal Biochem 169*(1), 142–150.

Krishnan, Y., and Bathe, M. (2012). Designer nucleic acids to probe and program the cell. *Trends Cell Biol 22*(12), 624–633.

Krishnan, Y., and Simmel, F.C. (2011). Nucleic acid based molecular devices. *Angew Chem Int Ed Engl 50*(14), 3124–3156.

Kuner, T., and Augustine, G.J. (2000). A genetically encoded ratiometric indicator for chloride: Capturing chloride transients in cultured hippocampal neurons. *Neuron 27*(3), 447–459.

Lange, P.F., Wartosch, L., Jentsch, T.J., and Fuhrmann, J.C. (2006). ClC-7 requires Ostm1 as a β-subunit to support bone resorption and lysosomal function. *Nature 440*(7081), 220–223.

LaPlante, J.M., Falardeau, J., Sun, M., Kanazirska, M., Brown, E.M., Slaugenhaupt, S.A., and Vassilev, P.M. (2002). Identification and characterization of the single channel function of human mucolipin-1 implicated in mucolipidosis type IV, a disorder affecting the lysosomal pathway. *FEBS Lett 532*(1–2), 183–187.

Lau, K.R., Evans, R.L., and Case, R.M. (1994). Intracellular Cl⁻ concentration in striated intralobular ducts from rabbit mandibular salivary glands. *Pflugers Arch 427*(1–2), 24–32.

Leisle, L., Ludwig, C.F., Wagner, F.A., Jentsch, T.J., and Stauber, T. (2011). ClC-7 is a slowly voltage-gated 2Cl⁻/1H⁺-exchanger and requires Ostm1 for transport activity. *EMBO J 30*(11), 2140–2152.

Li, P., Zhang, S., Fan, N., Xiao, H., Zhang, W., Wang, H., Tang, B., and Tang, B. (2014). Quantitative fluorescence ratio imaging of intralysosomal chloride ions with single excitation/dual maximum emission. *Chemistry 20*(37), 11760–11767.

López-Otín, C., and Bond, J.S. (2008). Proteases: Multifunctional enzymes in life and disease. *J Biol Chem 283*(45), 30433–30437.

Lukacs, G.L., Chang, X.B., Kartner, N., Rotstein, O.D., Riordan, J.R., and Grinstein, S. (1992). The cystic fibrosis transmembrane regulator is present and functional in endosomes: Role as a determinant of endosomal pH. *J Biol Chem 267*(21), 14568–14572.

Ma, T., Thiagarajah, J.R., Yang, H., Sonawane, N.D., Folli, C., Galietta, L.J., and Verkman, A.S. (2002). Thiazolidinone CFTR inhibitor identified by high-throughput screening blocks cholera toxin-induced intestinal fluid secretion. *J Clin Invest 110*(11), 1651–1658.

Majumdar, A., Capetillo-Zarate, E., Cruz, D., Gouras, G.K., and Maxfield, F.R. (2011). Degradation of Alzheimer's amyloid fibrils by microglia requires delivery of ClC-7 to lysosomes. *Mol Biol Cell 22*(10), 1664–1676.

Marandi, N., Konnerth, A., and Garaschuk, O. (2002). Two-photon chloride imaging in neurons of brain slices. *Pflügers Arch 445*(3), 357–365.

Markova, O., Mukhtarov, M., Real, E., Jacob, Y., and Bregestovski, P. (2008). Genetically encoded chloride indicator with improved sensitivity. *J Neurosci Methods 170*(1), 67–76.

Metzger, F., Repunte-Canonigo, V., Matsushita, S., Akemann, W., Diez-Garcia, J., Ho, C.S., Iwasato, T., Grandes, P., Itohara, S., Joho, R.H., and Knöpfel, T. (2002). Transgenic mice expressing a pH and Cl– sensing yellow-fluorescent protein under the control of a potassium channel promoter. *Eur J Neurosci 15*(1), 40–50.

Miyazaki, H., Shiozaki, A., Niisato, N., Ohsawa, R., Itoi, H., Ueda, Y., Otsuji, E., Yamagishi, H., Iwasaki, Y., Nakano, T., et al. (2008). Chloride ions control the G1/S cell-cycle checkpoint by regulating the expression of p21 through a p53-independent pathway in human gastric cancer cells. *Biochem Biophys Res Commun 366*(2), 506–512.

Modi, S., Bhatia, D., Simmel, F.C., and Krishnan, Y. (2010). Structural DNA nanotechnology: From bases to bricks, from structure to function. *J Phys Cehm Lett 1*(13), 13.

Modi, S., Nizak, C., Surana, S., Halder, S., and Krishnan, Y. (2013). Two DNA nanomachines map pH changes along intersecting endocytic pathways inside the same cell. *Nat Nanotechnol 8*(6), 459–467.

Modi, S., Souvik, M., Goswami, G.S., Gupta, D., Mayor, G.D., S., and Krishnan, Y. (2009). A DNA nanomachine that maps spatial and temporal pH changes inside living cells. *Nat Nanotechnol 4*(5), 325–330.

Muanprasat, C., Kaewmokul, S., and Chatsudthipong, V. (2007). Identification of new small molecule inhibitors of cystic fibrosis transmembrane conductance regulator protein: In vitro and in vivo studies. *Biol Pharm Bull 30*(3), 502–507.

Muanprasat, C., Sonawane, N.D., Salinas, D., Taddei, A., Galietta, L.J., and Verkman, A.S. (2004). Discovery of glycine hydrazide pore-occluding CFTR inhibitors: Mechanism, structure-activity analysis, and in vivo efficacy. *J Gen Physiol 124*(2), 125–137.

Munkonge, F., Alton, E.W., Andersson, C., Davidson, H., Dragomir, A., Edelman, A., Farley, R., Hjelte, L., McLachlan, G., Stern, M., and Roomans, G.M. (2004). Measurement of halide efflux from cultured and primary airway epithelial cells using fluorescence indicators. *J Cyst Fibros Off J Eur Cyst Fibros Soc 3*(Suppl 2), 171–176.

Novarino, G., Weinert, S., Rickheit, G., and Jentsch, T.J. (2010). Endosomal chloride-proton exchange rather than chloride conductance is crucial for renal endocytosis. *Science 328*(5984), 1398–1401.

Ohkuma, S., Moriyama, Y., and Takano, T. (1982). Identification and characterization of a proton pump on lysosomes by fluorescein-isothiocyanate-dextran fluorescence. *Proc Natl Acad Sci U S A 79*(9), 2758–2762.

Paige, J.S., Nguyen-Duc, T., Song, W., and Jaffrey, S.R. (2012). Fluorescence imaging of cellular metabolites with RNA. *Science 335*(6073), 1194.

Picollo, A., and Pusch, M. (2005). Chloride / proton antiporter activity of mammalian CLC proteins ClC-4 and ClC-5. *Nature 436*(7049), 420–423.

Piwon, N., Günther, W., Schwake, M., Bösl, M.R., and Jentsch, T.J. (2000). ClC-5 Cl$^-$ -channel disruption impairs endocytosis in a mouse model for Dent's disease. *Nature 408*(6810), 369–373.

Poenie, M. (1992). Measurements of intracellular calcium with fluorescent calcium indicators. In: *Intracellular Messengers*, A.A. Boulton, Baker, G.B., and Taylor, C.W., ed. pp. 129–174. Humana Press.

Puchelle, E., Gaillard, D., Ploton, D., Hinnrasky, J., Fuchey, C., Boutterin, M.C., Jacquot, J., Dreyer, D., Pavirani, A., and Dalemans, W. (1992). Differential localization of the cystic fibrosis transmembrane conductance regulator in normal and cystic fibrosis airway epithelium. *Am J Respir Cell Mol Biol 7*(5), 485–491.

Saha, S., Prakash, V., Halder, S., Chakraborty, K., and Krishnan, Y. (2015). A pH-independent DNA nanodevice for quantifying chloride transport in organelles of living cells. *Nat Nanotechnol 10*(7), 645–651.

Scheel, O., Zdebik, A.A., Lourdel, S., and Jentsch, T.J. (2005). Voltage-dependent electrogenic chloride/proton exchange by endosomal CLC proteins. *Nature 436*(7049), 424–427.

Schwartz, R.D., and Yu, X. (1995). Optical imaging of intracellular chloride in living brain slices. *J Neurosci Methods 62*(1–2), 185–192.

Scott, C.C., and Gruenberg, J. (2011). Ion flux and the function of endosomes and lysosomes: pH is just the start: The flux of ions across endosomal membranes influences endosome function not only through regulation of the luminal pH. *BioEssays 33*(2), 103–110.

Settembre, C., Fraldi, A., Medina, D.L., and Ballabio, A. (2013). Signals from the lysosome: A control centre for cellular clearance and energy metabolism. *Nat Rev Mol Cell Biol 14*(5), 283–296.

Smith, A.J., and Schwappach, B. (2010). Cell biology: Think vesicular chloride. *Science 328*(5984), 1364–1365.

Sonawane, N.D., Thiagarajah, J.R., and Verkman, A.S. (2002). Chloride concentration in endosomes measured using a ratioable fluorescent Cl- indicator: Evidence for chloride accumulation during acidification. *J Biol Chem 277*(7), 5506–5513.

Sonawane, N.D., and Verkman, A.S. (2003). Determinants of [Cl-] in recycling and late endosomes and Golgi complex measured using fluorescent ligands. *J Cell Biol 160*(7), 1129–1138.

Steinberg, B.E., Huynh, K.K., Brodovitch, A., Jabs, S., Stauber, T., Jentsch, T.J., and Grinstein, S. (2010). A cation counterflux supports lysosomal acidification. *J Cell Biol 189*(7), 1171–1186.

Surana, S., Bhat, J.M., Koushika, S.P., and Krishnan, Y. (2011). An autonomous DNA nanomachine maps spatiotemporal pH changes in a multicellular living organism. *Nat Commun 2*, 340.

Turk, V., Stoka, V., Vasiljeva, O., Renko, M., Sun, T., Turk, B., and Turk, D. (2012). Cysteine cathepsins: From structure, function and regulation to new frontiers. *Biochim Biophys Acta 1824*(1), 68–88.

Tyagi, S. (2009). Imaging intracellular RNA distribution and dynamics in living cells. *Nat Methods 6*(5), 331–338.

Van Dyke, R.W. (1993). Acidification of rat liver lysosomes: Quantitation and comparison with endosomes. *Am J Physiol 265*(4 Pt 1), C901–C917.

Verkman, A.S. (1990). Development and biological applications of chloride-sensitive fluorescent indicators. *Am J Physiol 259*(3 Pt 1), C375–C388.

Volpi, E.V., and Bridger, J.M. (2008). FISH glossary: An overview of the fluorescence in situ hybridization technique. *BioTechniques 45*, 385–386, 388, 390 passim.

Voss, F.K., Ullrich, F., Münch, J., Lazarow, K., Lutter, D., Mah, N., Andrade-Navarro, M.A., von Kries, J.P., Stauber, T., and Jentsch, T.J. (2014). Identification of LRRC8 heteromers as an essential component of the volume-regulated anion channel VRAC. *Science 344*(6184), 634–638.

Wachter, R.M., Elsliger, M.A., Kallio, K., Hanson, G.T., and Remington, S.J. (1998). Structural basis of spectral shifts in the yellow-emission variants of green fluorescent protein. *Structure 6*(10), 1267–1277.

Wachter, R.M., and Remington, S.J. (1999). Sensitivity of the yellow variant of green fluorescent protein to halides and nitrate. *Curr Biol 9*(17), R628–R629.

Wachter, R.M., Yarbrough, D., Kallio, K., and Remington, S.J. (2000). Crystallographic and energetic analysis of binding of selected anions to the yellow variants of green fluorescent protein. *J Mol Biol 301*(1), 157–171.

Waller-Evans, H., and Lloyd-Evans, E. (2015). Regulation of TRPML1 function. *Biochem Soc Trans 43*(3), 442–446.

Wang, X., Zhang, X., Dong, X.P., Samie, M., Li, X., Cheng, X., Goschka, A., Shen, D., Zhou, Y., Harlow, J., et al. (2012). TPC proteins are phosphoinositide-activated sodium-selective ion channels in endosomes and lysosomes. *Cell 151*(2), 372–383.

Wartosch, L., Fuhrmann, J.C., Schweizer, M., Stauber, T., and Jentsch, T.J. (2009). Lysosomal degradation of endocytosed proteins depends on the chloride transport protein ClC-7. *FASEB J 23*(12), 4056–4068.

Webster, P., Vanacore, L., Nairn, A.C., and Marino, C.R. (1994). Subcellular localization of CFTR to endosomes in a ductal epithelium. *Am J Physiol 267*(2 Pt 1), C340–C348.

Weinert, S., Jabs, S., Hohensee, S., Chan, W.L., Kornak, U., and Jentsch, T.J. (2014). Transport activity and presence of ClC-7/Ostm1 complex account for different cellular functions. *EMBO Rep 15*(7), 784–791.

Weinert, S., Jabs, S., Supanchart, C., Schweizer, M., Gimber, N., Richter, M., Rademann, J., Stauber, T., Kornak, U., and Jentsch, T.J. (2010). Lysosomal pathology and osteopetrosis upon loss of H+-driven lysosomal Cl- accumulation. *Science 328*(5984), 1401–1403.

Wöll, E., Gschwentner, M., Furst, J., Hofer, S., Buemberger, G., Jungwirth, A., Frick, J., Deetjen, P., and Paulmichl, M. (1996). Fluorescence-optical measurements of chloride movements in cells using the membrane-permeable dye diH-MEQ. *Pflugers Arch 432*(3), 486–493.

Yang, H., Shelat, A.A., Guy, R.K., Gopinath, V.S., Ma, T., Du, K., Lukacs, G.L., Taddei, A., Folli, C., Pedemonte, N., et al. (2003). Nanomolar affinity small molecule correctors of defective Delta F508-CFTR chloride channel gating. *J Biol Chem 278*(37), 35079–35085.

# 3 Endolysosomal Patch Clamping

## Approaches to Measure Vesicular Ion Channel Activities

Cheng-Chang Chen, Christian Grimm,
Christian Wahl-Schott, and Martin Biel

## CONTENTS

## 3.1  INTRODUCTION

The endolysosomal system is a series of membrane-bound organelles which is required for maintaining physiological functions of the cell, including transport of cargo molecules from the extracellular environment into the intracellular space (endocytosis) and *vice versa* (exocytosis and recycling). Endolysosomes are highly dynamic and belong to the smallest organelles in the cell. The size of these intracellular organelles is between 100 nm and 1,000 nm in diameter. Endolysosomal organelles are categorized into different subgroups including recycling endosomes (RE), early endosomes (EE), late endosomes (LE) and lysosomes (LY). It is widely accepted that phagosomes, autophagosomes, secretory vesicles, melanosomes (in melanocytes) and synaptic vesicles (in neurons) are also closely associated with the endolysosomal system. The endolysosomes can be classified by their specific membrane proteins, such as Ras-related proteins (Rab). For example, Rab11 is one of the most common membrane proteins of recycling endosomes; EEA1 and Rab5 proteins usually localize to early endosomes; Rab7 and Rab9 proteins are mainly localized on late endosomes and lysosomes. Likewise, different lipid compositions have also been assessed to identify individual stages of endolysosomes, e.g. phosphoinositides, such as phosphatidylinositol 3,5-bisphosphate [PI(3,5)P$_2$], are thought to be mainly localized to LE/LY, and phosphatidylinositol 3-phosphate (PI3P) and phosphatidylinositol 4,5-bisphosphate [PI(4,5)P$_2$] are primarily found on EE and the plasma membrane (Li et al., 2013). In the maturation pathway of endolysosomes, the pH in the lumen decreases gradually from neutral to acidic and from EE to LE/LY. After acidification of the luminal environment, endocytosed materials are degraded by hydrolytic cleavage in lysosomes.

The endolysosomal system plays a major role in intracellular vesicle trafficking, degradation and ion homoeostasis. These processes regulate important functions in different types of cells, i.e. migration of tumour cells or inflammatory and infection response in immune cells. An ever increasing number of studies suggest that endolysosomal membrane proteins are extremely critical for the function of the endolysosomal system. Dysfunction of these membrane proteins can impact or cause numerous human diseases, including neurodegenerative diseases, i.e. mucolipidosis type IV (MLIV) and Batten disease, metabolic diseases, infectious diseases and cancer.

Ion channels and transport proteins are embedded in membranes of endolysosomes and play essential roles in regulating ionic homeostasis and membrane potential of these organelles (Grimm et al., 2012a; Jentsch et al., 2005; Xu and Ren, 2015; Miao et al., 2015; Calcraft et al., 2009; Xiong and Zhu, 2016; Krogsaeter et al., 2018). In addition, calcium ions (Ca$^{2+}$) released from endolysosomes can act as a second messenger that regulates several fundamental functions in the cell, e.g., fusion and fission events of intracellular vesicles as well as vesicle trafficking. Characterizing the properties of endolysosomal ion channels thus not only allows a better under-standing of how organellar ion homeostasis is regulated, but also enables us to evalu-ate them as potential novel drug targets for different human diseases.

Electrophysiological methods are the most powerful techniques to investigate ion channels in detail. The conventional patch clamp approach is the gold standard tech-nique to characterize directly functional properties of ion channels localized in cell membranes. In this technique, a glass microelectrode (also referred to as pipette) filled with a solution (referred to as pipette or endolysosomal lumen solution) is used to form a tight seal with the surface membrane of the cell bathed in the bath solution or extra-cellular buffer. Then the conductance of the membrane is assessed by applying volt-age (voltage clamp) or injecting current (current clamp) through the pipette, under the control of an amplifier and determined according to Ohm's law. While this manual technique of conventional patch clamp has been very successful for characterizing ion channels on the plasma membrane of single cells, for channels expressed in intracellu-lar organelles, there are many challenges that limit the application of this conventional method. The first limitation is the size of intracellular organelles, with endolysosomes being particularly small (<1000 nm in diameter). Not only are endolysosomes difficult to identify under the microscope, but also they are smaller than the opening end of the typical glass patch pipette. The second challenge is how to isolate endolysosomes directly out of the target cell while maintaining the integrity of the organelles. The third challenge is the seal formation and then the rupturing of the endolysosomal mem-brane inside the patch pipette to form the most commonly used configuration of patch clamp recordings, the whole-endolysosome configuration.

Indirect electrophysiological methods have been employed to solve or circum-vent the above problems (Pitt et al., 2010; Brailoiu et al., 2010). These are (1) planar lipid bilayer recordings or (2) redirection of the endolysosomal protein to the plasma membrane for conventional patch clamping. In the bilayer recordings, purified ion channel proteins or membrane fractions containing the organelles are reconstituted into synthetic phospholipid bilayers. In the second method, the lysosomal targeting sequences of endolysosomal ion channels are mutated, resulting in lysosomal ion channels to be expressed predominantly on the plasma membrane instead of endoly-sosomal membranes. The main drawback of both methods is that the new mem-brane environment is fundamentally different from the endolysosomal membranes. In particular, the specific membrane composition and local membrane proteins are very different. The absence of possible interaction partners and cofactors may also increase the risk of incorrect channel gating phenomena or even change in conforma-tion of the channel structure. Recently, two direct electrophysiological approaches were developed to characterize endolysosomal ion channels directly on individual intact endolysosomes: (a) The solid base electrophysiology technique (Schieder et al., 2010a) and (b) a modified conventional patch clamp technique (Dong et al., 2008; Chen et al., 2017a).

### 3.1.1 Solid Base Electrophysiology

Recently, the endolysosomal planar patch clamp method was successfully applied to characterize endolysosomal two-pore channels (TPC) and endolysosomal members of the transient receptor potential superfamily of non-selective cation channels, i.e. mucolipins (TRPML) on intact endolysosomes, isolated, e.g., from fibroblasts that endogenously express the channel or HEK293 cell lines that stably express the channel (Schieder et al., 2010b; Chen et al., 2014; Grimm et al., 2014; Ruas et al., 2015). Solid-matrix planar glass chips were used in the Port-a-Patch system (Nanion, Munich) which represents a planar patch system, where isolated vesicles are attached to a small aperture (<1 μm in diameter) in a microstructured planar borosilicate chip. This glass chip with small aperture allows even small and native endolysosomes to be analyzed. A significant advantage of this approach is the combination of an automated patch clamp device with a pressure control system, which also provides a low-noise and zero-vibration environment. The purification of endolysosomes is the most crucial step of this method. The solid base electrophysiology allows floating cells and vesicles to be patched by an automatic pressure control system, which is essential to form a high-resistance seal (gigaseal) and to establish the whole-endolysosome recording configuration. However, purification requires multiple ultra-centrifugation steps which are relatively time-consuming. The other drawbacks are (1) no vision control by a microscope during measurements; (2) limited choices of solution compositions: high concentrations of luminal $Ca^{2+}$ and cytosolic $F^-$ are needed; (3) purification requires large amounts of cells ($>2 \times 10^7$) which can be a challenge for certain types of primary cells; and (4) no inside-out or outside-out patches can be established. Nevertheless, the application of the solid base endolysosomal patch clamp approach is advantageous when cells are growing only in suspension and not on glass coverslips, an essential prerequisite for the manual endolysosomal patch clamp approach. In addition, the possible bias towards patch clamping very large vesicles is less of a concern in the solid base endolysosomal patch clamp approach, which does not discriminate between smaller and larger vesicles, as long as they are larger than the aperture of the chip.

## 3.1.2 MODIFIED CONVENTIONAL PATCH CLAMPING

A modified conventional patch clamp technique has recently been applied in multiple studies to characterize various endolysosomal ion channels (TPCs, TRPMLs, BK, P2X4, TWIK2 and TMEM175), both endogenously and heterologously expressed in different cell types. This technique requires basic conventional glass-electrode-based patch clamp instrumentation. In brief, these include: (1) a microscope for visualization of cells and vesicles, (2) an anti-vibration table, (3) a micromanipulator for controlling the movement of glass pipette and (4) electronics for stimulation and recording.

(1) *Microscope.* For the manual isolation of intracellular organelles, it is important to be able to discriminate between plasma membrane, endolysosomal membrane and other cytoplasmic structures; hence phase-contrast microscopy is commonly applied instead of traditional bright-field microscopy.

(2) *Anti-vibration table.* Any vibrations can cause a drift of the patch pipette and the micromanipulator, which is often fatal to seals and recordings. A commercial heavy duty anti-vibration table is required. It needs to be set up in a highly stable area of the building. The air-float tabletop of the

anti-vibration table absorbs high-frequency vibrations. It is important that the air compressor of the table works properly. Frequent auto ON and OFF of the valve of the compressor damages the seals and can create extra noise during measurements.

(3) *Micromanipulator.* The major function of a micromanipulator in an endolysosomal patch-clamp setup is to control and finely tune the movement of the isolation-pipette so that the isolation of individual vesicles out of the cell can be achieved and to subsequently position the patch pipette tip onto the endolysosomal membrane. Minimizing vibration and minimizing drift are two main aspects of the manipulator. Precise horizontal movement in the x-y-plane is a critical requirement of micromanipulators used for the endolysosome isolation process.

(4) *Electronics.* The electronic requirements for endolysosomal patch clamping are identical to conventional patch clamping. A Faraday cage and electrical ground are essential to reduce the disruptive external noise and minimize the noise intrinsic to the system. Grounding all surfaces to minimize interference is especial. Patch clamp amplifiers and corresponding software are central components of the setup. As the endolysosomal capacitance and current amplitudes of endogenous endolysosomal ion channels are much smaller than those measured in regular whole-cell patch clamp experiments, the accuracy of capacitance compensation together with little background noise is very important.

The main critical feature of the modified conventional endolysosomal patch clamp method is the glass micropipette used to directly open up the plasma membrane to push the "enlarged" endolysosome out of the cell. This process is monitored using the microscope which provides a critical visual control. By application of pharmacological tools and specific membrane markers, the intact "enlarged (2–5 μm)" endolysosome of choice can be easily identified under the microscope. All classical configurations that have been applied to the conventional patch clamp recording of plasma membrane ion channels (e.g., whole-vesicle patch, inside-out patch and outside-out patch) are also applicable to the isolated organelles.

## 3.2 METHODOLOGY OF ENDOLYSOSOME PATCH-CLAMP ELECTROPHYSIOLOGY

This section will describe the concept and methodology of how to enlarge specific endolysosomes in different cell types. This method contains four essential steps: (1) the enlargement of one or more than one distinct endolysosomal subtypes, (2) the design and production of glass patch pipettes and isolation-pipettes, (3) the dissection of the intact endolysosomes out of the cell and into the bath solution and (4) the successful formation of a high-resistance seal between the pipette tip and the endolysosomal membrane and the establishment of the configuration of choice.

We have recently published the standard protocol of the modified conventional endolysosome patch clamp approach (Chen et al., 2017a). Hence, we also refer at this point to the information described in recent publications, including one particular study in which we introduced small molecules for patch clamping early endosomes (Chen et al., 2017b). Here, we provide the step-by-step protocols for patching specific endolysosomal types.

### 3.2.1 Cell Culture and Enlargement of Specific Types of Organelles

In principle, most cell types are suitable for manual endolysosomal patch clamping. There are three cellular features, which facilitate endolysosome patch clamping:

(1) *Cell adherence*: the interaction between cell surface and coverslip is an essential prerequisite of a successful endolysosome isolation. Epithelial cells, fibroblasts, hepatocytes, cardiomyocytes, macrophages and neurons are examples of cell types that have been successfully used for the manual endolysosomal patch clamp approach. On the contrary, less adherent or non-adherent cell types, e.g., red blood cells, are not suitable for this type of work. Importantly, colonies of 3–5 cells (with an overall cell confluence of ~30–50%) are better suited for endolysosomal patch clamping than individual cells. Furthermore, poly-L-lysine (1%) coating of the glass coverslips enhances the adherence of certain cell lines, such as transfected HEK293 and COS7 cells. Some primary cells, such as macrophages and neurons, attach very well on the coverslips even without poly-L-lysine coating. To coat the coverslips, autoclaved glass coverslips are submerged in a coating solution (0.1 mg/ml poly-L-lysine in 80 mM boric acid and 10 mM borate) for at least 24 hours at room temperature. After removing the poly-L-lysine solution by aspiration, the coverslips are rinsed three times with sterile distilled $H_2O$ and then stored in 80% ethanol at room temperature for up to 1 month. Before plating cells, the coated coverslips are placed individually into wells of 6-well plates or 24-well plates and allowed to dry for about 15 min under the laminar flow hood. Then the coverslips are rinsed twice with phosphate-buffered saline (PBS).

(2) *Size of the cytoplasm*: the cytoplasm highly impacts the enlargement of vesicles and their isolation. A small cell size with little cytoplasm limits the possibilities of vesicle enlargement according to (our) experience. Granules or particles in the cytoplasm strongly interfere with the isolation of the vesicles and the formation of gigaseals. Examples are melanocytes (containing melanosomes), myeloid cells (mast cells), dendritic cells and primary splenic macrophages which usually contain aged red blood cells in their cytoplasm. Such particles make the membrane surface of the vesicles rough, impeding the seal between the vesicle and the patch pipette. Also, there is an increased risk of unspecific seals between the patch pipette and unintended granules.

Different cell types and different endolysosomal enlargement agents have different optimal conditions in regard to time of treatment and concentrations to be used. It is therefore important to determine the optimal conditions before patch clamp experimentation.

### 3.2.1.1 Non-Selective Enlargement of Different Populations of Endolysosomal Vesicles

Endolysosomal ion channel currents are detectable in vacuolin-enlarged vacuoles (Dong et al., 2010; Cang et al., 2013; Sakurai et al., 2015; Chao et al., 2017; Bobak et al., 2017). These vacuoles can be of diverse origins. Vacuolin is known to increase the size of different kinds of endosomes and lysosomes (Chen et al., 2017b; Cerny et al., 2005). A treatment with 1 μM vacuolin-1 for 1–2 hours enlarges endolysosomes up to 2–5 μm in diameter, e.g., in HEK293 cells. Vacuolin-1 (Santa Cruz, Cat. No. sc-216045) can be dissolved in DMSO and stored at high concentration aliquots at −20°C for 6 months or at 4°C for 2–4 weeks. For endolysosomal vacuole enlargement, transfected and untransfected cells are treated with 1 μM vacuolin-1. Different cell types require different optimal incubation times with vacuolin-1. For native macrophages, it is 0.5–1 hour; for COS cells, 1–2 hours; for HEK293 cells, 1 hour (but overnight is also fine); for fibroblasts, cardiac myocytes and neurons, an overnight treatment with 2 μM vacuolin-1 is recommended. For each cell type and the specific treatment condition, without further labelling by specific endolysosomal membrane markers, the nature of the vacuolin-enlarged vacuoles used for endolysosomal patch clamping should be considered undefined. Nevertheless, vacuolin-1 is a highly efficient small molecule for the enlargement of endolysosomal organelles, although endogenous membrane proteins, lipids and cofactors of individual vacuoles in the endolysosomal system may differ greatly. The lipid and protein compositions of the enlarged vacuoles may also affect the function of organellar ion channels. It has been shown, for example, that $PI(3,5)P_2$ induces TRPML1-like or TPC2-like currents only in a subset of vacuolin-enlarged vacuoles (Dong et al., 2010; Wang et al., 2012), highlighting the possible impacts of lipid and protein compositions on the activation of these channels.

### 3.2.1.2 Specific Enlargement of Early Endosomes

To functionally characterize ion channels in early endosomal membranes with the patch clamp technique, it is essential to selectively enlarge early endosomes. Inhibition of Rab5 activity stimulates membrane fusion between early endosomes, which can be achieved by transfection with Rab5-Q79L, a dominant-negative Rab5 mutant. This manipulation can selectively enlarge early endosomes to up to 5 μm in diameter, allowing ion channels on the early endosomes to be examined by patch clamping (Cang et al., 2015). To transfect Rab5-Q79L into HEK293 cells or COS-1 cells, PolyJet (SignaGen Laboratories) or Turbofect (Thermo Fisher Scientific) can be used; Lipofectamine LTX (Invitrogen) or Lipofectamine 3000 (Invitrogen) should be used for neurons, glial cells or RAW264.7 macrophages (Cang et al., 2015). However, gene transfection in native cells, such as primary macrophages, is very difficult. Therefore, pharmacological tools have also been sought after. Vicenistatin, a natural compound that enhances homotypic fusion between early endosomes, has recently been reported as a possible small molecule tool for early endosome (Rab5-positive) enlargement, and the vacuoles produced by a treatment with 300 nM vicenistatin for 2 hours are suitable for patch clamping (Wang et al., 2017). Alternatively, a combined treatment with two small molecules, wortmannin and latrunculin B, also selectively enlarges Rab5-positive early endosomes but not Rab7-, LAMP1- or Rab11-positive vesicles (Chen et al., 2017b). Typically, cells are treated with 200 nM wortmannin in combination with 10 nM latrunculin B (e.g., 10–15 min for HEK293 cells; 20 min for peritoneal macrophages; 20 min for lung-tissue macrophages) prior to experimentation. The compounds are washed out before the patch clamp experiment. Wortmannin and latrunculin B can be purchased from Sigma-Aldrich (Cat. No. W1628 and L5288, respectively) and stored at −20°C for 2–4 months. Only freshly diluted compounds should be used.

### 3.2.1.3   Specific Enlargement of Late Endosomes/Lysosomes

To selectively record ion channel activities on LE/LY, inhibitors of PIKfyve, the kinase that converts PI3P to $PI(3,5)P_2$, can be used to specifically enlarge LE/LY. These include YM201636 (Grimm et al., 2014; Chen et al., 2017b) and apilimod (Wang et al., 2017). The treatment of YM201636 (800 nM/2 hours or 400 nM/overnight for HEK293 cells; 400 nM/1–2 hours for peritoneal macrophages; 400 nM/1–3 hours for lung macrophages; 800 nM/30 min or 400 nM/1 hour for alveolar macrophages) specifically enhances the size of LAMP1-positive LE/LY, but not Rab5-positive EE or Rab11-positive RE. Apilimod has been used at 1 μM for 8 hours to enlarge LE/LY in COS-1 cells. TPC2, TRPML and BK channel activities have been measured successfully using the PIKfyve inhibitor (YM201636 or apilimod). YM201636 (Chemdea CD0181) should be dissolved in DMSO and stored at high concentration aliquots at −20°C for 6 months or 4°C for 1–2 weeks.

### 3.2.1.4   Other Vacuole Enlargement Methods

Additionally, the incubation of cells with sucrose (50 mM) for 8–12 hours has been applied to enlarge LAMP1-positive lysosomal vacuoles for whole-lysosome patch clamping. Sucrose is taken up by cells through endocytosis but not degraded within the vacuoles, resulting in its accumulation inside vacuoles and osmotic swelling of the LAMP1- and LAMP2-positive lysosomes (DeCourcy and Storrie, 1991). The median diameter of the enlarged vacuoles can reach 1.3 μm (Bandyopadhyay et al., 2014). In a recent study, $Ca^{2+}$-activated $K^+$ outward currents through BK channels located on endolysosomal membranes of COS-1 cells have been measured by enlarging the vacuoles using a low concentration of sucrose (Wang et al., 2017).

### 3.2.2   Micromanipulator

Vacuole isolation and seal formation in manual whole-endolysosome patch clamp experiments require visual control by microscopy optics and mechanical control via a micromanipulator. We have used commercially available multi-micromanipulator systems, e.g., Sutter Instrument's MPC-200 or MPC-225, for this purpose. The manipulator needs to be fixed tightly to the microscope stage. Pipette instability may occur if the pipette is fixed incorrectly on the connector of the manipulator, which could seriously disturb the endolysosomal seal formation.

The z-axis angle of the diagonal mode movement of the micromanipulator should be set between 29 and 45 degrees according to the operation manual. It is important to have the correct DIP (Dual Inline Package; MP-225 operation manual) switch number corresponding to the diagonal mode movement angle (Sutter instrument, MP-200/225) for accurate movement along the horizontal plane. For successful whole-endolysosome patch clamping, either one or two manipulators may be used. With just one manipulator, the same manipulator is first used to operate the "isolation-pipette" for dissection and release of the enlarged endolysosomal vesicle, and then the isolation-pipette is replaced by the "patch pipette" for patch clamp recording of the isolated vacuole. With two manipulators, the added one may be used to hold the target cell or the isolated endolysosome, which can facilitate the stability of the dissection and the subsequent release of the endolysosomal vesicle.

### 3.2.3 MICROPIPETTES

One of the main challenges in endolysosomal patch clamping is the production of micropipettes. The optimal adjustment of the diameter as well as pipette thickness and glass type are critical. To establish a stable connection between pipette tip and endolysosomal membrane, the surface of the glass pipette tip should be flat and smooth enough to balance the membrane-glass adhesion energy ($\sim$1 mJ $\cdot$ m$^{-2}$) (Ursell et al., 2011). Besides, the isolated enlarged endolysosomes are surrounded by cytosolic materials spilled out from the cell, such as actin and microfilaments. Therefore, the optimal diameter of the pipette tip opening is around 0.2 μm (0.15–0.3 μm), which is not too wide to allow intact organelles to slip through the pipette tip, and not too narrow to be blocked by small particles released from the cell after vacuole isolation. To optimize the geometry of patch pipettes for endolysosomal patch clamping, a combination of the following equipment is recommended: (1) capillary glass with filament (borosilicate glass with filament, fire polished, outer diameter 1.5 mm, inner diameter 0.75 mm, length 10 cm), e.g., Sutter Instrument BF150-75-10; (2) a Flaming/Brown-type micropipette puller (Sutter Instrument, P-97) with 3.0 mm wide trough filament (Sutter Instrument, FT330B); (3) a microforge with platinum heater (Narishige, MF-830).

We recommend the following steps to program the puller:

- Switch on the P-97 puller (consider warming up for 15 min).
- Run a RAMP test with the capillary on the puller to determine a heat value (HEAT) that will start to melt the glass capillaries (consider daily variations depending on experimental conditions, e.g., room temperature, age of filament).
- Design a pulling program for the Sutter instrument puller with six individual pulling cycles using the HEAT, velocity (VEL) and time (TIME) parameters. The six pulling cycles with a total pulling time of around 17.0 sec will create a thick, smooth and even capillary wall of the pipette tip. The last two cycles determine the shape and geometry of the tip.
- After each final cycle of pulling, inspect the pipette with the microforge through the eyepiece. The diameter of the tip opening should be between 0.5 and 0.9 μm and completely flat without contaminants.
- If one side of the pipette wall is thicker than the other side, it will be bent after polishing. This also means that the capillary is not centred in the trough

filament and not positioned correctly to the air-jet hole of the puller (refer to the Sutter Instrument Pipette Cookbook P-97). Adjust these positions.

- If the tip of the pipette is too wide (>1 μm) or too thick, increase the HEAT parameter of the sixth cycle by 5 units or increase the VEL parameter by 1 unit. Pull a new capillary to examine the pipettes again. If the tip is too narrow and thin, reduce the parameters accordingly. Optimal HEAT and VEL parameters for the sixth cycle must be determined after each pulling process. The VEL parameter for the fifth cycle may be further adjusted if necessary. Even under optimal conditions, 50% of the pipettes are typically not suitable for endolysosomal patch clamping (e.g., due to too narrow/wide opening, uneven width or dust contaminants).

Heat polishing is required to smoothen the edges and generate the optimal geometry of the patch pipette tip, as well as to remove any contaminants left on the tip after pulling. This is achieved using the following steps:

- Set the temperature wheel of the Narishige MF-830 microforge to graduation level 80–85.
- With the pipette mounted on the microforge and the tip placed at about 3 mm above the heat filament, apply one or a series of brief heat pulses (0.5–1 sec) with the foot switch of the microforge, while monitoring the change of geometry of the pipette tip through the eyepiece.
- The desired tip opening diameter should be smaller than 0.3 μm, and the parallel inner wall should ideally be longer than 2 μm. If the pipette tip is bent or adapted a semicircle shape because of overheating, discard them and pull new ones. After polishing, the optimal recording pipettes usually have resistances of 5–8 MΩ when placed in high $K^+$, neutral pH bath and high $Na^+$, acidic pH pipette/luminal solutions (solution compositions described in the next section).
- Use the polished pipettes as soon as possible or store them in a closed clean box to prevent contamination from the environment (cannot be stored for longer than 4 hours). Older pipettes or pipettes that do not fulfil the criteria of desired tip geometry can be used as "isolation-pipettes" for isolating endolysosomal vacuoles.

### 3.2.4  PATCH CLAMPING

Pipette solutions were designed to mimic the luminal environment of endolysosomes with low pH (pH 4.5–4.6 for lysosomes; for endosomes 6.7), high $Na^+$ (~140 mM) and high $Ca^{2+}$ (~2 mM). A high concentration of $K^+$ (~140 mM) and neutral pH (pH 7.0–7.2) are commonly used in the bath solution. For optimal recording conditions, the luminal (lysosome) solution contains (in mM): 140 Na-MSA, 5 K-MSA, 2 Ca-MSA, 1 $CaCl_2$, 10 HEPES and 10 MES; the bath (cytosolic) solution is composed of: 140 K-MSA, 5 KOH, 4 NaCl, 0.39 $CaCl_2$, 1 EGTA and 20 HEPES. The pH is adjusted to 4.6 and 7.2 with MSA and KOH, respectively. The osmolality of the solutions is adjusted to 300 mOsm/l with glucose. Empirically, about 5–10 mOsm/l higher osmolality of the luminal (pipette) solution than the cytosolic solution has been found to facilitate proper maintenance of the surface tension of the isolated vacuole membrane and increases the stability of the formed seal. The solutions should be sterilized by passing through a 0.2-μm filter, after which they can be stored in 50-ml conical tubes at room temperature for 2–4 weeks. Osmolality and sterilization of the solutions are critical for endolysosomal patch clamping because endolysosomes are generally fragile, and contamination, as well as hypo-/hyper-osmotic stress, reduces the rate of successful patch clamp experiments. The osmolality of the bath solution can change significantly due to evaporation, especially under low-humidity conditions. Ideally, endolysosome patch clamp experiments should be done in 20–30 min after taking out the cells from the incubator.

### 3.2.4.1   Isolation Procedure

The first step of endolysosome patch clamping is the identification of a suitable cell with enlarged organelles of interest. For transfected cells, usually DNA constructs used for endolysosomal recordings contain coding the sequence for a GFP or YFP tag to allow identification of the organelles expressing the protein. In addition, endolysosomal membrane markers (Rab or LAMP proteins) with fluorescence tags are also used to help detect specific organelles for patch clamping as described above. For primary, untransfected cells, specific organellar enlargement procedures as described above are necessary to ensure selective isolation of vesicles of interest.

Steps for isolation of enlarged vacuoles:

- Evaluate cells under the microscope to determine whether the cells are healthy and adhere well to the coverslip. Cell confluence of ~30–50% provides enough space for dissection and release of vesicles. The vacuoles of interest should be large enough (>2 μm) for patch clamping.
- Transfer the coverslip onto the microscope chamber containing 1 ml of bath solution.
- Select the cell that contains enlarged vacuole of interest (diameter between 2 μm and 5 μm). Suitably enlarged endolysosomes are visible as clear and colourless vesicles under transmitted light in the microscope. It is preferred to choose enlarged vesicles that are near the edge of the cell and close to the side of the manipulator, rather than at the opposite side of the manipulator.
- Mount the "isolation-pipette" on the holder of the micromanipulator.
- Move the isolation-pipette downward until it touches the edge of the plasma membrane and also slightly touches the glass surface of the coverslip (Figure 3.1A).
- Rapidly move the isolation-pipette away horizontally (Figure 3.1A). This step should pull out a piece of the plasma membrane but not disrupt the enlarged endolysosome.
- Repeat the press and pull movement several times until the edge of the plasma membrane is clearly opened. This dissection process varies depending on the adherence and morphology of the cell. For example, HEK293 cells have a considerably high tensile strength and membrane toughness, which make it more difficult to disrupt the plasma membrane; on the

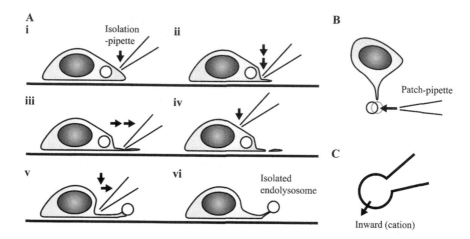

**FIGURE 3.1** Schematic showing the whole-endolysosome patch clamp process. (A) Sectional views illustrating the dissection and isolation of individual enlarged endolysosomal vacuole from a cell attached to a coverslip. The isolation-pipette is pressed against the edge of the cell near the enlarged target vacuole (i), hard-pressed until touching the coverslip (ii) and rapidly pulled away to cut apart the plasma membrane (iii). Then, the same isolation-pipette is moved up and forward to push against the cell membrane to slowly squeeze the target vacuole out of the cell (iv and v). The isolated vacuole will be exposed outside but still connected to the cell by a tiny bundle of cytosolic filaments (cytoskeleton) (vi). (B) A top view of the cell and the isolated enlarged vacuole with the patch pipette approaching. The vacuole is moved because of the slight solution flow from the patch pipette with positive pressure, which is released immediately when the patch pipette is close to the vacuole. A gigaseal should form within a few seconds. (C) The whole-endolysosomal configuration is achieved by application of ZAP pulses. Inward currents are defined as cations flowing out of the organelle lumen to the cytosol.

contrary, fibroblasts have a low tensile strength and membrane toughness and therefore are easier to be cut open. By using a phase-contrast micro-scope, the entire cell edge can be distinguished by the grey shade. The thickness of the cytoplasm at the opening is usually thinner (less contrast) than at the uncut membrane parts.

- Use the isolation-pipette to slowly push the endolysosome through the opening and away from the cell (Figure 3.1A). The process of release can be monitored under the microscope. Once the vacuole has been pushed out of the cell, its membrane appears brighter (thinner) than before release. Take care not to allow cytosolic debris or plasma membrane to stick to the isolated organelle, as this usually interferes with the seal or the formation of accurate whole-organelle configuration. The isolated organelle should ideally maintain a weak connection with the cell through cellular filaments (microtubule and microfilament), which helps stabilize the position of the isolated vacuole by avoiding vacuole drifting.

- Move the isolation-pipette away from the isolated endolysosome. Sometimes the isolated organelle may stick to the pipette tip, which can be avoided by moving the pipette 90 degrees up or down or vertically. An isolated endolysosome can stay at the same position with the same morphology for 2 min to 1 hour depending on the composition and osmolality of the bath solution and the condition of the organelle itself. The integrity of the organelle during and after the release process also depends on the tensile strength and membrane toughness.

### 3.2.4.2 Seal Formation

1. Use a freshly polished patch pipette and fill it with the luminal solution. Use just enough solution to cover the tip of the Ag-AgCl electrode and the pipette tip.
2. Rapidly flick the pipette several times to remove air bubbles.
3. Assemble the pipette onto the pipette holder.
4. Apply a positive air pressure ($\Delta p = p_{pipette} - p_{bath}$) to the lumen of the pipette. Start with overpressure ($\Delta p = 20$–$50$ mbar; $0.03$–$0.05$ ml of the syringe scale). This positive pressure is necessary to clean the tip of the pipette from dust and contaminants.
5. Move the pipette tip into contact with the bath solution using the micromanipulator.
6. Observe the pipette resistance determined by the test seal function of the amplifier, which is based on the current response to a rectangular voltage pulse (5 mV, 5 ms step). The current may go off scale immediately when the tip contacts the bath solution.
7. Cancel offset potentials between pipette and reference electrode, by adjusting the pipette offset control until the current is close to zero. Pipette resistance can then be monitored and this should be around 5–8 MΩ for the whole-endolysosomal recordings.
8. Once the pipette tip reaches the upper part of the isolated vacuole near the longitudinal axis of the edge of the vacuole, slowly move down until the isolated vacuole is moved slightly by the luminal solution flow (Figure 3.1B).
9. Release the pressure with the syringe, which will spontaneously generate a negative pressure that will pull a tiny amount of the bath solution into the pipette ($\Delta p = \sim-5$ mbar). The isolated vacuole will rebound and be sucked iinto the tip of the pipette immediately, and form a gigaseal within 3 sec. A successful gigaseal is recognized by current response to a test pulse (resistance >1 GΩ).
10. If the resistance is only around 500~1,000 MΩ, apply a series of fast-ramp protocols (−100 mV to +100 mV in 100 ms at 1-s intervals for 10–100 times). This may facilitate the seal formation and help obtain a gigaseal within 1–2 min. In addition, application of additional negative pressure (−20 to −50 mbar) may allow the establishment of a gigaseal in about 3 sec. However, the fast-ramp and pulse negative pressure may interrupt the integrity of the organelle.
11. If a gigaseal is not formed within 2 min, apply positive pressure and replace the patch pipette with a fresh one. Repeat the process from the beginning.

12. If a gigaseal is formed, slowly move the pipette together with the vacuole up (2–10 μm) and horizontally away from the cell (20–100 μm). This will prevent the impact from an unexpected movement (nm to μm) of the pipette tip by elastic force resulting from the process of assembling and rotating between the pipette and the electrode holder.

13. All kinds of patch-clamp configurations can be used after the gigaseal formation, e.g., whole-organelle mode for voltage/current clamp recordings (next section), organelle-attached mode for single channel recordings, or lumen-out mode for single channel recordings.

### 3.2.4.3 Whole-Organelle Mode

After the formation of a gigaseal, the fast capacitance cancellation (C-fast) is used to reduce the access resistance before breaking the patch. The only available approach to break the membrane to establish the whole-organelle configuration is ZAP, a high-voltage short pulse (200 μsec or 500 μsec). ZAP command can be set by the PatchMaster software (HEKA amplifier system) or the pClamp software (Axon amplifier system) from −500 mV up to −1,200 mV, decreasing by −100 mV or −200 mV step-by-step until the membrane is broken. It is recommended to wait 60 sec until the pressure across the membrane ($\Delta p$) reaches the steady-state before ZAP application. The capacitive transients of the test pulse will suddenly increase during the electrical access to the interior of the organelle. After that, C-slow and R-series controls on the amplifier are adjusted to cancel the transient, which will give estimates of the membrane capacitance (from 0.1 pF to 5 pF) and the series resistance (<100 MΩ). Inward currents are defined as the cation flow from the pipette (lumen) into the bath solution (cytosol) (Figure 3.1C).

## 3.3  RESULTS

The protocols of voltage and current clamp experiments in endolysosomal patch clamp are designed as in conventional patch clamp. The ramp and step protocols are designed in a similar way as in conventional patch clamp and can span a broad voltage range (e.g., −200 mV to +200 mV).

After breaking into the endolysosomal vesicle, slow transients indicate access to the lumen of the vacuole. Based on the transients, most parameters are obtained like in the conventional patch clamp. For typical whole-endolysosome recordings, the series resistance ranges from 20 MΩ to 100 MΩ, seal resistance ranges from 1 GΩ to 20 GΩ and the capacitance ranges from 0.1 pF to 5 pF.

In whole-intracellular organelle conformation, endolysosomal (cat)ion channel currents can be recorded directly on endolysosomal membranes. Nano-ampere TRPML3 currents are activated by applying TRPML3 agonists using the voltage-ramp protocol on intact LE/LY and EE isolated from HEK293 cells expressing TRPML3 (Figure 3.2A,B). Families of cation current traces obtained by applying a voltage step protocol on vacuolin-enlarged endolysosomes isolated from HEK293 cells expressing TPC2 are shown in Figure 3.2C. TWIK2 channels are constitutively active and therefore their potassium conductance can be measured in the absence of any ligand (Figure 3.2D–F). Current-clamp mode or single channel recording is also possible (Chen et al., 2017a).

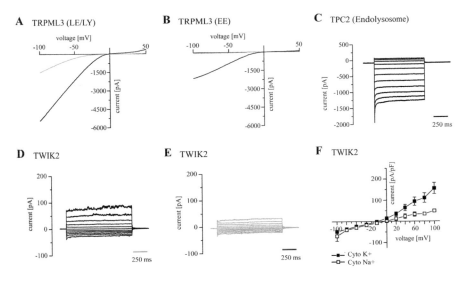

**FIGURE 3.2** Representative whole-organelle recordings (voltage clamp). Shown are selectively enlarged late endosome/lysosome (A), early endosome (B) and vacuolin-enlarged endolysosomes (C–F). Pipette solutions contained a high concentration of sodium (140 mM). Bath solutions contained a high concentration of potassium (140 mM) (A–D). In (A) and (B), voltage-ramp protocols (+50 mV to −100 mV in 500 ms, holding potential is 0 mV) were applied. In (C–F), voltage step protocols (−100 mV to +100 mV with a 20-mV step) were applied. Basal currents (grey) and ML-SA1 (black) evoked inwardly rectifying cation currents on LE/LY and EE from TRPML3-transfected HEK293 are shown in (A) and (B), respectively. PI(3,5)P$_2$-evoked inward cation currents were recorded on a vacuolin-enlarged endolysosome isolated from a HEK293 cell expressing TPC2 (C). Outward K$^+$ currents recorded on a vacuolin-enlarged endolysosome isolated from a HEK293 cell expressing TWIK2 (D). Currents were reduced when symmetrical Na$^+$ concentrations were used (E). (F) Current-voltage relationships for experiments are shown in (D) and (E).

Ion selectivity refers to the ability of a channel to permeate specific ions through cell membranes, which is fundamental for multiple important biological functions. Using specific solutions (e.g., bi-ionic solutions) and the equations shown in the Appendix, endolysosomal ion channel selectivity can be determined. The relative permeability to different cations can be calculated from the measured reversal potential using the Goldman–Hodgkin–Katz equation and solutions containing two or more cations (Appendix). To determine the relative permeability of TPC2 for monovalent cations relative to Na$^+$, bi-ionic solutions and equation III.1 in the Appendix were used (Chao et al., 2017). Before measuring the reversal potentials, all reversal potentials should be corrected for liquid junction potentials according to the solutions used in the experiment. The reversal potentials were obtained with a voltage-ramp protocol (−100 mV to +100 mV, 500 ms), using bath solutions containing 160 mM (pH 7.2, HEPES 5 mM) of the respective cations (Na$^+$, Li$^+$, K$^+$, Rb$^+$ and Cs$^+$), and a pipette solution containing 160 mM NaCl (pH 7.2, HEPES 5 mM). The recordings were started with symmetric Na$^+$ solutions (160 mM NaCl in both the pipette and bath), and then the bath solution was exchanged by the respective monovalent cation solution. The results indicate that the selectivity of wild-type TPC2 is comparable to the Eisenman selectivity sequence X: Na$^+$ > Li$^+$ > K$^+$ > Rb$^+$ > Cs$^+$. To estimate the pore diameter of TPC2, the relative permeability ratios of cations relative to Na$^+$ can be plotted against the size of the cations (referring to Stoke's diameter, e.g., the ionic radii of Li$^+$, K$^+$, Rb$^+$ and Cs$^+$ are 0.6, 1.33, 1.48 and 1.69 Å respectively). Fitting the following equation to the plot will then yield an estimation of the pore diameter:

$$\frac{P_{X^+}}{P_{Na^+}} = k\left(1 - \frac{a}{b}\right)^2$$

where $a$ is the diameter of the permeant cation, $k$ is a constant factor and $d$ is the pore diameter. In our recordings, the estimated pore diameter of wild-type TPC2 is 3.7 Å.

## 3.4  PERSPECTIVES AND CHALLENGES

Whole-endolysosome patch clamping is not only allowing the direct measurement of intracellular ion channel activities and characteristics but is also providing a way to study endolysosomal channel proteins in a more native context, compared to plasma membrane redistribution or lipid bilayer reconstitution experiments. In the future, it is highly desired to find ways to also patch clamp other intracellular vesicular structures such as lysosome-related organelles (LRO) or perhaps even synaptic vesicles or Golgi-derived vesicles.

By using whole-endolysosome patch clamp approaches, an increasing number of endolysosomal (cat)ion channels have been characterized in selectively enlarged organelles.

### 3.4.1  TRPML1

TRPML1–3 (transient receptor potential mucolipins 1, 2 and 3) constitute a family of endolysosomal cation channels with homology to the transient receptor potential superfamily. By using whole-endolysosome patch clamp, TRPMLs are described as inwardly rectifying, PI(3,5)P$_2$-sensitive, calcium-permeable, and non-selective cation channels. Loss-of-function mutations in the human TRPML1 gene result in the neurodegenerative lysosomal storage disease mucolipidosis type IV (MLIV). TRPML1 is ubiquitously expressed in the mammalian body. Endogenous TRPML1 currents have been shown, e.g., on vacuolin-enlarged endolysosomes and YM201636-enlarged LE/LY isolated from fibroblasts, bone marrow macrophages or peritoneal macrophages (Chen et al., 2017b; Dong et al., 2010). PI(3,5)P$_2$ binds and activates TRPML channels; PI(4,5)P$_2$, PI(3,4)P$_2$ and PI(3,4,5)P$_3$ also bind but inhibit PI(3,5)P$_2$-evoked TRPML1 currents; Golgi-specific PI(4)P or early endosome-specific PI(3)P have no effect (Zhang et al., 2012). Plasma membrane lipids and sphingomyelins also inhibit TRPML1 activity (Shen et al., 2012). Besides, oxidants specifically activate endolysosomal TRPML1 (Zhang et al., 2016). At physiological (lysosomal lumen) pH 4.6, higher amplitudes of TRPML1 currents are measured than at neutral pH (Dong et al., 2008). Synthetic agonists (e.g., SF-22, ML-SA1 or MK6-83) have been demonstrated to increase TRPML1 activity directly on endolysosomal membranes (Chen et al., 2014; Shen et al., 2012; Feng et al., 2014). Recently, organelle-selective patch clamp experiments directly prove that TRPML1 activity is only found in LE/LY, but not EE, e.g., in macrophages, proving the highly specific and organelle-selective expression pattern of TRPML1 as postulated before based on immunocytochemistry experiments (Chen et al., 2017b).

### 3.4.2 TRPML2

TRPML2 is less well characterized than TRPML1 and TRPML3. TRPML2 has been shown to be also activated by PI(3,5)P$_2$ and by small molecule ligands such as ML2-SA1, ML-SA1, SF-21, SF-41 or SF-81 on vacuolin-enlarged vacuoles or in calcium imaging and whole-cell patch clamp experiments using the plasma membrane variant of TRPML2 (Dong et al., 2010; Shen et al., 2012; Grimm et al., 2012b; Plesch et al., 2018). TRPML2 is not activated by oxidants (Shen et al., 2012). Unlike TRPML1, endogenous expression of TRPML2 and TRPML3 is restricted to certain cell types and tissues. There is no disease-causing mutation known in the TRPML2 gene so far.

### 3.4.3 TRPML3

The gain-of-function mutation A419P in murine TRPML3 results in a constitutively active channel variant causing the varitint-waddler phenotype (Grimm et al., 2007; Xu et al., 2007; Nagata et al., 2008). Endolysosomal TRPML3 currents are evoked by, e.g., PI(3,5)P$_2$, MK6-83, ML-SA1, SF-51, SN-2, SF-11 or SF-22 (Chen et al., 2014; Grimm et al., 2012b; Kim et al. 2007). In contrast to PI(3,5)P$_2$, other phosphoinositides (EE-rich PI(3)P; PM-rich PI(3,4)P$_2$, PI(4,5)P$_2$ and phosphatidylserine) have no effect on TRPML3 (Chen et al., 2017b). PM-specific PI(4,5)P$_2$, but not PI(3,4)P$_2$, inhibits ~50% of the activity of TRPML3. Endogenous TRPML3 activities were recorded directly on EE and LE/LY from CD11b+ lung-tissue macrophages but could not be detected in peritoneal macrophages (Chen et al., 2017b). Neutral pH 6.7 and high concentration of K$^+$ enhance TRPML3 activity while acidic pH 4.6 and high Na$^+$ in the luminal solution reduce it (Chen et al., 2017b). Taken together, the endogenous TRPML3 activity is inhibited by the acidic pH and the PM-rich phosphoinositide PI(4,5)P$_2$, but activated by the lysosome-enriched phosphoinositide PI(3,5)P$_2$ at the neutral pH, suggesting that TRPML3 activation may occur particularly in heterotypic fusion processes (e.g., acidic LE/LY spatiotemporally fusing with non-acidic organelles) or during the maturation process of endolysosomes (e.g., early endosomes or early-stage lysosomes). Large basal activities of TRPML3 in the absence of agonists are observed on LE/LY from overexpressing HEK293 cells, which occur possibly due to the presence of higher amounts of PI(3,5)P$_2$ in LE/LY compared to EE or PM or a higher channel density (Chen et al., 2017b).

### 3.4.4 TPC1

TPC1 and TPC2 are also non-selective, calcium-permeable cation channels in endolysosomes distantly related to the TRP superfamily on the one hand, and voltage-gated calcium channels on the other hand (Grimm et al., 2017a). Using whole-organelle patch clamp techniques, TPC1 has been measured and described as a voltage-gated cation channel that is activated by lysosome-specific $PI(3,5)P_2$ and alkaline pH (Cang et al., 2014). $PI(3,5)P_2$-evoked endogenous voltage-dependent TPC1 activities were observed on vacuolin-enlarged vesicles isolated from, e.g., cardiomyocytes and kidney cells, but not macrophages. A specific small molecule agonist for TPC1 is currently not available.

## 3.4.5  TPC2

There are no disease-related mutations reported for human TPC1 or TPC2 so far (Grimm et al., 2017b; Morgan and Galione, 2014). However, TPCs have been suggested to play a role in hair pigmentation, tumour migration, cholesterol trafficking and viral as well as bacterial toxin trafficking (Sakurai et al., 2015; Bellono et al., 2016; Nguyen et al., 2017). TPC2 currents have been measured on vacuolin-enlarged endolysosomes isolated from overexpressing cell lines or from cardiomyocytes, hepatocytes, fibroblasts and macrophages by using whole-organelle electrophysiological methods (Cang et al., 2013; Chao et al., 2017; Wang et al., 2012). TPC2 is a $Na^+$ and $Ca^{2+}$ permeable, voltage-independent cation channel (Schieder et al., 2010b; Ruas et al., 2015; Jha et al., 2014). It is activated by the phosphoinositide $PI(3,5)P_2$ and by NAADP while it is inhibited by ATP, Ned-19 and tetrandrine (Sakurai et al., 2015). ATP is known to bind to TPCs via the mTOR-ATP complex which regulates TPC activity directly (Cang et al., 2013; Chao et al., 2017). No specific lipophilic small molecule agonist for TPC2 is currently available.

## 3.4.6  K⁺ CHANNELS

Endolysosomal potassium channels were characterized directly on endolysosomes by using whole-endolysosome patch clamp approaches, such as TMEM175 (transmembrane protein 175) (Cang et al., 2015), TWIK2 (weakly inwardly rectifying potassium channel 2) (Bobak et al., 2017) and BK (big-conductance $Ca^{2+}$-activated potassium) (Wang et al., 2017; Zhong et al., 2016; Cao et al., 2015a). Unidentified background $K^+$ conductance was observed in endolysosomes isolated from macrophages and non-transfected HEK293 cells (Bobak et al., 2017; Cang et al., 2014), which were recently suggested to be mediated by TMEM175 and TWIK2. The potassium conductance of TMEM175 was further recorded on Rab5-Q79L-enlarged Rab5-positive endosomes isolated from neurons and glial cells, and on vacuolin-enlarged vacuoles from glial cells, RAW264.7 mouse macrophages and transiently transfected HEK293 cells. Voltage-independent outward TMEM175 currents and weakly rectifying outward TWIK2 currents may be observed under high cytosolic $K^+$ solutions on endolysosomes from all kinds of cells. These currents have been suggested to control endolysosomal pH and the membrane potential. Recently, it was shown that BK channels are not only present on the plasma membrane but also on endolysosome membranes by using the whole-organelle patch clamp technique. Endolysosomal BK channel activity was recorded in both excitable and non-excitable cells like, e.g., non-transfected COS-1, non-transfected HEK293, A7r5 smooth muscle cells, BECs (blood vascular endothelial cells), primary cortical neurons, INS-1 pancreatic cells, primary parietal cells and mouse embryonic fibroblasts (Wang et al., 2017).

### 3.4.7 OTHER ION CHANNELS

Luminal ATP (0.1 mM) at neutral pH activated cation currents of P2X4 on vacuolin-enlarged endolysosomes in whole-organelle patch clamping experiments (Huang et al., 2014; Cao et al., 2015b). Low luminal pH 4.6 inhibited endolysosomal P2X4 conductance significantly. Besides the channels described above, unidentified $H^+$ or $Cl^-$ conductance found on vacuolin-enlarged organelles remains to be elucidated on the molecular level (Cang et al., 2014).

## 3.5 APPENDIX: EXTENDED CONSTANT FIELD EQUATIONS

### I. GHK CURRENT EQUATION.

For solutions containing one permeant divalent cation and one or more permeant monovalent cations, the following GHK current equation can be used: (Eq. 13.47 from Jackson, 2006):

$$\frac{4F^2V}{RT}P_{dv}\left(\frac{[dv]_i\, e^{\frac{2VF}{RT}}-[dv]_o}{e^{\frac{V2F}{RT}}-1}\right)+\sum_i \frac{F^2V}{RT}P_{mvi}\left(\frac{[mv]_i\, e^{\frac{VF}{RT}}-[mv]_o}{e^{\frac{VF}{RT}}-1}\right)=0$$

*dv*: divalent
*mv*: monovalent
*i*: internal
*o*: external

Throughout, the term "internal" solution refers to the solution contained in the pipette (indexed as "i") and "external" or "outside" refers to the recording solution contained in the culture dish and is abbreviated by the index "o". Please note that for whole-cell recordings, the internal pipette solution corresponds to cytosolic solution, while in endolysosomal patch clamp it corresponds to the luminal solution. Likewise, in whole-cell patch clamp experiments, the external solution corresponds to extracellular solution, while in endolysosomal recordings it corresponds to cytosolic solution.

### II. DETERMINATION OF PERMEABILITY RATIOS FROM ABSOLUTE REVERSAL POTENTIAL FOR INTERNAL AND EXTERNAL SOLUTIONS CONTAINING MIXTURES OF TWO IONS.

### II.1. Internal and external solutions containing the same two permeant monovalents.

Example:

Permeable cations inside: $K^+$ and $Na^+$
Permeable cations outside: $K^+$ and $Na^+$

For solutions only containing permeant monovalent cations, only the right part of equation 1 (GHK current equation) is considered:

$$\sum_i \frac{F^2 V}{RT} P_{mvi} \left( \frac{[mv]_i \, e^{\frac{VF}{RT}} - [mv]_o}{e^{\frac{VF}{RT}} - 1} \right) = 0$$

$$P_{Na} \left( [Na]_i \, e^{\frac{VF}{RT}} - [Na]_o \right) + P_K \left( [K]_i \, e^{\frac{VF}{RT}} - [K]_o \right) = 0$$

$$\frac{P_{Na}}{P_K} = - \frac{[K]_i \, e^{\frac{VF}{RT}} - [K]_o}{[Na]_i \, e^{\frac{VF}{RT}} - [Na]_o}$$

## II.2. Internal and external solutions containing the same two permeant divalent cations.

Example:

Permeable cations inside: $Ca^{2+}$ and $Ba^{2+}$
Permeable cations outside: $Ca^{2+}$ and $Ba^{2+}$

For solutions only containing permeant divalent cations, only the left part of equation 1 is considered:

$$\sum_i \frac{4F^2 V}{RT} P_{dv} \left( \frac{[dv]_i \, e^{\frac{2VF}{RT}} - [dv]_o}{e^{\frac{V2F}{RT}} - 1} \right) = 0$$

$$P_{Ca} \left( [Ca]_i \, e^{\frac{2VF}{RT}} - [Ca]_o \right) + P_{Ba} \left( [Ba]_i \, e^{\frac{2VF}{RT}} - [Ba]_o \right) = 0$$

$$\frac{P_{Ba}}{P_{Ca}} = - \frac{[Ca]_i e^{\frac{2VF}{RT}} - [Ca]_o}{[Ba]_i e^{\frac{2VF}{RT}} - [Ba]_o}$$

## II.3. Internal and external solutions containing the same permeant monovalent and divalent cations.

Example:

Permeable cations inside: $Ca^{2+}$ and $Na^+$
Permeable cations outside: $Ca^{2+}$ and $Na^+$

Applying equation 1, we obtain:

$$\frac{4F^2V}{RT}P_{dv}\left(\frac{[dv]_i\,e^{\frac{2VF}{RT}}-[dv]_o}{e^{\frac{V2F}{RT}}-1}\right)+\sum_i\frac{F^2V}{RT}P_{mvi}\left(\frac{[mv]_i\,e^{\frac{VF}{RT}}-[mv]_o}{e^{\frac{VF}{RT}}-1}\right)=0$$

$$4P_{Ca}\left([Ca]_i\,e^{\frac{2VF}{RT}}-[Ca]_o\right)+P_{Na}\left([Na]_i\,e^{\frac{VF}{RT}}-[Na]_o\right)\left(e^{\frac{VF}{RT}}+1\right)=0$$

$$\frac{P_{Ca}}{P_{Na}}=-\left(e^{\frac{VF}{RT}}+1\right)\frac{\left([Na]_i\cdot e^{\frac{VF}{RT}}-[Na]_o\right)}{4\left([Ca]_i\,e^{\frac{2VF}{RT}}-[Ca]_o\right)}$$

III.  **DETERMINATION OF PERMEABILITY RATIOS FROM ABSOLUTE REVERSAL POTENTIAL FOR BI-IONIC SOLUTIONS.**

III.1.  **Internal solution contains one monovalent cation and external solution contains another different monovalent cation.**

Example:

Permeable cations inside: Only $K^+$
Permeable cations outside: Only $Na^+$

$$\sum_i\frac{F^2V}{RT}P_{mvi}\left(\frac{[mv]_i\,e^{\frac{VF}{RT}}-[mv]_o}{e^{\frac{VF}{RT}}-1}\right)=0$$

$$P_{Na}\left(0-[Na]_o\right)+P_K\left([K]_i\,e^{\frac{VF}{RT}}-0\right)=0$$

$$\frac{P_{Na}}{P_K}=\frac{[K]_i\,e^{\frac{VF}{RT}}}{[Na]_o}$$

III.2.  **Internal solution contains one divalent cation and external solution contains another different divalent cation.**

Example:

Permeable cations inside: Only $Ba^{2+}$
Permeable cations outside: Only $Ca^{2+}$

$$\frac{4F^2V}{RT} P_{dv} \left( \frac{[dv]_i \, e^{\frac{2VF}{RT}} - [dv]_o}{e^{\frac{V2F}{RT}} - 1} \right) = 0$$

$$P_{Ba} \frac{[Ba]_i \, e^{\frac{2VF}{RT}}}{\left( e^{\frac{VF}{RT}} + 1 \right)} + P_{Ca} \frac{-[Ca]_o}{\left( e^{\frac{VF}{RT}} + 1 \right)} = 0$$

$$\frac{P_{Ca}}{P_{Ba}} = \frac{[Ba]_i}{[Ca]_o} e^{\frac{2VF}{RT}}$$

When $[Ba]_i = [Ca]_i$

$$\frac{P_{Ca}}{P_{Ba}} = e^{\frac{2VF}{RT}}$$

## III.3.   Internal solution contains one monovalent cation and external solution contains one divalent cation.

Example:

Permeable cations inside: Only $Na^+$
Permeable cations outside: Only $Ca^{2+}$

$$\frac{4F^2V}{RT} P_{dv} \left( \frac{[dv]_i \, e^{\frac{2VF}{RT}} - [dv]_o}{e^{\frac{V2F}{RT}} - 1} \right) + \sum_i \frac{F^2V}{RT} P_{mvi} \left( \frac{[mv]_i \, e^{\frac{VF}{RT}} - [mv]_o}{e^{\frac{VF}{RT}} - 1} \right) = 0$$

$$4P_{Ca} \frac{0 - [Ca]_o}{\left( e^{\frac{VF}{RT}} + 1 \right)} + P_{Na} \left( [Na]_i \cdot e^{\frac{VF}{RT}} - 0 \right) = 0$$

$$4P_{Ca} \frac{[Ca]_o}{\left( e^{\frac{VF}{RT}} + 1 \right)} = P_{Na} [Na]_i \cdot e^{\frac{VF}{RT}}$$

$$\frac{P_{Ca}}{P_{Na}} = \frac{[Na]_i}{4[Ca]_o} \cdot e^{\frac{VF}{RT}} \left( e^{\frac{VF}{RT}} + 1 \right)$$

## IV.  DETERMINATION OF PERMEABILITY RATIOS FROM SHIFTS IN REVERSAL POTENTIAL FOR BI-IONIC SOLUTIONS UPON REPLACEMENT OF THE PERMEANT CATION IN THE EXTERNAL SOLUTION.

In Sections IV and V, derivation of permeability ratios from voltage shifts is presented. The experimental conditions for these calculations require the replacement of the extracellular solutions. For these experiments the internal solution remains the same and the reversal potential is determined for recording solution 1, which is subsequently replaced by a second recording solution. From these experiments, the absolute voltages and the voltage shift for the two solutions can be calculated. In the following, we outline how permeability ratios are calculated in such experiments. To do so, we first define the permeable cation contained in the pipette solutions and then define the permeable cations in solutions 1 and 2. We then derive the equation for the permeability ratio in question. The example presented in section IV deals with recording solutions containing only one permeant cation while examples presented in section V deal with recording solutions containing two permeant cations. Finally, the last example refers to a special case in which the internal solution incorporates two permeant cations, $Na^+$ and $Cs^+$. $Cs^+$ needs to be included in certain cells to block $K^+$ currents. In case the ion channel under investigation conducts $Cs^+$, this needs to be considered in the calculation of the permeability ratios. This is done for two particular cases for the determination of permeability ratios from absolute reversal potential and also from shifts in reversal potential upon replacement of the permeant ion in the recording solution.

### IV.1.  Replacement of the external solution containing one permeant monovalent by a second external solution containing a different permeant monovalent cation.

Example:
Permeable cations inside: Only $K^+$

Condition 1: Permeable cations outside: Only $Na^+$
Condition 2: Permeable cations outside: Only $X^+$

Condition 1:

$$\frac{P_{Na}}{P_K} = \frac{[K]_i \, e^{\frac{V_2 F}{RT}}}{[Na]_o}$$

Condition 2:

$$\frac{P_X}{P_K} = \frac{[K]_i \, e^{\frac{V_1 F}{RT}}}{[X]_o}$$

For both conditions, Equation III.1 is used.

Combine both equations to obtain the permeability ratio $P_{Na}/P_X$ from voltage shifts after substituting $[Na]_o$ for $[X]_o$:

$$\frac{\dfrac{P_{Na}}{P_K}}{\dfrac{P_X}{P_K}} = \frac{\dfrac{[K]_i e^{\frac{V_2 F}{RT}}}{[Na]_o}}{\dfrac{[K]_i e^{\frac{V_1 F}{RT}}}{[X]_o}}$$

$$\frac{P_{Na}}{P_K} \cdot \frac{1}{\dfrac{P_X}{P_K}} = \frac{[K]_i e^{\frac{V_2 F}{RT}}}{[Na]_o} \cdot \frac{1}{\dfrac{[K]_i e^{\frac{V_1 F}{RT}}}{[X]_o}}$$

$$\frac{P_{Na}}{P_K} \cdot \frac{P_K}{P_X} = \frac{[K]_i e^{\frac{V_2 F}{RT}}}{[Na]_o} \cdot \frac{[X]_o}{[K]_i e^{\frac{V_1 F}{RT}}}$$

$$\frac{P_{Na}}{P_X} = \frac{[X]_o}{[Na]_o} \cdot e^{\frac{(V_2 - V_1) F}{RT}}$$

For $[X]_o = [Na]_o$

$$\frac{P_{Na}}{P_X} = e^{\frac{(V_2 - V_1) F}{RT}}$$

$$\frac{P_{Na}}{P_X} = e^{\frac{\Delta V F}{RT}}$$

## IV.2.  Replacement of the external solution containing one permeant divalent by a second external solution containing a permeant monovalent cation.

Example:

Permeable cations inside: Only $X^+$

Condition 1: Permeable cations outside: Only $Ca^{2+}$
Condition 2: Permeable cations outside: Only $Na^+$

Condition 1:
  Use Equation III.3

$$\frac{P_{Ca}}{P_X} = \frac{[X]_i}{4[Ca]_o} e^{\frac{V_{Ca} F}{RT}} \left( e^{\frac{V_{Ca} F}{RT}} + 1 \right)$$

Condition 2:
Use equation III.1

$$\frac{P_{Na}}{P_X} = \frac{[X]_i e^{\frac{V_{Na1}F}{RT}}}{[Na]_o}$$

Combine both equations to obtain the permeability ratio $P_{Ca}/P_{Na}$ from voltage shifts after substituting $[Ca]_o$ for $[Na]_o$:

$$\frac{\frac{P_{Ca}}{P_X}}{\frac{P_{Na}}{P_X}} = \frac{[X]_i}{4[Ca]_o} e^{\frac{V_{Ca}F}{RT}} \left( e^{\frac{V_{Ca}F}{RT}} + 1 \right) \cdot \frac{1}{\frac{[X]_i e^{\frac{V_{Na}F}{RT}}}{[Na]_o}}$$

$$\frac{P_{Ca}}{P_X} \frac{P_X}{P_{Na}} = \frac{[X]_i}{4[Ca]_o} e^{\frac{V_{Ca}F}{RT}} \left( e^{\frac{V_{Ca}F}{RT}} + 1 \right) \cdot \frac{[Na]_o}{[X]_i e^{\frac{V_{Na}F}{RT}}}$$

$$\frac{P_{Ca}}{P_{Na}} = \frac{1}{4[Ca]_o} e^{\frac{V_{Ca}F}{RT}} \left( e^{\frac{V_{Ca}F}{RT}} + 1 \right) \cdot \frac{[Na]_o}{e^{\frac{V_{Na}F}{RT}}}$$

$$\frac{P_{Ca}}{P_{Na}} = \frac{[Na]_o}{4[Ca]_o} e^{\frac{V_{Ca}F}{RT}} e^{\frac{V_{Na}F}{RT}} \left( e^{\frac{V_{Ca}F}{RT}} + 1 \right)$$

$$\frac{P_{Ca}}{P_{Na}} = \frac{[Na]_o}{4[Ca]_o} e^{\frac{(V_{Ca}-V_{Na})F}{RT}} \left( e^{\frac{V_{Ca}F}{RT}} + 1 \right)$$

## IV.3. Replacement of the external solution containing one permeant divalent by a second external solution containing a different permeant divalent cation.

Example:
Permeable cations inside: Only $X^+$

Condition 1: Permeable cations outside: Only $Ca^{2+}$
Condition 2: Permeable cations outside: Only $Ba^+$

Condition 1:
Use Equation III.3

$$\frac{P_{Ca}}{P_X} = \frac{[X]_i}{4[Ca]_o} e^{\frac{V_{Ca}F}{RT}} \left( e^{\frac{V_{Ca}F}{RT}} + 1 \right)$$

Condition 2:
 Use Equation III.3

$$\frac{P_{Ba}}{P_X} = \frac{[X]_i}{4[Ba]_o} e^{\frac{V_{Ba}F}{RT}} \left( e^{\frac{V_{Ba}F}{RT}} + 1 \right)$$

Combine both equations to obtain the permeability ratio $P_{Ca}/P_{Ba}$ from voltage shifts after substituting $[Ca]_o$ for $[Ba]_o$:

$$\frac{P_{Ca}}{P_X} \frac{P_X}{P_{Ba}} = \frac{[X]_i}{4[Ca]_o} \frac{4[Ba]_o}{[X]_i} e^{\frac{V_{Ca}F}{RT}} e^{\frac{-V_{Ba}F}{RT}} \left( \frac{e^{\frac{V_{Ca}F}{RT}} + 1}{e^{\frac{V_{Ba}F}{RT}} + 1} \right)$$

$$\frac{P_{Ca}}{P_{Ba}} = \frac{[Ba]_o}{[Ca]_o} e^{\frac{\Delta VF}{RT}} \left( \frac{e^{\frac{V_{Ca}F}{RT}} + 1}{e^{\frac{V_{Ba}F}{RT}} + 1} \right)$$

## V. DETERMINATION OF PERMEABILITY RATIOS FROM SHIFTS IN REVERSAL POTENTIAL FOR INTERNAL AND EXTERNAL SOLUTIONS CONTAINING MIXTURES OF TWO IONS UPON REPLACEMENT OF ONE PERMEANT CATION IN THE EXTERNAL SOLUTION.

### V.1. Replacement of the external solution containing a mixture of Na⁺ and Ca²⁺ to a second external solution containing only Na⁺.
 Example:

Permeable cations inside: Only Na⁺
Condition 1: Permeable cations outside: Na⁺ and Ca²⁺
Condition 2: Permeable cations outside: Only Na⁺

Condition 1:
 Use Equation II.3 with $[Ca]_i = 0$

$$\left( e^{\frac{VF}{RT}} + 1 \right) \frac{\left( [Na]_i \cdot e^{\frac{VF}{RT}} - [Na]_o \right)}{4 \left( [Ca]_o - 0 \right)} = \frac{P_{Ca}}{P_{Na}}$$

Condition 2:
   Use the Nernst equation

$$\frac{[Na]_o}{[Na]_i} = e^{\frac{V_{Na}F}{RT}}$$

$$[Na]_o = [Na]_i\, e^{\frac{V_{Na}F}{RT}}$$

$$[Na]_i = [Na]_o\, e^{\frac{-V_{Na}F}{RT}}$$

Combine both equations to obtain the permeability ratio $P_{Ca}/P_{Na}$ from voltage shifts after substituting external solution containing $[Na]_o$ and $[Ca]_o$ for external solution containing only $[Na]_o$:

$$\frac{P_{Ca}}{P_{Na}} = \left(e^{\frac{V_{Ca}F}{RT}} + 1\right)\frac{\left([Na]_i\, e^{\frac{V_{Ca}F}{RT}} - [Na]_o\right)}{4[Ca]_o}$$

$$\frac{P_{Ca}}{P_{Na}} = \left(e^{\frac{V_{Ca}F}{RT}} + 1\right)\frac{\left([Na]_o\, e^{\frac{-V_{Na}F}{RT}}e^{\frac{V_{Ca}F}{RT}} - [Na]_o\right)}{4[Ca]_o}$$

$$\frac{P_{Ca}}{P_{Na}} = \left(e^{\frac{V_{Ca}F}{RT}} + 1\right)\frac{\left([Na]_o\, e^{\frac{\Delta VF}{RT}} - [Na]_o\right)}{4[Ca]_o}$$

$$\frac{P_{Ca}}{P_{Na}} = \left(e^{\frac{V_{Ca}F}{RT}} + 1\right)\left(e^{\frac{\Delta VF}{RT}} - 1\right)\frac{[Na]_o}{4[Ca]_o}$$

## V.2. Replacement of the external solution containing a mixture of NMDG and Ca²⁺ to a second external solution containing only NMDG.

Example:

Permeable cations inside: Only Na⁺
Condition 1: Permeable cations outside: NMDG and Ca²⁺
Condition 2: Permeable cations outside: Only NMDG

Condition 1:

For solution containing two permeant monovalent and one divalent cations, equation 1 yields:

$$-4P_{Ca}[Ca]_o + P_{Na}\left([Na]_i\, e^{\frac{V_{Ca}F}{RT}}\right)\left(e^{\frac{V_{Ca}F}{RT}}+1\right) - P_{NMDG}[NMDG]_o\left(e^{\frac{V_{Ca}F}{RT}}+1\right)=0$$

$$\frac{P_{Ca}}{P_{Na}} = \frac{[Na]_i}{4[Ca]_o}\, e^{\frac{V_{Ca}F}{RT}}\left(e^{\frac{V_{Ca}F}{RT}}+1\right) - \frac{[NMDG]_o}{4[Ca]_o}\frac{P_{NMDG}}{P_{Na}}\left(e^{\frac{V_{Ca}F}{RT}}+1\right)$$

$$\frac{P_{Ca}}{P_{Na}} = \left(\frac{[Na]_i}{4[Ca]_o}\, e^{\frac{V_{Ca}F}{RT}} - \frac{[NMDG]_o}{4[Ca]_o}\frac{P_{NMDG}}{P_{Na}}\right)\left(e^{\frac{V_{Ca}F}{RT}}+1\right)$$

Condition 2:

Use equation III.1

$$P_{Na}\left([Na]_i\, e^{\frac{V_{Na}F}{RT}}\right) - P_{NMDG}[NMDG]_o = 0$$

$$[Na]_i = \frac{P_{NMDG}}{P_{Na}}[NMDG]_o\, e^{\frac{-V_{Na}F}{RT}}$$

Combine both equations to obtain the permeability ratio $P_{Ca}/P_{Na}$ from voltage shifts after substituting external solution containing $[NMDG]_o$ and $[Ca]_o$ for external solution containing only $[NMDG]_o$:

$$\frac{P_{Ca}}{P_{Na}} = \left(\frac{P_{NMDG}}{P_{Na}}\frac{[NMDG]_o}{4[Ca]_o}\, e^{\frac{-V_{Na}F}{RT}}e^{\frac{V_{Ca}F}{RT}} - \frac{[NMDG]_o}{4[Ca]_o}\frac{P_{NMDG}}{P_{Na}}\right)\left(e^{\frac{V_{Ca}F}{RT}}+1\right)$$

$$\frac{P_{Ca}}{P_{Na}} = \left(\frac{P_{NMDG}}{P_{Na}}\frac{[NMDG]_o}{4[Ca]_o}\, e^{\frac{\Delta VF}{RT}} - \frac{[NMDG]_o}{4[Ca]_o}\frac{P_{NMDG}}{P_{Na}}\right)\left(e^{\frac{V_{Ca}F}{RT}}+1\right)$$

$$\frac{P_{Ca}}{P_{Na}} = \frac{P_{NMDG}}{P_{Na}}\frac{[NMDG]_o}{4[Ca]_o}\left(e^{\frac{VF}{RT}}-1\right)\left(e^{\frac{V_{Ca}F}{RT}}+1\right)$$

## ACKNOWLEDGEMENTS

This work was supported by funding from the German Research Foundation (SFB/TRR152 TP04 to C. G., TP06 to C. W.-S. and TP12 to M. B., as well as SFB870 TP05 to C. W.-S., TP10 to M.B. and TP15 to C. W.-S.) and funding by the NCL Foundation Hamburg to C. G.

# REFERENCES

Bandyopadhyay, D., Cyphersmith, A., Zapata, J. A., Kim, Y. J., Payne, C. K. (2014). Lysosome transport as a function of lysosome diameter. *PloS one*, 9(1), e86847.

Bellono, N. W., Escobar, I. E., Oancea, E. (2016). A melanosomal two-pore sodium channel regulates pigmentation. *Scientific Reports*, 6, 26570.

Bobak, N., Feliciangeli, S., Chen, C. C., Soussia, I. B., Bittner, S., Pagnotta, S., Ruck, T., Biel, M., Wahl-Schott, C., Grimm, C., Meuth, S. G., Lesage, F. (2017). Recombinant tandem of pore-domains in a Weakly Inward rectifying K+ channel 2 (TWIK2) forms active lysosomal channels. *Scientific Reports*, 7(1), 649.

Brailoiu, E., Rahman, T., Churamani, D., Prole, D. L., Brailoiu, G. C., Hooper, R., Taylor, C. W., Patel, S. (2010). An NAADP-gated two-pore channel targeted to the plasma membrane uncouples triggering from amplifying Ca2+ signals. *The Journal of Biological Chemistry*, 285(49), 38511–38516.

Calcraft, P. J., Ruas, M., Pan, Z., Cheng, X., Arredouani, A., Hao, X., Tang, J., Teboul, L., Chuang, K. T., Lin, P., Xiao, R., Wang, C., Zhu, Y., Lin, Y., Wyatt, C. N., Parrington, J., Ma, J., Evans, A. M., Galione, A., Zhu, M. X. (2009). NAADP mobilizes calcium from acidic organelles through two-pore channels. *Nature*, 459(7246), 596.

Cang, C., Aranda, K., Seo, Y. J., Gasnier, B., Ren, D. (2015). TMEM175 is an organelle K+ channel regulating lysosomal function. *Cell*, 162(5), 1101–1112.

Cang, C., Bekele, B., Ren, D. (2014). The voltage-gated sodium channel TPC1 confers endolysosomal excitability. *Nature Chemical Biology*, 10(6), 463.

Cang, C., Zhou, Y., Navarro, B., Seo, Y. J., Aranda, K., Shi, L., Battaglia-Hsu, S., Nissim, I., Clapham, D. E., Ren, D. (2013). mTOR regulates lysosomal ATP-sensitive two-pore Na+ channels to adapt to metabolic state. *Cell*, 152(4), 778–790.

Cao, Q., Zhong, X. Z., Zou, Y., Murrell-Lagnado, R., Zhu, M. X., Dong, X. P. (2015). Calcium release through P2X4 activates calmodulin to promote endolysosomal membrane fusion. *The Journal of Cell Biology*, 209(6), 879–894.

Cao, Q., Zhong, X. Z., Zou, Y., Zhang, Z., Toro, L., Dong, X. P. (2015). BK channels alleviate lysosomal storage diseases by providing positive feedback regulation of lysosomal Ca2+ release. *Developmental Cell*, 33(4), 427–441.

Cerny, J., Feng, Y., Yu, A., Miyake, K., Borgonovo, B., Klumperman, J., Meldolesi, J., McNiel, P. L., Kirchhausen, T. (2005). The small chemical vacuolin-1 inhibits Ca (2+)-dependent lysosomal exocytosis but not cell resealing. *EMBO Reports*, 6(9), 898.

Chao, Y. K., Schludi, V., Chen, C. C., Butz, E., Nguyen, O. P., Müller, M., Krüger, J., Kammerbauer, C., Ben-Johny, M., Vollmar, A. M., Berking, C., Biel, M., Wahl-Schott, C. A., Grimm, C. (2017). TPC2 polymorphisms associated with a hair pigmentation phenotype in humans result in gain of channel function by independent mechanisms. *Proceedings of the National Academy of Sciences of the United States of America*, 114(41), E8595–E8602.

Chen, C. C., Butz, E. S., Chao, Y. K., Grishchuk, Y., Becker, L., Heller, S., Slaugenhaupt, S. A., Biel, M., Wahl-Schott, C., Grimm, C. (2017). Small molecules for early endosome-specific patch clamping. *Cell Chemical Biology*, 24(7), 907–916.

Chen, C. C., Cang, C., Fenske, S., Butz, E., Chao, Y. K., Biel, M., Ren, D., Wahl-Schott, C., Grimm, C. (2017). Patch-clamp technique to characterize ion channels in enlarged individual endolysosomes. *Nature Protocols*, 12(8), 1639.

Chen, C. C., Keller, M., Hess, M., Schiffmann, R., Urban, N., Wolfgardt, A., Schaefer, M., Bracher, F., Biel, M., Wahl-Schott, C., Grimm, C. (2014). A small molecule restores function to TRPML1 mutant isoforms responsible for mucolipidosis type IV. *Nature Communications*, 5, 4681.

DeCourcy, K., Storrie, B. (1991). Osmotic swelling of endocytic compartments induced by internalized sucrose is restricted to mature lysosomes in cultured mammalian cells. *Experimental Cell Research*, 192(1), 52–60.

Dong, X. P., Cheng, X., Mills, E., Delling, M., Wang, F., Kurz, T., Xu, H. (2008). The type IV mucolipidosis-associated protein TRPML1 is an endolysosomal iron release channel. *Nature*, 455(7215), 992.

Dong, X. P., Shen, D., Wang, X., Dawson, T., Li, X., Zhang, Q., Cheng, X., Zhang, Y., Weisman, L. S., Delling, M., Xu, H. (2010). PI(3,5)P2 controls membrane trafficking by direct activation of mucolipin Ca 2+ release channels in the endolysosome. *Nature Communications*, 1, 38.

Feng, X., Xiong, J., Lu, Y., Xia, X., Zhu, M. X. (2014). Differential mechanisms of action of the mucolipin synthetic agonist, ML-SA1, on insect TRPML and mammalian TRPML1. *Cell Calcium*, 56(6), 446–456.

Grimm, C., Butz, E., Chen, C. C., Wahl-Schott, C., Biel, M. (2017a). From mucolipidosis type IV to Ebola: TRPML and two-pore channels at the crossroads of endo-lysosomal trafficking and disease. *Cell Calcium*, 67, 148–155.

Grimm, C., Chen, C. C., Wahl-Schott, C., Biel, M. (2017b). Two-pore channels: Catalyzers of endolysosomal transport and function. *Frontiers in Pharmacology*, 8, 45.

Grimm, C., Cuajungco, M. P., Van Aken, A. F., Schnee, M., Jörs, S., Kros, C. J., Ricci, A. J., Heller, S. (2007). A helix-breaking mutation in TRPML3 leads to constitutive activity underlying deafness in the varitint-waddler mouse. *Proceedings of the National Academy of Sciences of the United States of America*, 104(49), 19583–19588.

Grimm, C., Hassan, S., Wahl-Schott, C., Biel, M. (2012a). Role of TRPML and two-pore channels in endolysosomal cation homeostasis. *The Journal of Pharmacology and Experimental Therapeutics*, 342(2), 236–244.

Grimm, C., Holdt, L. M., Chen, C. C., Hassan, S., Müller, C., Jörs, S., Cuny, H., Kissing, S., Schröder, B., Butz, E., Northoff, B., Castonguay, J., Luber, C. A., Moser, M., Spahn, S., Lüllmann-Rauch, R., Fendel, C., Klugbauer, N., Griesbeck, O., Haas, A., Mann, M., Bracher, F., Teupser, D., Saftig, P., Biel, M., Wahl-Schott, C. (2014). High susceptibility to fatty liver disease in two-pore channel 2-deficient mice. *Nature Communications*, 5, 4699.

Grimm, C., Jörs, S., Guo, Z., Obukhov, A. G., Heller, S. (2012b). Constitutive activity of TRPML2 and TRPML3 channels versus activation by low extracellular sodium and small molecules. *The Journal of Biological Chemistry*, 287(27), 22701–22708.

Huang, P., Zou, Y., Zhong, X. Z., Cao, Q., Zhao, K., Zhu, M. X., Murrell-Lagnado, R., Dong, X. P. (2014). P2X4 forms functional ATP-activated cation channels on lysosomal membranes regulated by luminal pH. *The Journal of Biological Chemistry*, 289(25), 17658–17667.

Jackson, M. B. (2006). *Molecular and Cellular Biophysics*, Cambridge University Press.

Jentsch, T. J., Neagoe, I., Scheel, O. (2005). CLC chloride channels and transporters. *Current Opinion in Neurobiology*, 15(3), 319–325.

Jha, A., Ahuja, M., Patel, S., Brailoiu, E., Muallem, S. (2014). Convergent regulation of the lysosomal two-pore channel-2 by Mg2+, NAADP, PI (3, 5) P2 and multiple protein kinases. *The EMBO Journal*, 33(5), 501–511.

Kim, H. J., Li, Q., Tjon-Kon-Sang, S., So, I., Kiselyov, K., Muallem, S. (2007). Gain-of-function mutation in TRPML3 causes the mouse Varitint-Waddler phenotype. *The Journal of Biological Chemistry*, 282(50), 36138–36142.

Krogsaeter, E. K., Biel, M., Wahl-Schott, C., Grimm, C. (2018). The protein interaction networks of mucolipins and two-pore channels. *Biochimica et Biophysica Acta (BBA)-Molecular Cell Research*, 18667(7), 1111–1123.

Li, X., Wang, X., Zhang, X., Zhao, M., Tsang, W. L., Zhang, Y., Yau, R. G., Weisman, L. S., Xu, H. (2013). Genetically encoded fluorescent probe to visualize intracellular phosphatidylinositol 3, 5-bisphosphate localization and dynamics. *Proceedings of the National Academy of Sciences of the United States of America*, 110(52), 21165–21170.

Miao, Y., Li, G., Zhang, X., Xu, H., Abraham, S. N. (2015). A TRP channel senses lysosome neutralization by pathogens to trigger their expulsion. *Cell*, 161(6), 1306–1319.

Morgan, A. J., Galione, A. (2014). Two-pore channels (TPC s): Current controversies. *BioEssays: News and Reviews in Molecular, Cellular and Developmental Biology*, 36(2), 173–183.

Nagata, K., Zheng, L., Madathany, T., Castiglioni, A. J., Bartles, J. R., García-Añoveros, J. (2008). The varitint-waddler (Va) deafness mutation in TRPML3 generates constitutive, inward rectifying currents and causes cell degeneration. *Proceedings of the National Academy of Sciences of the United States of America*, 105(1), 353–358.

Nguyen, O. N. P., Grimm, C., Schneider, L. S., Chao, Y. K., Atzberger, C., Bartel, K., Watermann, A., Ulrich, M., Mayr, D., Wahl-Schott, C., Biel, M., Vollmar, A. M. (2017). Two-pore channel function is crucial for the migration of invasive cancer cells. *Cancer Research*, 77(6), 1427–1438.

Pitt, S. J., Funnell, T. M., Sitsapesan, M., Venturi, E., Rietdorf, K., Ruas, M., Ganesan, A., Gosain, R., Churchill, G. C., Zhu, M. X., Parrington, J., Galione, A., Sitsapesan, R. (2010). TPC2 is a novel NAADP-sensitive Ca2+ release channel, operating as a dual sensor of luminal pH and Ca2+. *The Journal of Biological Chemistry*, 285(45), 35039–35046.

Plesch, E., Chen, C. C., Butz, E., Rosato, A. S., Krogsaeter, E. K., Yinan, H., Bartel, K., Keller, M., Robaa, D., Teupser, D., Holdt, L. M., Vollmar, A. M., Sippl, W., Puertollano, R., Medina, D., Biel, M., Wahl-Schott, C., Bracher, F., Grimm, C. (2018). Selective agonist of TRPML2 reveals direct role in chemokine release from innate immune cells. *eLife*, 7, e39720.

Ruas, M., Davis, L. C., Chen, C. C., Morgan, A. J., Chuang, K. T., Walseth, T. F., Grimm, C., Garnham, C., Powell, T., Platt, N., Platt, F. M., Biel, M., Wahl-Schott, C., Parrington, J., Galione, A. (2015). Expression of Ca2+-permeable two-pore channels rescues NAADP signalling in TPC-deficient cells. *The EMBO Journal*, 34(13), 1743–1758.

Sakurai, Y., Kolokoltsov, A. A., Chen, C. C., Tidwell, M. W., Bauta, W. E., Klugbauer, N., Grimm, C., Wahl-Schott, C., Biel, M., Davey, R. A. (2015). Two-pore channels control Ebola virus host cell entry and are drug targets for disease treatment. *Science*, 347(6225), 995–998.

Schieder, M., Rötzer, K., Brüggemann, A., Biel, M., Wahl-Schott, C. (2010b). Characterization of two-pore channel 2 (TPCN2)-mediated Ca2+ currents in isolated lysosomes. *The Journal of Biological Chemistry*, 285(28), 21219–21222.

Schieder, M., Rötzer, K., Brüggemann, A., Biel, M., Wahl-Schott, C. (2010a). Planar patch clamp approach to characterize ionic currents from intact lysosomes. *Science Signaling*, 3(151), pl3–pl3.

Shen, D., Wang, X., Li, X., Zhang, X., Yao, Z., Dibble, S., Dong, X. P., Yu, T., Lieberman, A. P., Showalter, H. D., Xu, H. (2012). Lipid storage disorders block lysosomal trafficking by inhibiting a TRP channel and lysosomal calcium release. *Nature Communications*, 3, 731.

Ursell, T., Agrawal, A., Phillips, R. (2011). Lipid bilayer mechanics in a pipette with glass-bilayer adhesion. *Biophysical Journal*, 101(8), 1913–1920.

Wang, X., Zhang, X., Dong, X. P., Samie, M., Li, X., Cheng, X., Goschka, A., Shen, D., Zhou, Y., Harlow, J., Zhu, M. X., Clapham, D. E., Ren, D., Xu, H. (2012). TPC proteins are phosphoinositide-activated sodium-selective ion channels in endosomes and lysosomes. *Cell*, 151(2), 372–383.

Wang, W., Zhang, X., Gao, Q., Lawas, M., Yu, L., Cheng, X., Gu, M., Sahoo, N., Li, X., Li, P., Ireland, S., Meredith, A., Xu, H. (2017). A voltage-dependent K+ channel in the lysosome is required for refilling lysosomal Ca2+ stores. *The Journal of Cell Biology*, 216(6), 1715–1730.

Xiong, J., Zhu, M. X. (2016). Regulation of lysosomal ion homeostasis by channels and transporters. *Science in China (Life Sciences)*, 59(8), 777–791.

Xu, H., Delling, M., Li, L., Dong, X., Clapham, D. E. (2007). Activating mutation in a muco-
    lipin transient receptor potential channel leads to melanocyte loss in varitint–wad-
    dler mice. *Proceedings of the National Academy of Sciences of the United States of
    America*, 104(46), 18321–18326.
Xu, H., Ren, D. (2015). Lysosomal physiology. *Annual Review of Physiology*, 77, 57–80.
Zhang, X., Cheng, X., Yu, L., Yang, J., Calvo, R., Patnaik, S., Hu, X., Gao, Q., Yang, M.,
    Lawas, M., Delling, M., Marugan, J., Ferrer, M., Xu, H. (2016). MCOLN1 is a ROS
    sensor in lysosomes that regulates autophagy. *Nature Communications*, 7, 12109.
Zhang, X., Li, X., Xu, H. (2012). Phosphoinositide isoforms determine compartment-specific
    ion channel activity. *Proceedings of the National Academy of Sciences of the United
    States of America*, 109(28), 11384–11389.
Zhong, X. Z., Sun, X., Cao, Q., Dong, G., Schiffmann, R., Dong, X. P. (2016). BK chan-
    nel agonist represents a potential therapeutic approach for lysosomal storage diseases.
    *Scientific Reports*, 6, 33684.

# 4 TRPML Subfamily of Endolysosomal Channels
## Concepts and Methods

*Nicholas E. Karagas, Morgan A. Rousseau, and Kartik Venkatachalam*

## CONTENTS

## 4.1  INTRODUCTION

The mucolipin subgroup of the transient receptor potential superfamily of cation channels (TRPMLs) are evolutionarily conserved non-selective cation channels that function in endolysosomal membranes, and play key roles in the regulation of endocytosis, autophagy, and intracellular trafficking. Mammalian genomes encode three TRPML paralogs – TRPML1, TRPML2, and TRPML3 – that differ in tissue distribution and exhibit subtle, yet significant, differences in subcellular localization and molecular function. In humans, *MCOLN1*, which encodes TRPML1, is ubiquitously expressed, and loss-of-function mutations in this gene cause a paediatric-onset lysosomal storage disease called mucolipidosis type IV (MLIV) (Bargal et al., 2000; Bassi et al., 2000; Sun et al., 2000).

Owing to the significance of TRPMLs in human health and disease, much has been learned about the function of endosomal proteins in a variety of biological contexts. The effort to understand TRPML has been facilitated by the proliferation of many tools and techniques to study these channels. For example, robust models of MLIV exist in several genetically tractable organisms, and reliable protocols that leverage small molecules that modulate channel activity have been identified. These developments have aided researchers in elucidating the function of TRPMLs, which has contributed to the redefinition of endolysosomes as complex and dynamic organelles that serve myriad functions that extend well beyond the notion of these vesicles being the sites of macromolecular degradation. Additional studies have focused on the development of therapies that mitigate the pathology associated with MLIV and other related lysosomal diseases.

## 4.2   TRPMLS IN HEALTH AND DISEASE

Loss-of-function mutations in *MCOLN1*, which is located on chromosome 19p, lead to MLIV (Bargal et al., 2000; Bassi et al., 2000; Sun et al., 2000). The incidence of this disease is estimated to be 1 in 40,000 live births, but within the Ashkenazi Jewish population, the heterozygous carrier frequency is closer to 1:100, which points to a strong founder effect (Venkatachalam et al., 2015; Zeevi et al., 2007). The disease is found across other ethnicities as well, but the true frequencies in these cohorts are likely underrepresented due to misdiagnosis (Wakabayashi et al., 2011). Indeed, the manifestations of MLIV are very similar to those described in cerebral palsy. Whereas two mutations account for ~95% of Ashkenazi MLIV cases and lead to complete loss of gene expression, over 20 other mutations have been identified in total (Venkatachalam et al., 2015; Wakabayashi et al., 2011; Zeevi et al., 2007). Amongst the latter cohort are missense mutations that lead to intermediate phenotypes. As such, genotype–phenotype correlation is reasonably strong for MLIV.

Although appearing normal at birth, patients with MLIV present with a wide range of clinical symptoms early in post-natal development (Venkatachalam et al., 2015; Wakabayashi et al., 2011; Zeevi et al., 2007) (Figure 4.1). Severe psychomotor delay, characterized by intellectual disability and difficulty developing a variety of motor skills, is a prominent feature of MLIV. By adolescence and adulthood, most patients are unable to ambulate independently and suffer from cognitive impairment. Patients with MLIV also exhibit ophthalmological abnormalities including corneal opacity, which is considered a hallmark of the disease. The visual dysfunction apparent in MLIV is usually progressive and culminates in fulminant blindness. Although corneal clouding contributes to the loss of vision, the eventual onset of blindness is a consequence of progressive retinal degeneration. Degeneration in the central nervous system is not extensive, with patients manifesting neurological phenotypes early due to neurodevelopmental deficits, which is followed by a protracted

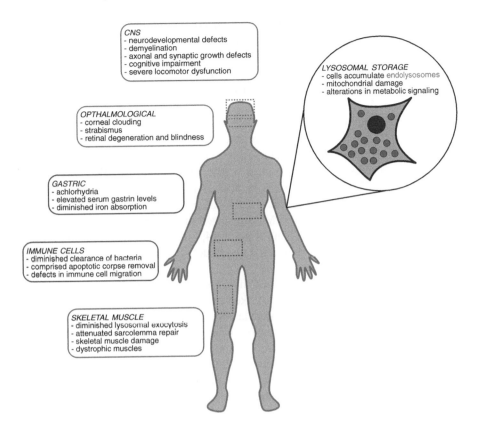

**FIGURE 4.1** Symptoms observed in MLIV patients. MLIV symptoms are categorized on the left on the basis of affected organ systems. Note that although the skeletal muscle and immune defects have been described in animal models, these alterations have not been directly examined in human patients. Nevertheless, the remarkable conservation of phenotypes across species suggests the existence of these defects in MLIV patients. The inset on the right depicts accumulation of endolysosomal vesicles (red) in virtually every cell of the patient. Other cellular phenotypes are also indicated.

phase of slow decline in central nervous system function. Intriguingly, neurological regression and seizures – defining features of the neural ceroid lipofuscinoses (NCL) cohort of lysosomal diseases (Bennett and Rakheja, 2013; Boustany, 2013) – have not been described in MLIV. Although the absence of seizures in diseases with lysosomal dysfunction is not unique to MLIV (Pastores and Maegawa, 2013), it remains to be determined whether the absence of seizures in MLIV reflects a potential role for TRPML1 in the onset of seizures in NCL patients. Another unusual feature of MLIV is the appearance of gastrointestinal ailments, which occur predominantly due to achlorhydria resulting from diminished secretion of gastric acid by parietal cells (Altarescu et al., 2002). Achlorhydria prevents adequate iron absorption in the gut, leading to iron deficiency and attendant anaemia. Patients also exhibit elevated levels of the hormone gastrin in the plasma, which has been used as a diagnostic criterion for MLIV.

Compared to *MCOLN1*, *MCOLN2* and *MCOLN3* exhibit relatively restricted tissue expression (Castiglioni et al., 2011; Cuajungco et al., 2016; Miao et al., 2015; Sun et al., 2015). Although human diseases with mutations in *MCOLN2* and *MCOLN3* have not been defined, naturally occurring gain-of-function mutations in murine *Mcoln3* cause the pathological varitint-waddler (Va) phenotype (Di Palma et al., 2002). The Va-associated mutation, A419P, has been shown to lock TRPML3 in the open state, resulting in constitutive channel activity and resistance to regulatory inhibition (Grimm et al., 2007; Kim et al., 2007; Nagata et al., 2008; Xu et al., 2007). Mice bearing this mutation are hypopigmented, deaf, and exhibit vestibular abnormalities that result in stereotypical wandering behaviour (Atiba-Davies and Noben-Trauth, 2007). The neurosensory phenotype results from degeneration of the sensory hair cells (Van Aken et al., 2008; Castiglioni et al., 2011; Nagata et al., 2008). The Va mutation in TRPML3 inspired the creation of analogous mutations in other TRPML proteins (Feng et al., 2014; Lev et al., 2010; Xu et al., 2007). These mutated channels are also constitutively active and have aided in the study of TRPML function.

TRPMLs also contribute to the pathophysiology of diseases that are not directly related to MLIV. Alzheimer's disease-linked mutations in presenilin-1 lead to elevated $Ca^{2+}$ release from endolysosomes via TRPML1 (Lee et al., 2015). Mitigating TRPML1 hyperactivation under these circumstances alleviates disease phenotypes. However, the role for TRPML1 in neurodegenerative diseases is likely more complex than initially envisioned since other studies have found that a decrease in TRPML1 activity is causally associated with Aβ1–42-dependent degeneration in Alzheimer's disease (Zhang et al., 2017b, 2017a). These findings are consistent with other reports that activation of TRPML1 is involved in the clearance of toxic Aβ aggregates in models of HIV infection (Bae et al., 2014). Furthermore, mutations in *VAC14* or *FIG4* – genes encoding proteins regulating levels of the endogenous TRPML agonist, phosphatidylinositol 3,5-bisphosphate – lead to Yunis-Varón syndrome and neurodegenerative motor neuron disease with features that mimic lysosomal storage (Lines et al., 2017; Zou et al., 2015). In these cases, reactivation of TRPML1 by synthetic agonists has been shown to ameliorate disease phenotypes. Notably, the importance of TRPMLs in health extends beyond the nervous system since the contribution of these channels to immune cell function highlights their involvement in preventing infections and/or immunodeficiency (Bretou et al., 2017; Dayam et al., 2015; Miao et al., 2015; Sun et al., 2015; Wong et al., 2017; Zhong et al., 2017).

## 4.3 BIOPHYSICAL AND MOLECULAR CHARACTERIZATION OF TRPMLS

TRPMLs are non-selective cation channels that exhibit inwardly rectifying currents (Dong et al., 2008; Feng et al., 2014; Grimm et al., 2007; Kim et al., 2007; Lev et al., 2010; Nagata et al., 2008; Xu et al., 2007). Mammalian TRPML1 and TRPML2 and *Drosophila* TRPML have all been found to be potentiated by low pH on the luminal side, which indicates that their activity increases as the vesicular environment acidifies during endolysosomal maturation (Dong et al., 2008; Feng et al., 2014; Lev et al., 2010). TRPML1 is optimally active at pH 4.5, which is also the pH of the mammalian lysosome. In contrast to the other isoforms, TRPML3 is inhibited by low pH, which is consistent with the activity of the channel in early endosomes before the lumen of the vesicles is acidified (Kim et al., 2008).

TRPMLs are activated by the endosomal phosphoinositide – phosphatidylinositol 3,5-bisphosphate ($PI(3,5)P_2$) (Dong et al., 2010; Feng et al., 2014). Interestingly, phosphatidylinositol 4, 5-bisphosphate ($PI(4,5)P_2$), which is abundant in the plasma membrane, inhibits TRPMLs indicating that these channels are inactivated at the plasma membrane. Being non-selective cation channels, TRPMLs are permeable to monovalent cations such as $Na^+$ as well as divalent cations such as $Ca^{2+}$ (Dong et al., 2008; Feng et al., 2014; Grimm et al., 2007; Kim et al., 2007; Lev et al., 2010; Nagata et al., 2008; Xu et al., 2007). Further validating the versatility of these channels, TRPML1 also permeates $Fe^{2+}$ and $Zn^{2+}$ with important consequences to cellular metabolism and gene transcription (Cuajungco and Kiselyov, 2017; Cuajungco et al., 2014; Dong et al., 2008; Eichelsdoerfer et al., 2010; Feng et al., 2014; Grimm et al., 2007; Kim et al., 2007; Kukic et al., 2013; Lev et al., 2010; Nagata et al., 2008; Xu et al., 2007).

As with other TRP channels, TRPMLs function as tetramers that can be either homo- or heteromultimeric (Curcio-Morelli et al., 2010; Venkatachalam and Montell, 2007; Venkatachalam et al., 2006; Zeevi et al., 2010). Förster resonance energy transfer (FRET) and immunoprecipitation assays have demonstrated that TRPML1 can form homomultimers or heteromultimers with either TRPML2 or TRPML3. Given that particular combinations of TRPMLs may possess different biophysical properties, the ability of TRPMLs to form heteromultimers may expand the functional diversity of these channels. Another shared feature is that each TRPML monomer is comprised of six membrane-spanning helices with N- and C-terminal domains residing in the cytosol (Venkatachalam and Montell, 2007). Recently, the first cryo-electron microscopy structures of TRPML proteins were described (Chen et al., 2017; Hirschi et al., 2017; Schmiege et al., 2017; Zhang et al., 2017c; Zhou et al., 2017). These studies correlate functional observations describing various regulatory mechanisms – such as the influence that $PI(3,5)P_2$ and pH have on channel activity – with structural information at the atomic level. Owing to the contributions of these studies, it is now understood that the TRPML1 agonist, ML-SA1, binds to a hydrophobic cavity that is *not* equivalent to the activating site on TRPV1 (Schmiege et al., 2017). The native ligand and inhibitor, $PI(3,5)P_2$ and $PI(4,5)P_2$, respectively, bind to the N-terminus of TRPMLs, and an intermediate domain couples ligand-binding to pore opening or closing (Chen et al., 2017; Hirschi et al., 2017). The intermediate domain is proposed to act as a 'gating pulley' in transferring the signal from the phosphoinositide to the channel pore (Hirschi et al., 2017). Additional identified features include the residues in the selectivity filter of TRPML1 that confer pH sensitivity (Chen et al., 2017), and a 'gating rod' on TRPML3 that connects to the pore loop and mediates the inhibition of this paralog by low pH (Zhou et al., 2017).

## 4.4  TISSUE AND SUBCELLULAR DISTRIBUTION OF TRPMLS

The lack of effective antibodies against TRPMLs, which is exacerbated by the low expression levels of these proteins, has hindered detailed examination of their tissue and subcellular distribution. Consequently, most studies investigating the location of these channels across tissues rely on mRNA quantification. These studies have revealed that *MCOLN1* is expressed in all tissues with relative enrichment in the brain, heart, kidney, liver, and spleen (Sun et al., 2000). Ubiquitous expression is conserved in evolution, as *Drosophila trpml* is also expressed at low levels in multiple tissues (Venkatachalam et al., 2008). In contrast to *MCOLN1*, expression of mammalian *MCOLN2* appears to be restricted to kidney and lymphoid tissues (Cuajungco et al., 2016; Samie et al., 2009; Sun et al., 2015). Indeed, the presence of TRPML2 in lymphoid organs informs a potential role in the function of immunity (Sun et al., 2015). In addition, there are long and short splice variants of TRPML2 – TRPML2lv and TRPML2sv, respectively – with the short variant exhibiting higher expression than the long variant (Samie et al., 2009). Interestingly, it appears that the expression of mucolipins is coordinated in certain contexts. For instance, expression of *Mcoln2*, but not *Mcoln3*, is diminished in mice lacking *Mcoln1*, which points to the existence of hierarchical control mechanisms that coordinate mucolipin gene expression (Samie et al., 2009). As is the case for *MCOLN2*, *MCOLN3* is expressed in the kidney and lymphoid organs. In addition, *MCOLN3* is expressed in the eyes, skin (melanocytes), and cochlea (hair cells). The pathological consequences of the aforementioned Va phenotype, including pigmentation abnormalities and deafness, are well-aligned with the tissue distribution of TRPML3 (Van Aken et al., 2008; Atiba-Davies and Noben-Trauth, 2007; Castiglioni et al., 2011; Miao et al., 2015; Nagata et al., 2008).

TRPMLs are endolysosomal membrane proteins. Fluorescently tagged TRPML1 is predominantly localized to late-endosomes and lysosomes as evidenced by colocalization with Rab7, lysosomal-associated membrane protein 1 (Lamp1), endolysosomal lipid LBPA, and LysoTracker (Manzoni et al., 2004; Thompson et al., 2007; Venkatachalam et al., 2006; Vergarajauregui and Puertollano, 2006). The TRPML1 ortholog in *Drosophila* also localizes to the membranes of late-endosomes and lysosomes (Venkatachalam et al., 2008; Wong et al., 2012). Human TRPML1 bears two di-leucine motifs that mediate the localization of the protein from the plasma membrane to endosomes (Venkatachalam et al., 2006; Vergarajauregui and Puertollano, 2006). Since expression of dominant-negative dynamin was sufficient to mislocalize TRPML1 to the cell surface, we envision that localization of TRPML1 to endolysosomal membrane requires internalization from the plasma membrane (Venkatachalam et al., 2006). However, TRPML1 can also be delivered to endocytic compartments directly from the *trans*-Golgi via a pathway mediated by adapter protein complex-1 (AP-1) (Vergarajauregui and Puertollano, 2006). The existence of multiple routes of endolysosomal delivery likely serves as a failsafe mechanism to ensure that TRPML1 reaches the endocytic compartment. Loss of *MCOLN1* or its orthologs in different species results in accumulation of endolysosomes, which is a defining feature of lysosomal storage diseases such as MLIV (Figure 4.1).

Given the physical interactions between TRPML1 and TRPML2, it stands to reason that the latter protein also localizes to late-endosomes (Venkatachalam et al., 2006). In addition, TRPML2 has been detected in long tubulovesicular compartments associated with GTPase ADP-ribosylation factor-6 (Arf-6) (Karacsonyi et al., 2007; Radhakrishna and Donaldson, 1997). Indeed, activation of Arf-6 has been shown to cause accumulation of TRPML2 in tubulovesicular structures where it colocalizes with major histocompatibility complex I and glycosylphosphatidylino-sitol-anchored proteins (Karacsonyi et al., 2007). Interactions with TRPML1 drive TRPML3 to the endolysosomal membrane (Venkatachalam et al., 2006). When overexpressed alone in cell culture models, murine TRPML3-YFP was found local-ized to the endoplasmic reticulum (ER) (Venkatachalam et al., 2006). Only upon coexpression with TRPML1 or TRPML2, which possess endolysosomal targeting motifs, was TRPML3 delivered to the vesicles, yet again pointing to a hierarchi-cal relationship between the channels. TRPML3 does appear to exhibit the greatest diversity in subcellular compartments. In addition to localizing to endolysosomal compartments, TRPML3 has also been shown to reside in the plasma membrane, early endosomes, and autophagosomal membranes (Kim et al., 2009; Martina et al., 2009; Miao et al., 2015).

## 4.5  ANIMAL MODELS OF MLIV

Evolutionarily, TRPMLs are highly conserved proteins with homologs identified in diverse lineages. Vertebrates encode multiple paralogs of TRPML – the mamma-lian and zebrafish genomes are marked by the expression of three and five TRPML encoding genes, respectively (Benini et al., 2013; Li et al., 2017). Two independently generated mouse models with *Mcoln1* deletions have been described (Chandra et al., 2011; Venugopal et al., 2007). Both models faithfully recapitulate various aspects of MLIV including neurodevelopmental and psychomotor defects, ophthalmologi-cal abnormalities and retinal degeneration, achlorhydria and elevated serum gastrin levels, and of course, diminished endolysosomal $Ca^{2+}$ release. The neurological phe-notypes of the $Mcoln1^{-/-}$ mice include diminished strength, shorter gait, and eventual paralysis of the hindlimbs. Remarkably, these mice also demonstrated MLIV phe-notypes on the cellular level including ubiquitous presence of endolysosomal inclu-sions. Zebrafish express two orthologs of human TRPML1, and their deletions elicit many of the features of MLIV including retinal and neuromuscular defects (Benini et al., 2013; Li et al., 2017).

The commonly studied invertebrates, *Drosophila melanogaster* and *Caenorhabditis elegans*, possess single TRPML encoding genes – *trpml* and *coe-lomocyte uptake defective-5* (*cup-5*), respectively (Fares and Greenwald, 2001; Venkatachalam et al., 2008). The worm *cup-5* mutants exhibit maternal-effect embryonic lethality and endolysosomal accumulation. Flies lacking *trpml* exhibit defects in completion of autophagy with a concomitant build-up of endolysosomes in a wide range of tissues, high rates of pupal lethality, age-dependent neurodegenera-tion, and locomotor impairment. The MLIV flies also exhibit defects in glutamater-gic synapse development and neurotransmission (Venkatachalam et al., 2008; Wong et al., 2015). Interestingly, the neurological phenotypes in the MLIV flies are a result of a complex interplay between neurons and phagocytic cells (Venkatachalam et al., 2008). First, cell autonomous endolysosomal defects in neurons led to accumula-tion of damaged mitochondria and diminished cell viability. A secondary, non-cell autonomous effect in phagocytic cells such as glia was triggered by the dying neu-rons and led to neuroinflammation. Remarkably, reintroduction of wild-type *trpml* in only the phagocytic cells was sufficient to significantly delay the locomotor defects and attendant lethality. These findings led to the intriguing proposal that bone marrow transplantation to introduce functional phagocytic cells such as microglia in patients lacking TRPML1 could delay the onset of MLIV – a concept that was successfully validated in a mouse model of MLIV (Walker and Montell, 2016).

In the yeast *Saccharomyces cerevisiae*, *yvc1* encodes a protein that possesses several striking functional similarities to TRPMLs at the level of protein sequence (~40% similarity with mammalian TRPMLs) (Denis and Cyert, 2002; Dong et al., 2010). Furthermore, in a manner similar to TRPML1, YVC1 is activated by PI(3,5)P$_2$ leading to the release of Ca$^{2+}$ from the yeast vacuole. In yeast lacking *yvc1*, expression of human TRPML1 led to a partial suppression of phenotypes (Dong et al., 2010). Conservation of function has also been demonstrated in *C. elegans* and *Drosophila*, where expression of human TRPML1 suppresses mutant phenotypes (Feng et al., 2014; Hersh et al., 2002; Treusch et al., 2004). Although the *C. elegans* mutant phenotype was suppressed by expression of human TRPML3 (Treusch et al., 2004), we have found that the phenotypes in *trpml*-deficient *Drosophila* larvae were not suppressed by the expression of human TRPML2 or TRPML3 (unpublished observations). Nevertheless, our observations argue in favour of fundamental and conserved biological roles for TRPML1 in eukaryotic cell biology.

## 4.6   CELLULAR FUNCTIONS OF TRPMLS

### 4.6.1   ENDOCYTOSIS AND AUTOPHAGY

The endocytic pathway is initiated at the plasma membrane, where molecularly defined regions of the bilayer are pinched inwards to form early endosomes via a pathway orchestrated with exquisite spatiotemporal precision (Kaksonen and Roux, 2018). Although likely inactive in that compartment, the delivery of TRPML1 to endosomes also occurs at the level of the plasma membrane, (Pryor et al., 2006) (Figure 4.2). The neutral extracellular pH as well as the abundance of PI(4,5)P$_2$ in the plasma membrane synergize to prevent TRPML activation at the cell surface (Dong et al., 2010; Feng et al., 2014). As TRPML1-bearing endosomes mature, the vacuolar ATPase (V-ATPase) pumps protons into the endolysosomal lumen such that the pH of the late-endosomal vesicles settles at ~4.5–5 in mammalian cells. In addition, activity of the Pikfyve/Vac14/Fig4 complex in late-endosomes leads to the generation of PI(3,5)P$_2$ (McCartney et al., 2014). The coincidence of low pH and PI(3,5) P$_2$ is necessary for TRPML1 activation. It is therefore not surprising that deletion of genes encoding the Pikfyve/Vac14/Fig4 complex leads to phenotypes that are remarkably similar to those observed in the absence of TRPMLs in both mammals and *Drosophila* (Rusten et al., 2006; Zolov et al., 2012).

Activation of TRPML1 has profound effects on the trafficking and fate of endolysosomal vesicles. The fusion of late-endosomes or autophagosomes with lysosomes are Ca$^{2+}$-dependent processes that depend upon luminal Ca$^{2+}$ released via endolysosomal channels such as TRPMLs (Pryor et al., 2000; Wong et al., 2012) (Figure 4.2). Therefore, TRPMLs participate in the heterotypic fusion of late-endosomes or amphisomes with lysosomes, which is important for the appropriate degradation of

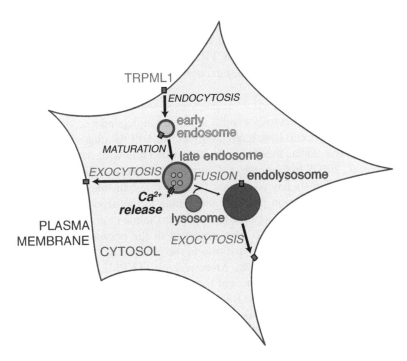

**FIGURE 4.2** Schematic diagram showing the functions of TRPML1 in endolysosomal vesicular trafficking. The route of TRPML1 (green rectangle) trafficking from the plasma membrane to endolysosomal vesicles is shown. Vesicular trafficking steps described in red letters require TRPML1 activity.

the material nucleated within those vesicles. Evidence from multiple model systems suggests that $Ca^{2+}$ efflux from the late-endosomes/amphisomes via TRPMLs promotes $Ca^{2+}$-dependent vesicle fusion (Schahcen et al., 2006; Vergarajauregui et al., 2008a; Wong et al., 2012). In *Drosophila*, loss of TRPML leads to attenuated late-endosome/amphisome–lysosome fusion leading to a build-up of these unfused vesicles (Venkatachalam et al., 2008; Wong et al., 2012). Similarly, in mammalian cells lacking TRPML1, fusion of vesicles in the autophagic pathway is delayed (Miedel et al., 2008; Vergarajauregui et al., 2008a). Consequently, markers of diminished endolysosomal and autophagic flux – accumulation of p62, polyubiquitinated proteins, and cellular waste destined for degradation – have been observed in TRPML-deficient human cells and model systems.

### 4.6.2 Regulation of Endolysosomal Exocytosis

In addition to mediating endosomal fusion, TRPMLs also regulate endolysosomal exocytosis – the process by which cells direct the traffic of vesicles to the plasma membrane for the release of endolysosomal contents into the extracellular space (Bretou et al., 2017; Cao et al., 2015; Cheng et al., 2014; Lima et al., 2012; Miao et al., 2015; Ravi et al., 2016; Sahoo et al., 2017; Samie et al., 2013; Zhong et al., 2016) (Figure 4.2). This notion is supported by evidence from studies demonstrating that gain-of-function mutations of mammalian TRPML1 cause an elevation in lysosomal trafficking to the plasma membrane in HEK293T cells and a predictable increase in the levels of TRPML1 at the plasma membrane (Dong et al., 2009). Furthermore, lysosomal exocytosis is impaired in MLIV (LaPlante et al., 2006).

Owing to the role of TRPMLs in exocytosis, many biological processes that require endolysosomal exocytosis exhibit a functional dependence on TRPMLs. In the murine macrophage cell line, RAW 264.7, delivery of the major histocompatibility complex II to the plasma membrane is diminished following *Mcoln1* knockdown (Thompson et al., 2007). In the context of immune cell function, TRPML1-dependent endolysosomal exocytosis has additional functions. For instance, focal exocytosis following TRPML1 activation provides membrane to the growing phagocytic cup during the internalization of apoptotic cell corpses (Samie et al., 2013). Diminished phagocytosis of apoptotic cells is also observed in the nervous system of *trpml*-deficient flies, where this defect contributes to the precipitous onset of neurodegeneration (Venkatachalam et al., 2008). More recently, TRPML1-mediated vesicular exocytosis has been shown to be critical for immune cell chemotaxis via a process requiring the actin cytoskeleton and Rac GTPases (Bretou et al., 2017; Dayam et al., 2017). TRPML1-mediated endolysosomal $Ca^{2+}$ release is required for the exocytosis of tubulovesicles for gastric acid in the parietal cells of the stomach (Sahoo et al., 2017). This cellular property of TRPML1 explains the achlorhydria that characterizes patients suffering from MLIV. The release of gastric acid-laden tubulovesicles in the parietal cell is triggered by an elevation of cytosolic cyclic AMP (cAMP) and the subsequent activation of protein kinase A (PKA) (Sahoo et al., 2017). These data indicate that cAMP and PKA are capable of triggering TRPML1-dependent endolysosomal exocytosis. Although the exact mechanism underlying TRPML1 activation by PKA remains undefined, these findings are aligned with a previous study that PKA phosphorylates TRPML1 (Vergarajauregui et al., 2008b). It also remains to be seen whether the crosstalk between cAMP–PKA–TRPML1 relates to other processes requiring TRPML1-dependent vesicle release. Conversely, it would be worth investigating whether TRPML1 plays a role in other pathways that require cAMP- and PKA-dependent exocytosis.

From a mechanistic perspective, the role of TRPML1 activation in endolysosomal exocytosis is especially intriguing in the context of situations that are marked by dramatic elevations in cytosolic $Ca^{2+}$. For instance, TRPML1-mediated exocytosis is required for the repair of skeletal muscle membrane (also called sarcolemma), following damage that is a consequence of normal muscle function or following acute injury (Cheng et al., 2014). Indeed, *Mcoln1*$^{-/-}$ mice exhibit muscle degeneration that is attributed to diminished sarcolemma repair. It is well known that skeletal muscle fibres exhibit dramatic elevations in cytosolic $Ca^{2+}$ during contraction, which will only be amplified if the sarcolemma were damaged. In this framework, it stands to reason that the role of TRPML1 in endolysosomal exocytosis is not related to elevation of cytosolic $Ca^{2+}$ *per se*. We envision that specific steps in the endolysosomal trafficking process require the TRPML1 channel in a manner that cannot be explained by global cytosolic $Ca^{2+}$ elevations although a role for localized $Ca^{2+}$ elevations remains a possibility.

### 4.6.3 Bidirectional Interactions with the Mechanistic Target of Rapamycin Complex 1 (mTORC1) Signalling

By mediating the fusion of vesicles carrying material destined for degradation, TRPML1 influences several signalling modalities in the cell. Diminished lysosomal degradation of proteins in the absence of TRPMLs results in diminished activity of mTORC1 – a master regulator of anabolism and protein synthesis (Sancak et al., 2010; Venkatachalam et al., 2013; Wong et al., 2012, 2015; Zoncu et al., 2011). Normally, lysosomal degradation of proteins and the consequent increase in the availability of free amino acids activate mTORC1, which in turn prevents the necessity for endolysosomes and autophagosomes during periods of amino acid sufficiency (Efeyan et al., 2012). However, cells lacking functional TRPMLs are characterized by attenuated endolysosomal protein degradation and the consequent paucity of free amino acids leading to low mTORC1 activity (Venkatachalam et al., 2013; Wong et al., 2012, 2015) (Figure 4.3). In *Drosophila*, the decrease in mTORC1 activation in cells lacking *trpml* can be restored by ectopic supplementation of a high protein diet or the genetic reactivation of mTORC1. In addition to the effects of TRPML activation on the bioavailability of amino acids that activate mTORC1, endolysosomal $Ca^{2+}$ release via TRPML1 can also directly activate mTORC1 via calmodulin (Li et al., 2016; Sun et al., 2018). Thus, the activity of TRPML1 influences mTORC1 activity through multiple pathways.

Pointing to a bidirectional relationship between mTORC1 and TRPML1, the activation of mTORC1 influences TRPML1-mediated endolysosomal $Ca^{2+}$ release. The reciprocal relationship likely reflects an intricate feedback loop since starvation activates TRPML1-mediated endolysosomal $Ca^{2+}$ response via mTORC1 (Onyenwoke et al., 2015; Wang et al., 2015). This model is consistent with mTORC1 negatively regulating the activity of TRPML1 channels. Besides decreasing channel conductance, the activation of mTORC1 in *Drosophila* leads to elevated localization of TRPML at the plasma membrane (Wong et al., 2012). Mislocalization of TRPML in the plasma membrane would be expected to compromise the function of the channels due to the

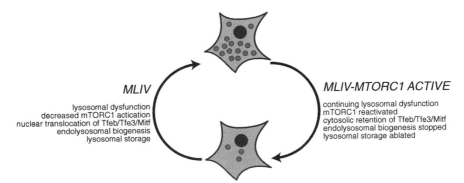

**FIGURE 4.3** Schematic diagram showing the role played by mTORC1 in endolysosomal accumulation in cells lacking TRPML1. Steps on the left depict the alterations in MLIV cells that underlie lysosomal storage. Reactivation of mTORC1 in those cells mitigates lysosomal storage despite continuing lysosomal dysfunction.

fact that plasma membrane-enriched $PI(4,5)P_2$ negatively influences the activity of *Drosophila* TRPML (Feng et al., 2014). These studies also indicate that starvation-induced decrease in mTORC1 activity stimulates TRPML1, which in turn would restore mTORC1 activity via a combination of direct $Ca^{2+}$-dependent and indirect amino acid-dependent processes.

### 4.6.4 REGULATION OF ENDOLYSOSOMAL BIOGENESIS

Pioneering studies have demonstrated that expression of many genes encoding endolysosomal proteins is under the transcriptional control of Tfeb/Mitf/Tfe3 (Bouché et al., 2016; Martina et al., 2014; Palmieri et al., 2011; Ploper and De Robertis, 2015; Ploper et al., 2015; Sardiello et al., 2009; Settembre et al., 2011). Pointing to functional relationships between endolysosomal biogenesis and growth-inducing kinases – mTORC1 and AKT – both kinases phosphorylate and inactivate Tfeb leading to diminished endolysosomal gene expression (Martina et al., 2012; Roczniak-Ferguson et al., 2012; Settembre et al., 2012). Since *MCOLN1* is under the control of Tfeb/Mitf/Tfe3-mediated endolysosomal gene expression (Medina et al., 2011; Sardiello et al., 2009; Wang et al., 2015), low mTORC1 activity during starvation also promotes the transcriptional upregulation of *MCOLN1*. This high-level regulatory pathway likely synergizes with direct activation of TRPML1 in cells characterized by diminished mTORC1 function. The activation of TRPML1 eventually leads to the restoration of mTORC1 kinase activity and termination of the feedback loop. This model also explains the endolysosomal accumulation observed in cells characterized by diminished TRPML function – absence of TRPML function results in decreased mTORC1 activity and disinhibition of Tfeb/Mitf/Tfe3-dependent endolysosomal biogenesis. Indeed, ectopic stimulation of mTORC1 with a high protein diet or genetic manipulations mitigates the endolysosomal storage phenotype in *trpml*-deficient tissues in *Drosophila* (Wong et al., 2012, 2015). Alternatively, it has been proposed that endolysosomal $Ca^{2+}$ released via TRPML1 activates the $Ca^{2+}$-responsive phosphatase calcineurin, which in turn, dephosphorylates Tfeb and promotes its translocation into the nucleus (Medina et al., 2015). The consequences of TRPML1 activity on both Tfeb inactivation via mTORC1 *and* Tfeb activation via calcineurin point to the complexities of endolysosomal biogenesis that will likely be resolved in future studies.

### 4.6.5 REGULATION OF TRACE METAL BIOLOGY

Although the permeability to $Ca^{2+}$ underpins many of the biological functions of TRPML1, the permeability to trace cations such as $Fe^{2+}$ and $Zn^{2+}$ also fulfil important roles (Cuajungco and Kiselyov, 2017; Cuajungco et al., 2014; Dong et al., 2008; Eichelsdoerfer et al., 2010; Feng et al., 2014; Grimm et al., 2007; Kim et al., 2007; Kukic et al., 2013; Lev et al., 2010; Nagata et al., 2008; Xu et al., 2007). Given that iron is delivered to the cell via endocytosis or autophagic degradation of iron-containing proteins, a role for TRPML1 in the regulation of $Fe^{2+}$-dependent processes can be envisioned (Mills et al., 2010). Indeed, impaired myelination in mice lacking *Mcoln1* is attributed to alterations in iron levels in the brain (Grishchuk et al., 2015).

In addition to $Fe^{2+}$, there is also evidence that TRPML influences $Zn^{2+}$ metabolism, including the observation that $Zn^{2+}$ also accumulates in endolysosomes upon loss of TRPML1 (Cuajungco and Kiselyov, 2017; Cuajungco et al., 2014; Dong et al., 2008; Eichelsdoerfer et al., 2010; Feng et al., 2014; Grimm et al., 2007; Kim et al., 2007; Kukic et al., 2013, 2014; Lev et al., 2010; Nagata et al., 2008; Xu et al., 2007). However, unlike with $Fe^{2+}$, direct measurements of $Zn^{2+}$ conductance have not been conducted, leaving to possibility that TRPML1 may regulate $Zn^{2+}$ transport indirectly.

### 4.6.6 CROSSTALK BETWEEN LYSOSOMES AND OTHER ORGANELLES

Multiple lines of evidence support the notion of functional crosstalk between lysosomes and other cellular organelles, in particular the ER and mitochondria (Plotegher and Duchen, 2017; Repnik and Turk, 2010; Ronco et al., 2015). Interestingly, TRPMLs could be important participants in interorganellar communication, and loss of TRPMLs has a strikingly adverse impact on mitochondrial health, which may contribute significantly to the aetiology of MLIV (Jennings et al., 2006; Venkatachalam et al., 2008). Conversely, mammalian TRPML1 responds to oxidative stress that can originate from damaged or stressed mitochondria (Ravi et al., 2016; Zhang et al., 2016). In addition, $Ca^{2+}$ dynamics of the lysosomes and ER exhibit functional relationships via a process requiring TRPML1 (Garrity et al., 2016; Kilpatrick et al., 2016). It would be interesting to evaluate whether phenotypes associated with MLIV and other lysosomal diseases involve aberrant crosstalk between endolysosomes and ER.

## 4.7 METHODS TO STUDY TRPML TRAFFICKING AND FUNCTION

The purpose of the following sections is to provide an overview of some of the tools and resources that may be used to study the localization, trafficking, and channel function of TRPMLs. As evidenced by the extensive contribution of TRPMLs to endolysosomal function, many of the protocols described below can also be utilized to study the properties of these vesicles in general.

### 4.7.1 VISUALIZATION OF FUNCTIONALLY RELEVANT VESICLES

Human TRPML1 and its orthologs in other species localize to late-endocytic and lysosomal compartments, which by the virtue of low luminal pH can be visualized by LysoTracker – a fluorescent dye that accumulates in acidic organelles. Mammalian and invertebrate TRPML1 decorate the periphery of LysoTracker-positive vesicles (Venkatachalam et al., 2006, 2008). An important caveat that needs to be considered when using LysoTracker is that despite being useful for evaluating the abundance, shape, and size of acidic vesicles, the dye cannot be used to distinguish between late-endosomes, lysosomes, and other acidic vesicles. Furthermore, neither early endosomes nor autophagosomes can be detected using LysoTracker since these structures are not acidic.

To overcome the limitations of LysoTracker, co-labelling with specific-protein markers is also required. For instance, Rab5 and Rab7, which localize to the early- and late-endosomes, respectively, may be used as markers. Other markers of early endosome include HRS and EEA1, and late-endosomes/lysosomes include proteins such as LAMP1 and LAMP3 (Manzoni et al., 2004; Thompson et al., 2007; Venkatachalam et al., 2006). Lysosomes can be visualized using fluorescently tagged substrates for lysosomal enzymes such as cathepsin (e.g. Magic Red cathepsin L substrate) (Johnson et al., 2016). Autophagosomes are detected by labelling with fluorescently tagged Atg proteins or LC3, whereas amphisomes, which are generated by the fusion of autophagosomes and endosomes (Tanida et al., 2008), can be identified by appropriate co-labelling. In addition to these fluorescent techniques, autophagosomes, endosomes, amphisomes, and lysosomes can be effectively discriminated by electron microscopy, and have been shown to accumulate in cells lacking TRPMLs (Wong et al., 2012). Unfortunately, the absence of effective antibodies against TRPML proteins has prevented visualization of natively expressed proteins, which can be circumvented by examining the expression of ectopic expression of tagged TRPMLs.

The sample protocol provided below can be used to visualize LysoTracker staining in cells from a variety of tissues or organisms. Figure 4.4 shows a representative image of primary fibroblasts from control and two different MLIV patients. These data demonstrate the accumulation of LysoTracker-labelled vesicles in MLIV fibroblasts.

1. Dissect tissues or prepare cells that express tagged TRPML variants.
2. While still alive, incubate the tissues/cells with LysoTracker Red (Molecular Probes: 2 mM for *Drosophila* fat bodies, although other tissues may require different concentration) added to full-growth cell culture medium for the desired amount of time (usually 30 minutes).
3. Wash samples once with phosphate-buffered saline (PBS).
4. Fix tissues/cells in 4% paraformaldehyde PBS for a minimum of 30 minutes at room temperature.

nuclei (DAPI) LysoTracker

CONTROL             MLIV                 MLIV
FIBROBLASTS         FIBROBLASTS 1        FIBROBLASTS 2

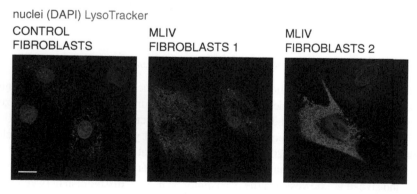

**FIGURE 4.4** LysoTracker staining in control and MLIV fibroblasts. Confocal images of fibroblasts from control or MLIV patients labelled with DAPI (blue) and LysoTracker (red). Scale bar shown in the panel on the left depicts 10 μm and applies to all panels. MLIV fibroblasts 1 and 2 refer to cells from two separate MLIV patients. The cells shown here were obtained from the Coriell Institute for Medical Research.

5. Wash samples thrice with 0.1%-Triton X-100 PBS.
6. Incubate samples with primary antibodies against the tag on TRPMLs in 0.1%-Triton X-100 PBS + 5% donkey serum at 4°C overnight.
7. Wash samples thrice with 0.1%-Triton X-100 PBS.
8. Incubate samples with appropriate Alexa Fluor-conjugated secondary antibodies at room temperature for 2.5 hours.
9. Wash samples thrice with 0.1%-Triton X-100 PBS.
10. Mount samples on glass slide using VECTASHIELD with DAPI (Vector Labs).
11. Image using confocal microscope.

### 4.7.2  Ca²⁺ IMAGING TO ASSAY TRPML FUNCTION

The activity of mammalian and *Drosophila* TRPML channels has been evaluated using the endolysosomal-patch clamp technique (Dong et al., 2008; Feng et al., 2014). Given that TRPMLs release endolysosomal $Ca^{2+}$, imaging changes in cytosolic $Ca^{2+}$ concentration ($[Ca^{2+}]$) also inform alterations in TRPML activity. In this context, TRPML activity can be evaluated either by measuring changes in bulk cytosolic $[Ca^{2+}]$ using $Ca^{2+}$ sensors such as fura-2 or by tagging TRPML proteins with genetically encoded $Ca^{2+}$ indicators (GECIs) such as GCaMPs (Kilpatrick et al., 2016; Shen et al., 2012; Wong et al., 2012, 2017).

Fura-2 is maximally excited at 340 nm when bound to $Ca^{2+}$ or 380 nm when unbound, and always emits maximally at 510 nm (Paredes et al., 2008). Therefore, the ratio of fura-2 emission at 510 nm following excitation at 340 nm and 380 nm, respectively, is a function of cytosolic free $[Ca^{2+}]$. Since fura-2 measurements are inherently ratiometric, potential sources of error such as varying concentration of dye in individual cells are of limited concern.

The use of GECIs provides an alternative and potentially more sophisticated way to measure intracellular $[Ca^{2+}]$, for instance, by targeting to subcellular compartments or genetically defined cell types. The popular GECIs, GCaMPs, are comprised of circularly permutated GFP and calmodulin, with the latter binding to free $Ca^{2+}$ and thereupon imposing an increase in the fluorescence of the former (Nakai et al., 2001). The power of GECIs is realized upon targeting to specific organelles, which allows for unprecedented spatiotemporal resolution of $Ca^{2+}$ measurements (Mao et al., 2008; Pologruto et al., 2004). Indeed, by tagging the termini of TRPMLs with derivatives of GCaMP, $Ca^{2+}$ in the vicinity of the channel can be detected in a cell type or tissue of interest in any genetically tractable organism. This approach allows measurement of $Ca^{2+}$ changes in the vicinity of endolysosomes when the GCaMP is tagged to TRPML proteins (Samie et al., 2013; Wong et al., 2017). It is, however, important to bear in mind that TRPML-GCaMP can detect $Ca^{2+}$ in the vicinity of the channel even if the actual source of the cations is not TRPML. As long as adequate free $Ca^{2+}$ can diffuse to the GCaMP moiety, this signal will be reported by an increase in fluorescence.

Provided below are two adaptable protocols to image endolysosomal $Ca^{2+}$ release. The first protocol describes a procedure to detect $[Ca^{2+}]$ in the bulk cytosol using fura-2 and the second protocol describes a more specialized approach that reflects

$Ca^{2+}$ signals in the vicinity of endolysosomal membranes. We have also provided a brief primer on pharmacological approaches to manipulate TRPML activity, which is of tremendous utility when examining endolysosomal $Ca^{2+}$ release.

### 4.7.3   Protocol 1: Fura-2

1. If using cultured cells, the experiment is performed on glass bottom culture dishes or cover slips. If the cells are transfected with specific constructs, $Ca^{2+}$ imaging should not be performed <24 hours post-transfection.

2. For loading the cells or tissues with fura-2, the acetoxymethyl (AM) ester fura-2 (Invitrogen: 10 μM) should be applied for a duration ranging from 30 minutes to 1 hour. The fura-2-AM should be dissolved in a buffer containing: 125 mM NaCl, 5 mM KCl, 10 mM $MgSO_4$, 10 mM $KH_2PO_4$, 1 mM $CaCl_2$, 5.5 mM glucose, and 5 mM HEPES; pH 7.4. The duration of fura-2 loading might have to be determined empirically for the cells/tissues being used. During this step, it is important to keep the cells covered so as to prevent exposure to light, which may bleach the fura-2 signal. Some cell lines are inherently harder to load with fura-2, due to the presence of organic anionic transporters that extrude the dye (for example, S2 cells from *Drosophila*). In these cases, the anionic transport can be blocked by the inclusion of 5 mM probenecid in the buffer.

3. After the completion of the loading phase, remove the buffer containing fura-2-AM and replace with fresh buffer. At this point, the fura-2-AM will be de-esterified by endogenous esterases in the cytosol into fura-2, which is inherently membrane-impermeable and will remain in the cytosol. De-esterification should be complete in ~30 minutes after removal of fura-2-AM.

4. Using an appropriate $Ca^{2+}$ imaging set-up and a wide-field fluorescence microscope, the ratio of emission intensities at 510 nm, following excitation at 340 nm and 380 nm, will provide an indication of cytosolic free $[Ca^{2+}]$. To convert the ratio to $[Ca^{2+}]$, an appropriate calibration using known $Ca^{2+}$ standards would be needed.

5. Different pharmacological agents can be used to trigger the movement of $Ca^{2+}$ across organellar membranes and/or the plasma membrane in order to gain insights into the biological processes of interest.

### 4.7.4   Protocol 2: GCaMP

1. Mammalian cells or animal tissues expressing TRPML1-GCaMP5G or *Drosophila* TRPML-GCaMP5G can be used to measure $[Ca^{2+}]$ in the endosomal periphery. If isolated from an animal, TRPML-GCaMP5-expressing cells should be first allowed to adhere to glass bottom dishes coated with concanavalin A.

2. After a few washes with full-growth cell culture medium, the cells are ready for imaging using a wide-field fluorescence imaging system.

3. GCaMP5G emission following excitation at 490 nm may be interpreted as a measure of cytosolic [$Ca^{2+}$].

4. After subtracting baseline, the GCaMP5G signals may be expressed as real-time fluorescence relative to intensity at the beginning of the run.

### 4.7.5 Pharmacological Manipulation of TRPML Function

There are several compounds that either directly or indirectly influence the activity of TRPML channels, and therefore, permit the rapid investigation of channel function in a multitude of contexts. The first TRPML inhibitor, mucolipin synthetic inhibitor 1 (ML-SI1), also known as GW-405833, was originally found to be a selective partial agonist of the endocannabinoid receptors, CB2 and CB1, having a weaker affinity for the latter (Clayton et al., 2002). In addition to its action on endocannabinoid receptors, ML-SI1 is an antagonist of TRPML1 (Samie et al., 2013; Wang et al., 2015). Since the description of ML-SI1, newer generation TRPML1 antagonists with relatively higher specificity have been developed (Kilpatrick et al., 2016; Samie et al., 2013). These compounds are particularly valuable because many conventional cation channel blockers are not effective inhibitors of TRPML1. Given that TRPML channels are activated by PI(3,5)P$_2$, inhibitors of the enzyme involved in the biogenesis of this endolysosomal phosphoinositide – Pikfyve – are indirect inhibitors of TRPML activity. In this context, YM201636 and apilimod are Pikfyve inhibitors that inhibit TRPML-mediated endolysosomal $Ca^{2+}$ release (Dong et al., 2010; Lee et al., 2015; Wong et al., 2017). Direct TRPML agonists have also been described. First in this class was a compound named mucolipin synthetic agonist 1 (ML-SA1) (Shen et al., 2012). Other drugs that act on TRPML1, as well as TRPML2 and TRPML3, have also been described (Chen et al., 2014; Grimm et al., 2010, 2012). The utility of these drugs is highlighted by the fact that they are all cell-permeable and can be added to the extracellular media to influence channel activity within cells. Alternatively, we have found that mixing these drugs into fly food is an effective approach to inhibit the activity of TRPML in *Drosophila* (unpublished observations).

## 4.8  CONCLUSIONS

Here, we have provided an overview of the biological functions of TRPMLs and described several methods that can be used to further study these intriguing channels. Over the last few decades, the effort to understand the molecular underpinnings of MLIV has yielded a wealth of information about the function of TRPMLs. Given the availability of numerous models and techniques to study these proteins, we expect the field will continue to expand and provide fresh biologic insights. We hope this review serves as a reliable guide for those interested in contributing to research in this direction.

## ACKNOWLEDGEMENTS

The authors would like to thank Dr. Ching-On Wong for useful discussions. N.E.K. was funded by the National Center for Advanced Translational Sciences of the

NIH under award numbers TL1TR000369 and UL1TR000371. K.V. is funded by the NIH grants R01NS081301 and R21AG061646. The authors declare no conflicts of interest.

# REFERENCES

van Aken, A.F.J., Atiba-Davies, M., Marcotti, W., Goodyear, R.J., Bryant, J.E., Richardson, G.P., Noben-Trauth, K., and Kros, C.J. (2008). TRPML3 mutations cause impaired mechano-electrical transduction and depolarization by an inward-rectifier cation current in auditory hair cells of varitint-waddler mice. *J. Physiol. 586*(22), 5403–5418.

Altarescu, G., Sun, M., Moore, D.F., Smith, J.A., Wiggs, E.A., Solomon, B.I., Patronas, N.J., Frei, K.P., Gupta, S., Kaneski, C.R., et al. (2002). The neurogenetics of mucolipidosis type IV. *Neurology 59*(3), 306–313.

Atiba-Davies, M., and Noben-Trauth, K. (2007). TRPML3 and hearing loss in the varitint-waddler mouse. *Biochim. Biophys. Acta Mol. Basis Dis. 1772*(8), 1028–1031.

Bae, M., Patel, N., Xu, H., Lee, M., Tominaga-Yamanaka, K., Nath, A., Geiger, J., Gorospe, M., Mattson, M.P., and Haughey, N.J. (2014). Activation of TRPML1 clears intraneuronal A in preclinical models of HIV infection. *J. Neurosci. 34*(34), 11485–11503.

Bargal, R., Avidan, N., Ben-Asher, E., Olender, Z., Zeigler, M., Frumkin, A., Raas-Rothschild, A., Glusman, G.., Lancet, D., and Bach, G. (2000). Identification: Of the gene causing mucolipidosis type IV. *Nat. Genet. 26*, 118–121.

Bassi, M.T., Manzoni, M., Monti, E., Pizzo, M.T., Ballabio, A., and Borsani, G. (2000). Cloning of the gene encoding a novel integral membrane protein, mucolipidin-and identification of the two major founder mutations causing mucolipidosis type IV. *Am. J. Hum. Genet. 67*(5), 1110–1120.

Benini, A., Bozzato, A., Mantovanelli, S., Calvarini, L., Giacopuzzi, E., Bresciani, R., Moleri, S., Zizioli, D., Beltrame, M., and Borsani, G. (2013). Characterization and expression analysis of mcoln1.1 and mcoln1.2, the putative zebrafish co-orthologs of the gene responsible for human mucolipidosis type IV. *Int. J. Dev. Biol. 57*(1), 85–93.

Bennett, M.J., and Rakheja, D. (2013). The neuronal ceroid-lipofuscinoses. *Dev. Disabil. Res. Rev. 17*(3), 254–259.

Bouché, V., Espinosa, A.P., Leone, L., Sardiello, M., Ballabio, A., and Botas, J. (2016). *Drosophila* Mitf regulates the V-ATPase and the lysosomal-autophagic pathway. *Autophagy 12*(3), 484–498.

Boustany, R.-M.N. (2013). Lysosomal storage diseases – The horizon expands. *Nat. Rev. Neurol. 9*(10), 583–598.

Bretou, M., Sáez, P.J., Sanséau, D., Maurin, M., Lankar, D., Chabaud, M., Spampanato, C., Malbec, O., Barbier, L., Muallem, S., et al. (2017). Lysosome signaling controls the migration of dendritic cells. *Sci. Immunol. 2*(16), eaak9573.

Cao, Q., Zhong, X.Z., Zou, Y., Zhang, Z., Toro, L., and Dong, X.-P. (2015). BK channels alleviate lysosomal storage diseases by providing positive feedback regulation of lysosomal Ca2+ release. *Dev. Cell 33*(4), 427–441.

Castiglioni, A.J., Remis, N.N., Flores, E.N., and García-Añoveros, J. (2011). Expression and vesicular localization of mouse Trpml3 in stria vascularis, hair cells, and vomeronasal and olfactory receptor neurons. *J. Comp. Neurol. 519*(6), 1095–1114.

Chandra, M., Zhou, H., Li, Q., Muallem, S., Hofmann, S.L., and Soyombo, A.A. (2011). A role for the Ca2+ channel TRPML1 in: Gastric acid secretion, based on analysis of knockout mice. *Gastroenterology 140*, 857–867.e1.

Chen, C.-C., Keller, M., Hess, M., Schiffmann, R., Urban, N., Wolfgardt, A., Schaefer, M., Bracher, F., Biel, M., Wahl-Schott, C., and Grimm, C. (2014). A small molecule restores function to TRPML1 mutant isoforms responsible for mucolipidosis type IV. *Nat. Commun. 5*, 4681.

Chen, Q., She, J., Zeng, W., Guo, J., Xu, H., Bai, X., and Jiang, Y. (2017). Structure of mammalian endolysosomal TRPML1 channel in nanodiscs. *Nature 550*(7676), 415–418.

Cheng, X., Zhang, X., Gao, Q., Ali Samie, M., Azar, M., Tsang, W.L., Dong, L., Sahoo, N., Li, X., Zhuo, Y., et al. (2014). The intracellular Ca2+ channel MCOLN1 is required for sarcolemma repair to prevent muscular dystrophy. *Nat. Med. 20*(10), 1187–1192.

Clayton, N., Marshall, F.H., Bountra, C., and O'Shaughnessy, C.T. (2002). CB1 and CB2 cannabinoid receptors are implicated in inflammatory pain. *Pain 96*(3), 253–260.

Cuajungco, M.P., Basilio, L.C., Silva, J., Hart, T., Tringali, J., Chen, C.-C., Biel, M., and Grimm, C. (2014). Cellular zinc levels are modulated by TRPML1-TMEM163 interaction. *Traffic 15*(11), 1247–1265.

Cuajungco, M.P., and Kiselyov, K. (2017). The mucolipin-1 (TRPML1) ion channel, transmembrane-163 (TMEM163) protein, and lysosomal zinc handling. *Front. Biosci. (Landmark Ed.) 22*, 1330–1343.

Cuajungco, M.P., Silva, J., Habibi, A., and Valadez, J.A. (2016). The mucolipin-2 (TRPML2) ion channel: A tissue-specific protein crucial to normal cell function. *Pflug. Arch. Eur. J. Physiol. 468*(2), 177–192.

Curcio-Morelli, C., Zhang, P., Venugopal, B., Charles, F.A., Browning, M.F., Cantiello, H.F., and Slaugenhaupt, S.A. (2010). Functional multimerization of mucolipin channel proteins. *J. Cell. Physiol. 222*(2), 328–335.

Dayam, R.M., Saric, A., Shilliday, R.E., and Botelho, R.J. (2015). The phosphoinositide-gated lysosomal Ca 2+ channel, TRPML1, is required for phagosome maturation. *Traffic 16*(9), 1010–1026.

Dayam, R.M., Sun, C.X., Choy, C.H., Mancuso, G., Glogauer, M., and Botelho, R.J. (2017). The lipid kinase PIKfyve coordinates the neutrophil immune response through the activation of the Rac GTPase. *J. Immunol. 199*(6), 2096–2105.

Denis, V., and Cyert, M.S. (2002). Internal Ca 2+ release in yeast is triggered by hypertonic shock and mediated by a TRP channel homologue. *J. Cell Biol. 156*(1), 29–34.

Dong, X.-P., Cheng, X., Mills, E., Delling, M., Wang, F., Kurz, T., and Xu, H. (2008). The type IV mucolipidosis-associated protein TRPML1 is an endolysosomal iron release channel. *Nature 455*(7215), 992–996.

Dong, X., Shen, D., Wang, X., Dawson, T., Li, X., Zhang, Q., Cheng, X., Zhang, Y., Weisman, L.S., Delling, M., and Xu, H. (2010). PI(3,5)P2 controls membrane trafficking by direct activation of mucolipin Ca2+ release channels in the endolysosome. *Nat. Commun. 1*, 1–11.

Dong, X., Wang, X., Shen, D., Chen, S., Liu, M., Wang, Y., Mills, E., Cheng, X., Delling, M., and Xu, H. (2009). Activating mutations of the TRPML1 channel revealed by proline-scanning mutagenesis. *J. Biol. Chem. 284*(46), 32040–32052.

Efeyan, A., Zoncu, R., and Sabatini, D.M. (2012). Amino acids and mTORC1: From lysosomes to disease. *Trends Mol. Med. 18*(9), 524–533.

Eichelsdoerfer, J.L., Evans, J.A., Slaugenhaupt, S.A., and Cuajungco, M.P. (2010). Zinc dyshomeostasis is linked with the loss of mucolipidosis IV-associated TRPML1 ion channel. *J. Biol. Chem. 285*(45), 34304–34308.

Fares, H., and Greenwald, I. (2001). Regulation of endocytosis by CUP-5, the Caenorhabditis elegans mucolipin-1 homolog. *Nat. Genet. 28*(1), 64–68.

Feng, X., Huang, Y., Lu, Y., Xiong, J., Wong, C.-O., Yang, P., Xia, J., Chen, D., Du, G., Venkatachalam, K., et al. (2014). *Drosophila* TRPML forms PI(3,5)P 2 -activated cation channels in both endolysosomes and plasma membrane. *J. Biol. Chem. 289*(7), 4262–4272.

Garrity, A.G., Wang, W., Collier, C.M., Levey, S.A., Gao, Q., and Xu, H. (2016). The endoplasmic reticulum, not the pH gradient, drives calcium refilling of lysosomes. *eLife 5*, e15887.

Grimm, C., Cuajungco, M.P., van Aken, A.F.J., Schnee, M., Jors, S., Kros, C.J., Ricci, A.J., and Heller, S. (2007). A helix-breaking mutation in TRPML3 leads to constitutive activity underlying deafness in the varitint-waddler mouse. *Proc. Natl. Acad. Sci. U.S.A. 104*(49), 19583–19588.

Grimm, C., Jors, S., Guo, Z., Obukhov, A.G., and Heller, S. (2012). Constitutive activity of TRPML2 and TRPML3 channels versus activation by low extracellular sodium and small molecules. *J. Biol. Chem. 287*(27), 22701–22708.

Grimm, C., Jörs, S., Saldanha, S.A., Obukhov, A.G., Pan, B., Oshima, K., Cuajungco, M.P., Chase, P., Hodder, P., and Heller, S. (2010). Small molecule activators of TRPML3. *Chem. Biol. 17*(2), 135–148.

Grishchuk, Y., Pena, K.A., Coblentz, J., King, V.E., Humphrey, D.M., Wang, S.L., Kiselyov, K.I., and Slaugenhaupt, S.A. (2015). Impaired myelination and reduced brain ferric iron in the mouse model of mucolipidosis IV. *Dis. Model. Mech. 8*(12), 1591–1601.

Hersh, B.M., Hartwieg, E., and Horvitz, H.R. (2002). The Caenorhabditis elegans mucolipin-like gene cup-5 is essential for viability and regulates lysosomes in multiple cell types. *Proc. Natl. Acad. Sci. U.S.A. 99*(7), 4355–4360.

Hirschi, M., Herzik Jr, M.A., Wie, J., Suo, Y., Borschel, W.F., Ren, D., Lander, G.C., and Lee, S.-Y. (2017). Cryo-electron microscopy structure of the lysosomal calcium-permeable channel TRPML3. *Nature 550*(7676), 411–414.

Jennings, J.J., Zhu, J., Rbaibi, Y., Luo, X., Chu, C.T., and Kiselyov, K. (2006). Mitochondrial aberrations in mucolipidosis Type IV. *J. Biol. Chem. 281*(51), 39041–39050.

Johnson, D.E., Ostrowski, P., Jaumouillé, V., and Grinstein, S. (2016). The position of lysosomes within the cell determines their luminal pH. *J. Cell Biol. 212*(6), 677–692.

Kaksonen, M., and Roux, A. (2018). Mechanisms of clathrin-mediated endocytosis. *Nat. Rev. Mol. Cell Biol. 19*(5), 313–326.

Karacsonyi, C., Miguel, A.S., and Puertollano, R. (2007). Mucolipin-2 localizes to the Arf6-associated pathway and regulates recycling of GPI-APs. *Traffic 8*(10), 1404–1414.

Kilpatrick, B.S., Yates, E., Grimm, C., Schapira, A.H., and Patel, S. (2016). Endo-lysosomal TRP mucolipin-1 channels trigger global ER $Ca^{2+}$ release and $Ca^{2+}$ influx. *J. Cell Sci. 129*(20), 3859–3867.

Kim, H.J., Li, Q., Tjon-Kon-Sang, S., So, I., Kiselyov, K., and Muallem, S. (2007). Gain-of-function mutation in TRPML3 causes the mouse Varitint-waddler phenotype. *J. Biol. Chem. 282*(50), 36138–36142.

Kim, H.J., Li, Q., Tjon-Kon-Sang, S., So, I., Kiselyov, K., Soyombo, A.A., and Muallem, S. (2008). A novel mode of TRPML3 regulation by extracytosolic pH absent in the varitint-waddler phenotype. *EMBO J. 27*(8), 1197–1205.

Kim, H.J., Soyombo, A.A., Tjon-Kon-Sang, S., So, I., and Muallem, S. (2009). The Ca(2+) channel TRPML3 regulates membrane trafficking and autophagy. *Traffic 10*(8), 1157–1167.

Kukic, I., Kelleher, S.L., and Kiselyov, K. (2014). Zn2+ efflux through lysosomal exocytosis prevents Zn2+-induced toxicity. *J. Cell Sci. 127*(14), 3094–3103.

Kukic, I., Lee, J.K., Coblentz, J., Kelleher, S.L., and Kiselyov, K. (2013). Zinc-dependent lysosomal enlargement in TRPML1-deficient cells involves MTF-1 transcription factor and ZnT4 (Slc30a4) transporter. *Biochem. J. 451*(2), 155–163.

LaPlante, J.M., Sun, M., Falardeau, J., Dai, D., Brown, E.M., Slaugenhaupt, S.A., and Vassilev, P.M. (2006). Lysosomal exocytosis is impaired in mucolipidosis type IV. *Mol. Genet. Metab. 89*(4), 339–348.

Lee, J.-H., McBrayer, M.K., Wolfe, D.M., Haslett, L.J., Kumar, A., Sato, Y., Lie, P.P.Y., Mohan, P., Coffey, E.E., Kompella, U., et al. (2015). Presenilin 1 maintains lysosomal Ca2+ homeostasis via TRPML1 by regulating vATPase-mediated lysosome acidification. *Cell Rep. 12*(9), 1430–1444.

Lev, S., Zeevi, D.A., Frumkin, A., Offen-Glasner, V., Bach, G., and Minke, B. (2010). Constitutive activity of the human TRPML2 channel induces cell degeneration. *J. Biol. Chem. 285*(4), 2771–2782.

Li, H., Pei, W., Vergarajauregui, S., Zerfas, P.M., Raben, N., Burgess, S.M., and Puertollano, R. (2017). Novel degenerative and developmental defects in a zebrafish model of mucolipidosis type IV. *Hum. Mol. Genet. 26*(14), 2701–2718.

Li, R.-J., Xu, J., Fu, C., Zhang, J., Zheng, Y.G., Jia, H., and Liu, J.O. (2016). Regulation of mTORC1 by lysosomal calcium and calmodulin. *eLife 5.*

Lima, W.C., Leuba, F., Soldati, T., and Cosson, P. (2012). Mucolipin controls lysosome exocytosis in Dictyostelium. *J. Cell Sci. 125*(9), 2315–2322.

Lines, M.A., Ito, Y., Kernohan, K.D., Mears, W., Hurteau-Miller, J., Venkateswaran, S., Ward, L., Khatchadourian, K., McClintock, J., Bhola, P., et al. (2017). Yunis-Varón syndrome caused by biallelic VAC14 mutations. *Eur. J. Hum. Genet. 25*(9), 1049–1054.

Manzoni, M., Monti, E., Bresciani, R., Bozzato, A., Barlati, S., Bassi, M.T., and Borsani, G. (2004). Overexpression of wild-type and mutant mucolipin proteins in mammalian cells: Effects on the late endocytic compartment organization. *FEBS Lett. 567*(2–3), 219–224.

Mao, T., O'Connor, D.H., Scheuss, V., Nakai, J., and Svoboda, K. (2008). Characterization and subcellular targeting of GCaMP-type genetically-encoded calcium indicators. *PloS one 3*(3), e1796.

Martina, J.A., Chen, Y., Gucek, M., and Puertollano, R. (2012). MTORC1 functions as a transcriptional regulator of autophagy by preventing nuclear transport of TFEB. *Autophagy 8*(6), 903–914.

Martina, J.A., Diab, H.I., Lishu, L., Jeong, A., Patange, L., Raben, S., N., and Puertollano, R. (2014). The nutrient-responsive transcription factor TFE3 promotes autophagy, lysosomal biogenesis, and clearance of cellular debris. *Sci. Signal. 7*(309), ra9–ra9.

Martina, J.A., Lelouvier, B., and Puertollano, R. (2009). The calcium channel Mucolipin-3 is a novel regulator of trafficking along the endosomal pathway. *Traffic 10*(8), 1143–1156.

McCartney, A.J., Zhang, Y., and Weisman, L.S. (2014). Phosphatidylinositol 3,5-bisphosphate: Low abundance, high significance. *BioEssays 36*(1), 52–64.

Medina, D.L., Fraldi, A., Bouche, V., Annunziata, F., Mansueto, G., Spampanato, C., Puri, C., Pignata, A., Martina, J.A., Sardiello, M., et al. (2011). Transcriptional activation of lysosomal exocytosis promotes cellular clearance. *Dev. Cell 21*(3), 421–430.

Medina, D.L., Di Paola, S., Peluso, I., Armani, A., De Stefani, D., Venditti, R., Montefusco, S., Scotto-Rosato, A., Prezioso, C., Forrester, A., et al. (2015). Lysosomal calcium signalling regulates autophagy through calcineurin and TFEB. *Nat. Cell Biol. 17*(3), 288–299.

Miao, Y., Li, G., Zhang, X., Xu, H., and Abraham, S.N. (2015). A TRP channel senses lysosome neutralization by pathogens to trigger their expulsion. *Cell 161*(6), 1306–1319.

Miedel, M.T., Rbaibi, Y., Guerriero, C.J., Colletti, G., Weixel, K.M., Weisz, O.A., and Kiselyov, K. (2008). Membrane traffic and turnover in TRP-ML1-deficient cells: A revised model for mucolipidosis type IV pathogenesis. *J. Exp. Med. 205*(6), 1477–1490.

Mills, E., Dong, X.-P., Wang, F., and Xu, H. (2010). Mechanisms of brain iron transport: Insight into neurodegeneration and CNS disorders. *Future Med. Chem. 2*(1), 51–64.

Nagata, K., Zheng, L., Madathany, T., Castiglioni, A.J., Bartles, J.R., and Garcia-Anoveros, J. (2008). The varitint-waddler (Va) deafness mutation in TRPML3 generates constitutive, inward rectifying currents and causes cell degeneration. *Proc. Natl. Acad. Sci. U.S.A. 105*(1), 353–358.

Nakai, J., Ohkura, M., and Imoto, K. (2001). A high signal-to-noise Ca2+ probe composed of a single green fluorescent protein. *Nat. Biotechnol. 19*(2), 137–141.

Onyenwoke, R.U., Sexton, J.Z., Yan, F., Diaz, M.C.H., Forsberg, L.J., Major, M.B., and Brenman, J.E. (2015). The mucolipidosis IV Ca2+ channel TRPML1 (MCOLN1) is regulated by the TOR kinase. *Biochem. J. 470*(3), 331–342.

Di Palma, F., Belyantseva, I.A., Kim, H.J., Vogt, T.F., Kachar, B., and Noben-Trauth, K. (2002). Mutations in Mcoln3 associated with deafness and pigmentation defects in varitint-waddler (Va) mice. *Proc. Natl. Acad. Sci. U.S.A. 99*(23), 14994–14999.

Palmieri, M., Impey, S., Kang, H., di Ronza, A., Pelz, C., Sardiello, M., and Ballabio, A. (2011). Characterization of the CLEAR network reveals an integrated control of cellular clearance pathways. *Hum. Mol. Genet. 20*(19), 3852–3866.

Paredes, R.M., Etzler, J.C., Watts, L.T., Zheng, W., and Lechleiter, J.D. (2008). Chemical calcium indicators. *Methods 46*(3), 143–151.

Pastores, G.M., and Maegawa, G.H.B. (2013). Neuropathic lysosomal storage disorders. *Neurol. Clin. 31*(4), 1051.

Ploper, D., and De Robertis, E.M. (2015). The MITF family of transcription factors: Role in endolysosomal biogenesis, Wnt signaling, and oncogenesis. *Pharmacol. Res. 99*, 36–43.

Ploper, D., Taelman, V.F., Robert, L., Perez, B.S., Titz, B., Chen, H.-W., Graeber, T.G., von Euw, E., Ribas, A., and De Robertis, E.M. (2015). MITF drives endolysosomal biogenesis and potentiates Wnt signaling in melanoma cells. *Proc. Natl. Acad. Sci. U.S.A. 112*(5), E420–E429.

Plotegher, N., and Duchen, M.R. (2017). Crosstalk between lysosomes and mitochondria in Parkinson's disease. *Front. Cell Dev. Biol. 5*, 110.

Pologruto, T.A., Yasuda, R., and Svoboda, K. (2004). Monitoring neural activity and [Ca2+] with genetically encoded Ca2+ indicators. *J. Neurosci. 24*(43), 9572–9579.

Pryor, P.R., Mullock, B.M., Bright, N.A., Gray, S.R., and Luzio, J.P. (2000). The role of intra-organellar Ca(2+) in late endosome-lysosome heterotypic fusion and in the reformation of lysosomes from hybrid organelles. *J. Cell Biol. 149*(5), 1053–1062.

Pryor, P.R., Reimann, F., Gribble, F.M., and Luzio, J.P. (2006). Mucolipin-1 is a lysosomal membrane protein required for intracellular lactosylceramide traffic. *Traffic 7*(10), 1388–1398.

Radhakrishna, H., and Donaldson, J.G. (1997). ADP-ribosylation factor 6 regulates a novel plasma membrane recycling pathway. *J. Cell Biol. 139*(1), 49–61.

Ravi, S., Peña, K.A., Chu, C.T., and Kiselyov, K. (2016). Biphasic regulation of lysosomal exocytosis by oxidative stress. *Cell Calcium 60*(5), 356–362.

Repnik, U., and Turk, B. (2010). Lysosomal–mitochondrial cross-talk during cell death. *Mitochondrion 10*(6), 662–669.

Roczniak-Ferguson, A., Petit, C.S., Froehlich, F., Qian, S., Ky, J., Angarola, B., Walther, T.C., and Ferguson, S.M. (2012). The transcription factor TFEB links mTORC1 signaling to transcriptional control of lysosome homeostasis. *Sci. Signal. 5*(228), ra42–ra42.

Ronco, V., Potenza, D.M., Denti, F., Vullo, S., Gagliano, G., Tognolina, M., Guerra, G., Pinton, P., Genazzani, A.A., Mapelli, L., et al. (2015). A novel Ca2+-mediated crosstalk between endoplasmic reticulum and acidic organelles: Implications for NAADP-dependent Ca2+ signalling. *Cell Calcium 57*(2), 89–100.

Rusten, T.E., Rodahl, L.M.W., Pattni, K., Englund, C., Samakovlis, C., Dove, S., Brech, A., and Stenmark, H. (2006). Fab1 phosphatidylinositol 3-phosphate 5-kinase controls trafficking but not silencing of endocytosed receptors. *Mol. Biol. Cell 17*(9), 3989–4001.

Sahoo, N., Gu, M., Zhang, X., Raval, N., Yang, J., Bekier, M., Calvo, R., Patnaik, S., Wang, W., King, G., et al. (2017). Gastric acid secretion from parietal cells is mediated by a Ca 2+ efflux channel in the tubulovesicle. *Dev. Cell 41*(3), 262–273.e6.

Samie, M., Wang, X., Zhang, X., Goschka, A., Li, X., Cheng, X., Gregg, E., Azar, M., Zhuo, Y., Garrity, A.G., et al. (2013). A TRP channel in the lysosome regulates large particle phagocytosis via focal exocytosis. *Dev. Cell 26*(5), 511–524.

Samie, M.A., Grimm, C., Evans, J.A., Curcio-Morelli, C., Heller, S., Slaugenhaupt, S.A., and Cuajungco, M.P. (2009). The tissue-specific expression of TRPML2 (MCOLN-2) gene is influenced by the presence of TRPML1. *Pflug. Arch. Eur. J. Physiol. 459*(1), 79–91.

Sancak, Y., Bar-Peled, L., Zoncu, R., Markhard, A.L., Nada, S., and Sabatini, D.M. (2010). Ragulator-rag complex targets mTORC1 to the lysosomal surface and is necessary for its activation by amino acids. *Cell 141*(2), 290–303.

Sardiello, M., Palmieri, M., di Ronza, A., Medina, D.L., Valenza, M., Gennarino, V.A., Di Malta, C., Donaudy, F., Embrione, V., Polishchuk, R.S., et al. (2009). A gene network regulating lysosomal biogenesis and function. *Science 325*(5939), 473–477.

Schaheen, L., Dang, H., and Fares, H. (2006). Basis of lethality in C. elegans lacking CUP-5, the mucolipidosis Type IV orthologue. *Dev. Biol. 293*(2), 382–391.

Schmiege, P., Fine, M., Blobel, G., and Li, X. (2017). Human TRPML1 channel structures in open and closed conformations. *Nature 550*(7676), 366–370.

Settembre, C., Di Malta, C., Polito, V.A., Arencibia, M.G., Vetrini, F., Erdin, S., Erdin, S.U., Huynh, T., Medina, D., Colella, P., et al. (2011). TFEB links autophagy to lysosomal biogenesis. *Science 332*(6036), 1429–1433.

Settembre, C., Zoncu, R., Medina, D.L., Vetrini, F., Erdin, S., Erdin, S., Huynh, T., Ferron, M., Karsenty, G., Vellard, M.C., et al. (2012). A lysosome-to-nucleus signalling mechanism senses and regulates the lysosome via mTOR and TFEB. *EMBO J. 31*(5), 1095–1108.

Shen, D., Wang, X., Li, X., Zhang, X., Yao, Z., Dibble, S., Dong, X., Yu, T., Lieberman, A.P., Showalter, H.D., and Xu, H. (2012). Lipid storage disorders block lysosomal trafficking by inhibiting a TRP channel and lysosomal calcium release. *Nat. Commun. 3*, 731.

Sun, L., Hua, Y., Vergarajauregui, S., Diab, H.I., and Puertollano, R. (2015). Novel role of TRPML2 in the regulation of the innate immune response. *J. Immunol. 195*(10), 4922–4932.

Sun, M., Goldin, E., Stahl, S., Falardeau, J.L., Kennedy, J.C., Acierno, J.S., Bove, C., Kaneski, C.R., Nagle, J., Bromley, M.C., et al. (2000). Mucolipidosis type IV is caused by mutations in a gene encoding a novel transient receptor potential channel. *Hum. Mol. Genet. 9*(17), 2471–2478.

Sun, X., Yang, Y., Zhong, X.Z., Cao, Q., Zhu, X.-H., Zhu, X., and Dong, X.-P. (2018). A negative feedback regulation of MTORC1 activity by the lysosomal Ca$^{2+}$ channel MCOLN1 (mucolipin 1) using a CALM (calmodulin)-dependent mechanism. *Autophagy 14*(1), 38–52.

Tanida, I., Ueno, T., and Kominami, E. (2008). LC3 and autophagy. In: *Methods in Molecular Biology (Clifton, N.J.)*, pp. 77–88.

Thompson, E.G., Schaheen, L., Dang, H., and Fares, H. (2007). Lysosomal trafficking functions of mucolipin-1 in murine macrophages. *BMC Cell Biol. 8*, 54.

Treusch, S., Knuth, S., Slaugenhaupt, S.A., Goldin, E., Grant, B.D., and Fares, H. (2004). Caenorhabditis elegans functional orthologue of human protein h-mucolipin-1 is required for lysosome biogenesis. *Proc. Natl. Acad. Sci. U.S.A. 101*(13), 4483–4488.

Venkatachalam, K., Hofmann, T., and Montell, C. (2006). Lysosomal localization of TRPML3 depends on TRPML2 and the mucolipidosis-associated protein TRPML1. *J. Biol. Chem. 281*(25), 17517–17527.

Venkatachalam, K., Long, A.A., Elsaesser, R., Nikolaeva, D., Broadie, K., and Montell, C. (2008). Motor deficit in a Drosophila model of mucolipidosis Type IV due to defective clearance of apoptotic cells. *Cell 135*(5), 838–851.

Venkatachalam, K., and Montell, C. (2007). TRP channels, Annu Rev Biochem 76, 387–417.

Venkatachalam, K., Wong, C.-O., and Montell, C. (2013). Feast or famine: Role of TRPML in preventing cellular amino acid starvation. *Autophagy 9*(1), 98–100.

Venkatachalam, K., Wong, C.-O., and Zhu, M.X. (2015). The role of TRPMLs in endolysosomal trafficking and function. *Cell Calcium 58*(1), 48–56.

Venugopal, B., Browning, M.F., Curcio-Morelli, C., Varro, A., Michaud, N., Nanthakumar, N., Walkley, S.U., Pickel, J., and Slaugenhaupt, S.A. (2007). Neurologic, gastric, and opthalmologic pathologies in a murine model of mucolipidosis Type IV. *Am. J. Hum. Genet. 81*(5), 1070–1083.

Vergarajauregui, S., Connelly, P.S., Daniels, M.P., and Puertollano, R. (2008a). Autophagic dysfunction in mucolipidosis type IV patients. *Hum. Mol. Genet. 17*(17), 2723–2737.

Vergarajauregui, S., Oberdick, R., Kiselyov, K., and Puertollano, R. (2008b). Mucolipin 1 channel activity is regulated by protein kinase A-mediated phosphorylation. *Biochem. J. 410*(2), 417–425.

Vergarajauregui, S., and Puertollano, R. (2006). Two di-leucine motifs regulate trafficking of mucolipin-1 to lysosomes. *Traffic 7*(3), 337–353.

Wakabayashi, K., Gustafson, A.M., Sidransky, E., and Goldin, E. (2011). Mucolipidosis type IV: An update. *Mol. Genet. Metab. 104*(3), 206–213.

Walker, M.T., and Montell, C. (2016). Suppression of the motor deficit in a mucolipidosis type IV mouse model by bone marrow transplantation. *Hum. Mol. Genet. 25*(13), ddw132, 2752–2761.

Wang, W., Gao, Q., Yang, M., Zhang, X., Yu, L., Lawas, M., Li, X., Bryant-Genevier, M., Southall, N.T., Marugan, J., et al. (2015). Up-regulation of lysosomal TRPML1 channels is essential for lysosomal adaptation to nutrient starvation. *Proc. Natl. Acad. Sci. U.S.A. 112*(11), E1373–E1381.

Wong, C.-O., Gregory, S., Hu, H., Chao, Y., Sepúlveda, V.E., He, Y., Li-Kroeger, D., Goldman, W.E., Bellen, H.J., and Venkatachalam, K. (2017). Lysosomal degradation is required for sustained phagocytosis of bacteria by macrophages. *Cell Host Microbe 21*(6), 719–730.

Wong, C.-O., Li, R., Montell, C., and Venkatachalam, K. (2012). Drosophila TRPML is required for TORC1 activation. *Curr. Biol. 22*(17).

Wong, C.-O., Palmieri, M., Li, J., Akhmedov, D., Chao, Y., Broadhead, G.T., Zhu, M.X., Berdeaux, R., Collins, C.A., Sardiello, M., and Venkatachalam, K. (2015). Diminished MTORC1-dependent JNK activation underlies the neurodevelopmental defects associated with lysosomal dysfunction. *Cell Rep. 12*(12), 2009–2020.

Xu, H., Delling, M., Li, L., Dong, X., and Clapham, D.E. (2007). Activating mutation in a mucolipin transient receptor potential channel leads to melanocyte loss in varitint-waddler mice. *Proc. Natl. Acad. Sci. U. S. A. 104*(46), 18321–18326.

Zeevi, D.A., Frumkin, A., and Bach, G. (2007). TRPML and lysosomal function. *Biochim. Biophys. Acta Mol. Basis Dis. 1772*(8), 851–858.

Zeevi, D.A., Lev, S., Frumkin, A., Minke, B., and Bach, G. (2010). Heteromultimeric TRPML channel assemblies play a crucial role in the regulation of cell viability models and starvation-induced autophagy. *J. Cell Sci. 123*(18), 3112–3124.

Zhang, L., Fang, Y., Cheng, X., Lian, Y., Xu, H., Zeng, Z., and Zhu, H. (2017a). TRPML1 participates in the progression of Alzheimer's disease by regulating the PPARγ/AMPK/Mtor signalling pathway. *Cell. Physiol. Biochem. 43*(6), 2446–2456.

Zhang, L., Fang, Y., Cheng, X., Lian, Y.-J., Xu, H., Zeng, Z.-S., and Zhu, H. (2017b). Curcumin exerts effects on the pathophysiology of Alzheimer's disease by regulating PI(3,5)P2 and transient receptor potential mucolipin-1 expression. *Front. Neurol. 8*, 531.

Zhang, S., Li, N., Zeng, W., Gao, N., and Yang, M. (2017c). Cryo-EM structures of the mammalian endo-lysosomal TRPML1 channel elucidate the combined regulation mechanism. *Protein Cell 8*(11), 834–847.

Zhang, X., Cheng, X., Yu, L., Yang, J., Calvo, R., Patnaik, S., Hu, X., Gao, Q., Yang, M., Lawas, M., et al. (2016). MCOLN1 is a ROS sensor in lysosomes that regulates autophagy. *Nat. Commun. 7*, 12109.

Zhong, X.Z., Sun, X., Cao, Q., Dong, G., Schiffmann, R., and Dong, X.-P. (2016). BK channel agonist represents a potential therapeutic approach for lysosomal storage diseases. *Sci. Rep. 6*, 33684.

Zhong, X.Z., Zou, Y., Sun, X., Dong, G., Cao, Q., Pandey, A., Rainey, J.K., Zhu, X., and Dong, X.-P. (2017). Inhibition of transient receptor potential channel mucolipin-1 (TRPML1) by lysosomal adenosine involved in severe combined immunodeficiency diseases. *J. Biol. Chem. 292*(8), 3445–3455.

Zhou, X., Li, M., Su, D., Jia, Q., Li, H., Li, X., and Yang, J. (2017). Cryo-EM structures of the human endolysosomal TRPML3 channel in three distinct states. *Nat. Struct. Mol. Biol. 24*(12), 1146–1154.

Zolov, S.N., Bridges, D., Zhang, Y., Lee, W.-W., Riehle, E., Verma, R., Lenk, G.M., Converso-Baran, K., Weide, T., Albin, R.L., et al. (2012). In vivo, Pikfyve generates PI(3,5)P2, which serves as both a signaling lipid and the major precursor for PI5P. *Proc. Natl. Acad. Sci. U. S. A. 109*(43), 17472–17477.

Zoncu, R., Bar-Peled, L., Efeyan, A., Wang, S., Sancak, Y., and Sabatini, D.M. (2011). mTORC1 senses lysosomal amino acids through an inside-out mechanism that requires the vacuolar H+-ATPase. *Science 334*(6056), 678–683.

Zou, J., Hu, B., Arpag, S., Yan, Q., Hamilton, A., Zeng, Y.-S., Vanoye, C.G., and Li, J. (2015). Reactivation of lysosomal Ca2+ efflux rescues abnormal lysosomal storage in FIG4-deficient cells. *J. Neurosci. 35*, 6801–6812.

# 5 Investigating the Role of Two-Pore Channel 2 (TPC2) in Zebrafish Neuromuscular Development

*Sarah E. Webb, Jeffrey J. Kelu, and Andrew L. Miller*

## CONTENTS

## 5.1 INTRODUCTION

Over the last decade, the rapid progress in the development, improvement and/ or commercialization of a range of different techniques, including molecular and genetic methodologies (Cong et al., 2013; Jinek et al., 2013) and imaging strategies (Carroni and Saibil, 2016; Meyer et al., 2008), as well as the development of novel pharmacological agents (Naylor et al., 2009), has encouraged the discovery of new proteins and advanced our knowledge of their function in cells, tissues and whole organisms. A key example is the identification and subsequent characterization of the two-pore channel (TPC) family (Calcraft et al., 2009). TPCs were identified during a search for a nicotinic acid adenine dinucleotide phosphate (NAADP) receptor. NAADP at concentrations as low as nanomolar amounts were known to stimulate the release of significant amounts of $Ca^{2+}$ in a highly localized manner in sea urchin (*Strongylocentrotus purpuratus* and *Lytechinus pictus*) egg homogenate (Lee and Aarhus, 1995) and in live sea urchin eggs (Aarhus et al., 1996), in starfish (*Asterina pectinifera*) oocytes (Santella et al., 2000) and in various mammalian cell types, including mouse pancreatic acinar cells (Cancela et al., 1999) and human Jurkat T-lymphocytes (Berg et al., 2000). The intracellular $Ca^{2+}$ stores involved in generating these highly localized signals were reported to be distinct from the endoplasmic reticulum (ER) (Genazzani and Galione, 1996; Lee and Aarhus, 1995; Patel et al., 2001), and they were identified as being lysosome-related acidic organelles (Churchill et al., 2002; Kinnear et al., 2004). At this time, it was also reported that in rat arterial smooth muscle cells, lysosomal $Ca^{2+}$ stores are closely associated with regions of the sarcoplasmic reticulum (SR) expressing ryanodine receptors (RyR), and it was suggested that localized $Ca^{2+}$ signals from the lysosomes might stimulate or "trigger" long-range $Ca^{2+}$ signalling by $Ca^{2+}$-induced $Ca^{2+}$ release (CICR) via RyR in the SR (Kinnear et al., 2004). The molecular identity of the NAADP receptor was subsequently identified as being a voltage-gated cation channel, and it was called the two-pore channel or TPC (Calcraft et al., 2009; Galione et al., 2009). Since then, it has been reported that there is bidirectional $Ca^{2+}$ signalling between the ER and acidic organelles. Thus, in addition to $Ca^{2+}$ released from acidic organelles triggering the release of $Ca^{2+}$ from the ER via inositol 1,4,5-trisphosphate ($IP_3$) receptors ($IP_3R$) and RyR (Morgan et al., 2011), $Ca^{2+}$ released from the ER can also activate and/or modulate NAADP-regulated channels (Morgan et al., 2013).

So far, three TPC isoforms have been identified in animals; TPC1 and TPC3 are localized on endosomal membranes, whereas TPC2 is localized on lysosomal membranes. The genes of all three TPCs (*TPCNs*) are reported to be expressed in most vertebrates although *TPCN3* is not expressed in humans, chimps, mice or rats

(Calcraft et al., 2009). Sea urchins are also reported to have all three TPC genes, but the sea squirts, *Ciona savignyi* and *Ciona intestinalis*, only express an isoform of *TPCN2* that has no introns, and *TPCN3*. In addition, some insects such as bees, beetles and silkworms express *TPCN1* but not *TPCN2* or *TPCN3*, whereas mosquitoes and flies do not express any of the *TPCN* genes. A *TPCN* gene has also been found in several plant species, including *Arabidopsis*, tobacco and rice. This was originally named *TPC1*, but it is actually distinct from all of the animal *TPCN* gene sequences (Calcraft et al., 2009). Due to the diversity of species expressing *TPC* genes, it was suggested that they might be part of an ancient gene family, and that certainly for vertebrates (if not other species), they likely have an important function (Calcraft et al., 2009). Indeed, in the last 10 years since the initial report describing TPCs, they (particularly TPC2) have been demonstrated to play an important role in embryonic development and differentiation, and in various aspects of mature cell function.

With regards to the role of TPCs in cell function, reports indicate that TPC2 plays a role in store-operated $Ca^{2+}$ entry in MEG01 megakaryoblasts and HEK-293 cells (López et al., 2012); regulates β-adrenoceptor signalling in isolated cardiac ventricular myocytes and in intact hearts in mice (Capel et al., 2015); controls pigmentation in human melanocytic MNT-1 cells by regulating the amount of melanin produced (Ambrosio et al., 2016); and plays a role in the contraction of smooth muscle isolated from guinea pig bladder (Tugba Durlu-Kandilci et al., 2010). In addition, both TPC1 and TPC2 are reported to play a role in stimulus-secretion coupling in isolated mouse pancreatic β-cells (Arredouani et al., 2015), and regulate autophagy in human and rodent cardiomyocytes (García-Rúa et al., 2016). Thus, TPCs appear to control a range of functions depending on the cell type.

Due to their important role in normal cell function, TPCs have also been implicated in a number of diseases when their activity is attenuated or blocked. For example, mice in which TPC2 alone or TPC1 and TPC2 were knocked out are highly susceptible to fatty liver disease (Grimm et al., 2014) and mature-onset obesity (Lear et al., 2015), respectively. TPC1 and TPC2 have also been demonstrated to play an important role in Ebola infection by controlling the entry and intracellular trafficking of the virus in human macrophages (Sakurai et al., 2015), and reports suggest that TPCs might play a role in the pathogenesis of neurodegenerative diseases such as Parkinson's disease (Hockney et al., 2015; Rivero-Ríos et al., 2016) and Alzheimer's disease (Ezeani and Omabe, 2016), as well as various cancers (Jahidin et al., 2016; Nguyen et al., 2017). Thus, the more we discover and understand about the function of TPCs, the more likely we are of developing novel treatment strategies for these diseases (Marchant and Patel, 2015).

In our laboratory, we are interested in the role of TPCs (particularly TPC2) in development. It has been reported that TPCs (or NAADP signalling) are important mediators of differentiation in a variety of cell types (Parrington and Tunn, 2014). These include neurons (Brailoiu et al., 2005, 2006), skeletal muscle cells (Aley et al., 2010), osteoclasts (Notomi et al., 2012), keratinocytes (Park et al., 2015) and embryonic stem cells (Zhang et al., 2013). Many of these experiments were conducted in isolated cells in culture. However, we use intact normally developing zebrafish embryos in our research, and over the last few years, we have provided some of the first evidence that TPC2 plays a key role in the development, coordination and maturation of early neuromuscular activity in a vertebrate *in vivo* (Kelu et al., 2015, 2017, 2018). Most recently, we have reported the expression of *arc1*-like (a putative enzyme for generating NAADP) and endogenous levels of NAADP during the development of slow muscle cells (SMCs) in zebrafish (Kelu et al., 2019). In this chapter, we discuss the techniques used when investigating the role of TPC2 in zebrafish neuromuscular development.

## 5.2   INVESTIGATING THE LOCALIZATION OF TPC2 IN ZEBRAFISH SLOW MUSCLE AND PRIMARY MOTOR NEURONS

The localization of TPC2 in zebrafish SMCs has been studied using immunolabelling in both intact embryos and in isolated primary cell cultures (Kelu et al., 2015, 2017, 2018). This same technique has also been used to demonstrate the localization of other $Ca^{2+}$ channels in the SMCs of intact zebrafish embryos, including $IP_3R$ and RyR (Brennan et al., 2005; Cheung et al., 2011; Hirata et al., 2007).

When immunolabelling intact embryos, the basic technique is very similar to that used when immunolabelling cells in culture. Thus, embryos are fixed and permeabilized, followed by, antibody incubation and wash steps similar to those used for cells in culture. However, some aspects of the methodology are different due to the large size and multi-cellular nature of the embryos being labelled. For example, all the incubation steps are conducted for longer periods of time. Thus, while cells in culture might be fixed (e.g., with paraformaldehyde) for just a few minutes at room temperature, embryos must be fixed for longer (i.e., typically overnight at 4°C). In addition, prior to fixation, embryos are anaesthetized with MS-222 (Topic Popovic et al., 2012) before being transferred to fixative, and the paraformaldehyde is warmed to ~28°C (the optimal temperature for zebrafish embryos; Kimmel et al., 1995), in order to help prevent/reduce the contraction of the trunk musculature during fixation. Although MS-222 does not paralyse the muscle directly (Attili and Hughes, 2014), the aim of this step is to render the larvae unconscious so that the muscles are in a somewhat relaxed state upon immersion in the fixative. Thus, following immunolabelling, any changes in the pattern of localization observed should be due to differences in the expression of the protein, rather than alterations in the contraction state of the trunk musculature. Another difference between isolated cells in culture and intact embryos is that for the latter, dimethylsulphoxide (DMSO) is added to all the buffers (permeabilization, block and wash) in order to increase the permeability of cell membranes and thus allow antibodies to penetrate deep within the embryonic tissues (Capriotti and Capriotti, 2012; de Ménorval et al., 2012). Furthermore, whereas cells tend to be incubated with primary and secondary antibodies for a relatively short period of time (e.g., ~1 h at room temperature), embryos are incubated with antibodies for longer (i.e., for ~4–6 h at room temperature, or overnight at 4°C; Kelu et al., 2015, 2017). Similar to cells, embryos are incubated with antibodies sequentially. Thus, for dual-immunolabelling, which is useful for determining where TPC2 is localized with respect to the SMCs, we incubate embryos first with our anti-TPC2 antibody (custom-made by Covalab UK Ltd., Cambridge, UK; raised in rabbit), then with an F59 anti-myosin heavy chain (MHC) antibody (raised in mouse; Devoto et al., 1996), then with an Atto 647N-tagged goat anti-rabbit IgG and finally with an Alexa Fluor 488-tagged goat anti-mouse IgG, with each antibody incubation being overnight at 4°C. Because the secondary antibodies were both raised in goat, the block buffer should contain goat serum, as this helps to reduce the chance of non-specific labelling due to the secondary antibodies. Thus, to dual-immunolabel embryos for TPC2 and the MHC, the protocol might take 5 days (or more), when compared with cells in culture, which might take just one day. At the end of immunolabelling, like cells in culture, the embryos can be mounted prior to visualization via confocal microscopy. AF1 mountant and Prolong Gold or Prolong Diamond (with or without DAPI) have been shown to work well for mounting zebrafish embryos (Kelu et al., 2015, 2017; Missinato et al., 2018; Pineda et al., 2006; Pipalia et al., 2016; Shi et al., 2017). However, in order for the trunk musculature to be mounted as flat as possible so that it lies horizontal to the plane of the coverslip, the head and yolk need to be excised with tungsten needles and discarded first (Kelu et al., 2015, 2017). Preparing trunk tissue in a sequential manner following a developmental time-line allows us to visualize the localization and progression of the organization of TPC2 as the SMCs develop. The protocol used to dual-immunolabel TPC2 and the MHC in intact zebrafish embryos is described in Section 5.6.1.

In addition to labelling intact embryos with the anti-TPC2 antibody, primary cultures of SMCs have also been prepared and then immunolabelled with the same antibody (Kelu et al., 2015). This avoids the high level of background fluorescence, which can be problematic following immunolabelling of intact embryos. When primary cell cultures of zebrafish SMCs are prepared, however, the subcellular localization of TPC2 is better-defined. However, when cells are isolated for primary culture, they require some time to adhere to a coverslip. Therefore, if trunk cells are isolated from embryos at 24 h post-fertilization (hpf), they might require at least 24 h to attach to coverslips, which means that they are no longer at 24 hpf. It has been suggested that the localization pattern of TPC2 in SMCs after 24 h and 48 h in culture is approximately the same as that observed in the SMCs of intact embryos at ~18–20 hpf and ~20–24 hpf, respectively (Kelu et al., 2015). This suggests that during the preparation of muscle cell cultures, the trunk cells undergo a certain amount of dedifferentiation. In an attempt to reduce the dedifferentiation to a minimum, various dissection and culture protocols have been tested. Thus, in addition to dissecting embryos at ~16 hpf and culturing the trunk cells on uncoated glass coverslips for 24 h or 48 h (Kelu et al., 2015), more recently embryos have been dissected at ~48 hpf and the isolated cells have been cultured for just 1 h on laminin-coated coverslips (Kelu et al., 2017). In both cases, a cell incubation temperature of ~28°C was used. With these methods, the localization of TPC2 with respect to the lysosomes (immunolabelled with an anti-LAMP1 antibody), or with respect to $IP_3R$ or RyR in the SR, was demonstrated (Kelu et al., 2015, 2017). In addition, the close localization of TPC2 (in the lysosomes) with the adjacent sarcomeric I-band and (to a lesser extent) the M-line, and the localization of TPC2 in the nucleus and peri-nuclear region of SMCs were demonstrated (Kelu et al., 2015, 2017). In these mixed cell cultures, the SMCs were identified from their morphology (i.e., they are mononucleate, whereas fast muscle cells – FMCs – are multinucleate; Roy et al., 2001). In addition, at the developmental stages when the cells were prepared, SMCs (but not FMCs) express the MHC (Devoto et al., 1996) and so can also be identified via immunolabelling.

The protocols used to prepare primary muscle cell cultures from the trunk of zebrafish embryos at 17 hpf, and then dual-immunolabel TPC2 and the MHC in these cells, are described in Sections 5.6.2 and 5.6.3, respectively.

In one series of experiments, SMCs dissected from embryos at 48 hpf were dual-immunolabelled with antibodies to TPC2 and RyR (or to IP3R type III and RyR) for subsequent dual-colour stimulated emission depletion (STED) super-resolution microscopy (Hell and Wichmann, 1994). In these experiments, the immunolabelling procedure was exactly the same as that used for the other zebrafish cell culture labelling experiments, using Atto 647N-tagged and Alexa Fluor 488-tagged secondary antibodies. These 647 nm and 488 nm dyes have distinct excitation and emission spectra and both have been reported to demonstrate good STED efficiency (Nishimune et al., 2016; Willig et al., 2007). Dual-colour STED imaging demonstrated that there were "nano-gaps" of ~50–90 nm between TPC2 clusters and distinct RyR punctae. As this distance was within a hypothetical limit (Fameli et al., 2014), this suggests that $Ca^{2+}$ released via TPC2 might act as a trigger to stimulate $Ca^{2+}$-induced $Ca^{2+}$ release in the SR via activation of the RyR (Kelu et al., 2017; Morgan et al., 2013). Unfortunately, TPC2 and IP3R type III could not be dual-immunolabelled as these antibodies were both raised in rabbits. However, when the RyR and IP3R type III were dual-immunolabelled and imaged via dual-STED, no distinct gaps between the two were observed.

Most recently the localization of TPC2 in primary motor neurons has also been investigated. Due to the high background fluorescence in intact embryos, however, this has only been tested in primary cell cultures. In this case, SAIGFF213A;UAS:GFP double-transgenic embryos (Muto et al., 2011), which specifically express GFP in the spinal neurons, were dissected at ~18 hpf, and the dissociated trunk cells were cultured on laminin-coated coverslips at ~28°C for 24 h (Kelu et al., 2018). Primary motor neurons were identified via the expression of GFP and their distinctive morphology. In addition, they were shown to express TPC2, LAMP1 and IP3R types I and II but not IP3R type III. If the SAIGFF213A;UAS:GFP double-transgenic embryos are not available, then wild-type embryos can be dissected and dual-immunolabelled with antibodies to TPC2 and the motor axon-specific antibody, znp-1 (Flanagan-Steet et al., 2005; Kelu et al., 2018; Trevarrow et al., 1990). For all the immunolabelling experiments, whether in intact embryos or primary cells in culture, secondary antibody controls should be conducted in order to confirm that any labelling observed is only due to the secondary antibody binding to the primary antibody (Burry, 2011).

## 5.3   INVESTIGATING THE ROLE OF TPC2 IN SMC DEVELOPMENT

The role of TPC2 in the differentiation of SMCs and PMNs in intact zebrafish embryos has been investigated using various approaches. Functional TPC2 protein was inhibited in embryos by gene knock down, gene knock out or pharmacological means, after which the effect of this inhibition was determined by monitoring: (1) the pattern of $Ca^{2+}$ signals generated specifically in the SMCs or the PMNs; and (2) the subsequent morphology of the cells. We describe each of the inhibition and read-out methodologies in the following sections.

## 5.3.1  Use of Morpholino Oligonucleotides to Knock Down TPC2 Expression/Activity

Over the last decade, antisense morpholino (MO) oligonucleotide technology has been one of the main molecular knock down approaches used to study gene function in the oocytes or embryos of a range of different species, including the Atlantic killifish (*Fundulus heteroclitus*), zebrafish (*Danio rerio*), medaka (*Oryzias latipes*), sea star (*Patiria miniata*), starfish (*Patiria pectinifera*), African clawed frog (*Xenopus laevis*), chick (*Gallus gallus*) and mouse (*Mus musculus*), due to their ease of delivery and the high level of efficacy in attenuating the expression of specific genes (Bestman and Cline, 2013; Blum et al., 2015; Hong et al., 2016; Norris and Streit, 2014; Notch et al., 2011; Oulhen et al., 2014; Saito et al., 2017; Siddall et al., 2002). MOs are short chains of approximately 25 morpholine subunits that carry a neutral charge, and they are highly stable and water-soluble (Summerton and Weller, 1997). They are also nuclease-resistant, which means they are not degraded to form toxic degradation products in cells; this makes them active through the first few days in development, and the effects only diminish with the dilution of [MO] during the successive rounds of cell division (Bill et al., 2009). MOs function via a steric blocking mechanism; they bind to the target mRNA via complementary base pairing, and thereby knock down the expression of a specific protein (Blum et al., 2015; Lawson and Wolfe, 2011). Typically, MOs work in two ways, they either block the initiation of translation in the cytosol or they modify the pre-mRNA splicing in the nucleus; they do not act by degrading their target RNA molecules (Blum et al., 2015; Lawson and Wolfe, 2011). By understanding the distinct modes of action of these different types of MO, it is possible to evaluate the efficiency of each. Translation-blocking MOs can be evaluated by assessing the expression of protein after MO knock down by either western blotting or immunolabelling methods using specific antibodies. In contrast, splice-inhibiting MOs can be evaluated by assessing the expression level of transcripts via either the reverse transcription polymerase chain reaction (RT-PCR) or *in situ* hybridization (Blum et al., 2015; Lawson and Wolfe, 2011).

Early studies with MOs suggested that they are both specific and efficacious (Nasevicius and Ekker, 2000). However, it was later discovered that ~15–20% of MO usage had an undesired, sequence-unspecific off-targeting effect, which led to developmental defects such as the formation of smaller heads and eyes resulting in craniofacial deformities, as well as somite and notochord abnormalities (Ekker and Larson, 2001). Initially such MO off-targeting effects were largely attributed to the injection of high doses (i.e., >5 ng) of MO, which were suggested to trigger non-specific binding in a different RNA target (Ekker and Larson, 2001). Robu et al. (2007) demonstrated that some of the off-targeting effects resulted from the activation of the p53 pathway. It was therefore crucial to address the off-targeting issue whenever the MO technology was to be applied. An effective means that has been proposed to help alleviate these off-targeting effects is by co-knock down of p53, i.e., by injecting the MO for the specific gene of interest along with a *p53*-MO (Bill et al., 2009; Robu et al., 2007). The *p53*-MO was suggested to be innocuous as it does not interfere with the penetrance of gene-specific phenotypes, and therefore does not affect the efficacy of gene-specific MOs. Furthermore, p53 knock down does not induce any significant defects *per se*, as p53 has been shown to be largely dispensable for normal embryonic development, certainly in fish and mice (Storer and Zon, 2010). Alternatively, it was suggested that injecting embryos with different doses of the MO of interest, followed by the examination of *p53* expression (as an indicator of off-target effects) via qPCR, might help identify the maximal dose of the MO that could be used where the off-target response is minimal (Stainier et al., 2015).

To study the function of *tpcn2* during zebrafish development, two *TPCN2*-MOs were designed and utilized: a translation-blocking MO (*TPCN2*-MO-T) and a splice-interfering MO (*TPCN2*-MO-S; Figure 5.1; Kelu et al., 2015, 2017, 2018). These targeted the translation start site (i.e., ATG codon) of the mature *tpcn2* mRNA, and the exon 2–intron 2 splice junction of the *tpcn2* pre-mRNA, respectively (Figure 5.1Ai,Bi; Kelu et al., 2015, 2017). In addition, a *p53*-MO was always co-injected with the *TPCN2*-MOs at 1.5:1 ratio to alleviate any potential off-targeting effects (Kelu et al., 2015, 2017, 2018). Furthermore, a standard control-MO (which is an irrelevant oligo sequence that causes no observable change in embryonic phenotype) or the *p53*-MO alone was injected to control for specificity. The efficacy of the *TPCN2*-MO-T was evaluated via immunolabelling with the custom-made zebrafish TPC2 antibody described above (Section 5.2; Figure 5.1Aii; Kelu et al., 2015), whereas the *TPCN2*-MO-S was evaluated via RT-PCR and gel electrophoresis (Figure 5.1Bii,Biii; Kelu et al., 2017). In the case of immunolabelling, a striated pattern of TPC2 expression (see white arrowheads in Figure 5.1Aii) was seen in the slow muscle fibres (outlined with white dashed lines in Figure 5.1Aii) in whole-mount control embryos at ~24 hpf. In contrast, after TPC2-knock down using the *TPCN2*-MO-T, the expression of TPC2 in the slow muscle fibres was much reduced as shown by the distinct lack of fluorescence after immunolabelling (Figure 5.1Aii). These results helped to confirm the specificity of the custom-made TPC2 antibody and verify the action of the translation-blocking MO. With regard to RT-PCR, primers were designed to flank *tpcn2* exons 1–3 (i.e., using the F and R primers shown in Figure 5.1Bii). Gel electrophoresis then revealed that two aberrantly spliced *tpcn2* mRNA transcripts were detected in the *TPCN2*-MO-S-injected embryos that corresponded to either the inclusion of intron 2 or the exclusion of exon 2 (Figure 5.1Biii). This resulted in an increase and decrease of the *tpcn2* transcript size in the morphants, respectively, when compared with the controls (Figure 5.1Biii). These data thus verified the action of the splice-interfering MO. The morphants were subsequently shown to have attenuated $Ca^{2+}$ signalling in the developing myotome, as well as induce defects in myogenesis and motility (Kelu et al., 2015, 2017). The *TPCN2*-MOs were also shown to disrupt the normal ipsilateral correlation and contralateral anti-correlation of the $Ca^{2+}$ signals generated in the caudal primary (CaP) motor neurons (Kelu et al., 2018).

Currently, the zebrafish community are developing a series of guidelines or standard protocols, which aims to validate the specificity of MOs (Stainier et al., 2017). These include: (1) conducting immunolabelling or RT-PCR experiments to check the efficiency of MO knock down; (2) making use of a standard control-MO (or a five-base mismatch-MO), to demonstrate a normal phenotype for (and continued significant biological activity in) cells, tissues and organs, and to account for any developmental delay that might be observed; (3) making use of a *p53*-MO (to suppress p53 activity) in order to circumvent some of the non-specific phenotypes that

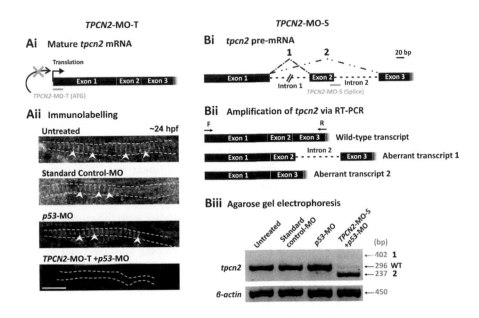

**FIGURE 5.1** Design and validation of the *TPCN2* morpholino (MO) oligonucleotides. (Ai) The mature mRNA of zebrafish *tpcn2*, showing exons 1–3, and the target locus for the translation-blocking *TPCN2*-MO-T. Binding of the *TPCN2*-MO-T to the start codon inhibits the translation of the transcript. (Aii) The action of the *TPCN2*-MO-T was validated by immunolabelling. Embryos at ~24 hpf were fixed, and dual-immunolabelled using the custom-made zebrafish TPC2 antibody (Kelu et al., 2015), to visualize endogenous TPC2, and the F59 antibody to identify the SMCs. Labelled embryos were then mounted and imaged using laser scanning confocal microscopy. In the single optical sections of SMCs shown (see the white dashed lines), a characteristic, striated pattern of TPC2 expression (see white arrowheads) was observed in embryos that were untreated, or else injected with either the standard control-MO or the *p53*-MO. In contrast, the expression of TPC2 was much reduced in SMCs of embryos injected with the *TPCN2*-MO-T (+*p53*-MO). The F59 antibody labelling is not shown. (Bi) The pre-mRNA of zebrafish *tpcn2*, showing exons 1–3, introns 1 and 2 and the target locus for the splice-interfering *TPCN2*-MO-S. The binding of the *TPCN2*-MO-S to the exon 2–intron 2 splice junction was predicted to result in two potential aberrant splicing patterns, as indicated by the dotted lines 1 and 2. (Bii) The wild-type *tpcn2* transcript (with exons 1–3 alone) showing the design of the forward (F) and reverse (R) primers for performing RT-PCR. Two possible aberrant *tpcn2* transcripts, showing either the inclusion of intron 2 (labelled aberrant transcript 1), or the exclusion of exon 2 (labelled aberrant transcript 2), resulted from the splice-blocking action of the *TPCN2*-MO-S. (Biii) The action of the *TPCN2*-MO-S was validated by RT-PCR. The F+R primers were used to amplify the *tpcn2* locus, followed by agarose gel electrophoresis. This showed the presence of the two aberrant transcripts (1 and 2) in the morphants injected with *TPCN2*-MO-S (+ *p53*-MO). *β-actin* was used as an internal control. In panels (Ai), (Bi) and (Bii), all the diagrams were drawn to scale, and the scale bar is 20 bp. In panel (Aii), the scale bar is 10 μm. (Panel (Biii) is reproduced with permission, from "Ca²⁺ release via two-pore channel type 2 (TPC2) is required for slow muscle cell myofibrillogenesis and myotomal patterning in intact zebrafish embryos" by Kelu, J.J., Webb, S.E., Parrington, J., Galione, A., and Miller, A.L., 2017. *Developmental Biology 425*, 109–129, Elsevier.)

might arise; (4) using two or more non-overlapping MOs that are designed to target independent regions of the gene of interest, and to check if they give rise to the same phenotype; (5) comparing the phenotypes of morphants with corresponding known mutants (if possible); and (6) conducting rescue experiments by co-injecting a form of mRNA that is not recognized by the gene-specific MO (Blum et al., 2015; Eisen and Smith, 2008; Lawson and Wolfe, 2011; Stainier et al., 2017).

To test the specificity of our *TPCN2*-MO-T, a *tpcn2* rescue construct was prepared that contained silent mutations in the target sequence, which meant that it could not be recognized by the *TPCN2*-MO-T (Kelu et al., 2015). The mutant *tpcn2* mRNA was generated via *in vitro* transcription using a linearized DNA template obtained from the *tpcn2* rescue construct. Rescue experiments were conducted by microinjecting 1-cell stage zebrafish embryos into the yolk with the *TPCN2*-MO-T, after which they were immediately injected into the blastodisc with the mutant *tpcn2* mRNA. The "rescued" embryos were shown to have a partial (but significant) recovery with regard to the $Ca^{2+}$ signals generated in the developing myotome and spinal cord, as well as with regard to myogenesis and motility (Kelu et al., 2015, 2017, 2018).

### 5.3.2  CRISPR/Cas9 Gene-Editing to Generate *TPCN2* Knock Out Mutants

Over the last few decades, a variety of site-specific nuclease technologies have been developed to perform genetic analysis and gene-editing both in cells in culture and in embryos (Komor et al., 2017). Within the last decade, the clustered regulatory interspaced short palindromic repeat/Cas9 endonuclease (CRISPR/Cas9; Cong et al., 2013; Jinek et al., 2012) has emerged as being the most popular gene-editing technique, due to its relative simplicity, cost-effectiveness and efficiency (Komor et al., 2017; Li et al., 2016; Singh et al., 2017).

CRISPR was first described as being a series of short direct repeats interspaced with short sequences in the *E. coli* genome (Ishino et al., 1987). Subsequent studies revealed the detection of the CRISPR loci in numerous bacteria and archea species, where it was predicted to be responsible for DNA repair or regulation (Makarova et al., 2002; Mojica et al., 2000). More recently it was suggested that the CRISPR/Cas type II system requires only a single protein (i.e., Cas9), for RNA-guided DNA recognition and cleavage. Indeed, the simplicity of this system greatly facilitated its development into the gene-editing tool that is so popular today (Doudna and Charpentier, 2014). To increase the simplicity of the system further, the tracrRNA:crRNA duplex, which guides the Cas protein to cleave the target DNA, was engineered as a single guide RNA (gRNA; Cong et al., 2013; Jinek et al., 2012). Thus, a 20-nucleotide sequence at the 5' end of the gRNA determines the specificity of DNA targeting by Watson-Crick base pairing, whereas a double-stranded structure at the 3' end binds to the Cas (nuclease) protein (Cong et al., 2013; Jinek et al., 2012). By changing the 20-nucleotide so-called "guide" sequence, the CRISPR/Cas9 can be programmed to target virtually any DNA sequence of interest, as long as it is adjacent to a protospacer adjacent motif (PAM), which is crucial for the binding of and subsequent cleavage by the Cas protein. To date, the *Streptococcus pyogenes* Cas9 (SpCas9) is the best-characterized and most popular CRISPR nuclease in use, and its PAM nucleotide sequence requirement is "NGG", where "N" can be A/T/C/G. As this sequence occurs on average once every 8–12 base pairs (bp) in the reference human genome (Cong et al., 2013; Hsu et al., 2014), this indicates the wide range of genomic sites that are amenable to editing. In addition, the success of the CRISPR/Cas9 system stems from its ability to induce site-specific double-stranded breaks in DNA, which then trigger either non-homologous end joining (NHEJ) repair or gene replacement by homology-directed repair (HDR; Hsu et al., 2014). During NHEJ repair, stochastic insertions or deletions (indels) of nucleotides occur at the site of gene-editing, and this frequently leads to the induction of frameshift mutations. Indeed, it has been reported that CRISPR/Cas9-mediated mutations via NHEJ repair can reach efficiencies of ~20–60% (Maruyama et al., 2015). As NHEJ-induced DNA repair is error-prone in the sense that it induces stochastic indel events, this method is extensively employed in loss-of-function studies. In contrast, HDR requires the incorporation of an exogenous DNA fragment, i.e., a donor template, and so this method allows for knock-in of specific mutations such as codon replacement and reporter insertions. However, the efficiency of HDR-mediated incorporation is typically very low (i.e., <5%; Chu et al., 2015).

CRISPR/Cas9 technology has been applied in a vast array of cells and organisms including the zebrafish to successfully target, edit or modify the genome (Chang et al., 2013; Hwang et al., 2013; Irion et al., 2014; Jao et al., 2013; Kimura et al., 2014; Li et al., 2016; Singh et al., 2017; Varshney et al., 2015a,b). During our exploration of the role of TPC2 in the neuromuscular development of zebrafish, a 23-bp *tpcn2* gRNA target sequence contained within exon 9 of *tpcn2* (i.e., which encodes part of the first homologous domain of the ion transporting six-transmembrane-segments of TPC2) (Zhu et al., 2010; Figure 5.2A) was selected using CRISPRdirect (a web server for identifying rational CRISPR/Cas9 targets; http://crispr.dbcls.jp/; Naito et al., 2015). This target sequence was chosen because: (1) a nucleotide BLAST of the seed sequence (i.e., the 12-bp sequence located 5' of the PAM; Cong et al., 2013; Jinek et al., 2012) indicated an absence of potential off-targets; and (2) it was shown to contain the AvaI restriction site (underlined in the sequence in Figure 5.2A), which was useful for the evaluation of mutation efficiency.

To construct the *tpcn2* gRNA, a linear DNA template was first amplified from the gRNA scaffold vector via PCR (Kelu et al., 2017), using short oligonucleotides as primers. The forward primer contained the T7 promoter (for *in vitro* transcription), followed by the 20-bp *tpcn2* gRNA target sequence (excluding the PAM) and then the 5' portion of the gRNA scaffold, whereas the reverse primer contained only the 3' portion of the gRNA scaffold. The *tpcn2* gRNA was then synthesized via *in vitro* transcription and purified using phenol/chloroform extraction. Similarly, the Cas9 mRNA was synthesized via *in vitro* transcription using the linearized DNA template obtained from the pT3TS plasmid vector (Jao et al., 2013), and then purified. To perform gene-editing, a mixture of the *tpcn2* gRNA and Cas9 mRNA was co-injected into the blastodisc of wild-type zebrafish embryos at the 1-cell stage (Figure 5.2Bi; Kelu et al., 2017). To evaluate the mutation efficiency in the injected embryos ($F_0$), the restriction endonuclease digestion assay was performed. Several injected embryos were sacrificed at ~24 hpf, and the genomic DNA was extracted. The target region was then amplified via PCR using a primer pair flanking *tpcn2*

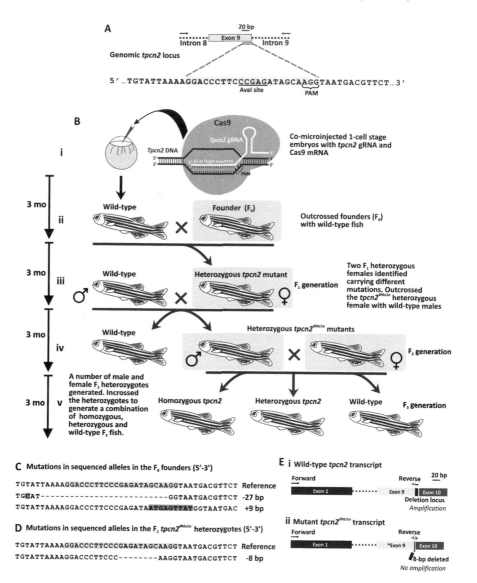

**FIGURE 5.2** CRISPR/Cas9-induced mutagenesis of *tpcn2*. (A) The genomic locus of zebrafish *tpcn2*, showing exon 9, introns 8 and 9, and the 23-bp target sequence of the *tpcn2* gRNA. (B) The workflow of the CRISPR/Cas9-induced mutagenesis of *tpcn2*. (Bi) Wild-type embryos were co-injected with *tpcn2* gRNA and Cas9 mRNA at the 1-cell stage; some embryos were then sacrificed to evaluate the mutation efficiency via the restriction endo-nuclease digestion assay, while the rest were raised to adulthood (i.e., ~3 months old). (Bii) Founder fish ($F_0$) were identified via the restriction endonuclease digestion assay, and the *tpcn2* mutant alleles in these fish were characterized via Sanger sequencing analysis. The founder fish were then outcrossed with wild-type fish to test for germline transmission of the *tpcn2* mutation in the $F_1$ generation. (Biii) Two $F_1$ heterozygous females that carried different germline transmitted *tpcn2* mutant alleles were identified by Sanger sequencing analysis. The single heterozygous female that was shown to carry the *tpcn2*^dhkz1a^ mutation was then further

**FIGURE 5.2 (CONTINUED)**
outcrossed with wild-type males to obtain a number of $F_2$ heterozygous male and female fish. (Biv) By incrossing the $F_2$ *tpcn2^{dhkzla}* heterozygotes, (Bv) a combination of homozygotes, heterozygotes and wild-type fish were obtained in the $F_3$ generation. The process of generating the *tpcn2^{dhkzla}* mutant line took ~12 months to complete. (C,D) Sanger sequencing analysis (C) of two representative mutant alleles found in the $F_0$ founder fish, and (D) of the germline transmitted *tpcn2^{dhkzla}* mutant allele, which was identified in one of the $F_1$ heterozygous females. (E) RT-PCR was performed to validate the *tpcn2^{dhkzla}* mutant at the RNA level. (Ei) The wild-type *tpcn2* transcript showing exons 1, 9 and 10, with the design of the forward (F) and reverse (R) primers used for RT-PCR. The target sequence of the reverse primer spans the 8-bp locus that is deleted in the *tpcn2^{dhkzla}* mutant transcript. (Eii) The *tpcn2^{dhkzla}* mutant transcript showing exon 1, the mutated exon 9 and exon 10. The inaccessibility of the reverse primer to the deletion locus in the *tpcn2^{dhkzla}* mutant transcript leads to amplification failure. In panels (A) and (E), all the diagrams were drawn to scale; scale bar, 20 bp. (Panels (A), (C), (D), (Ei) and (Eii) are reproduced with permission, from "Ca$^{2+}$ release via two-pore channel type 2 (TPC2) is required for slow muscle cell myofibrillogenesis and myotomal patterning in intact zebrafish embryos" by Kelu, J.J., Webb, S.E., Parrington, J., Galione, A., and Miller, A.L., 2017. *Developmental Biology 425*, 109–129, Elsevier.)

exon 9 (Figure 5.2A), after which the amplicons were restriction-digested using AvaI and separated via agarose gel electrophoresis. Finding the ratio of the intensity of the undigested band and the two digested bands on the gel indicates the proportion of mutated *versus* wild-type *tpcn2* alleles in the injected embryos. The *tpcn2* mutations were further characterized using TOPO cloning followed by Sanger sequencing analysis, and were shown to contain both insertions and deletions from within the *tpcn2* locus (Figure 5.2C; Kelu et al., 2017).

The remaining injected embryos were raised to adulthood, and the founder fish were identified using the restriction endonuclease digestion assay, by excising the tip of the caudal fin as a source of DNA. The founders were then outcrossed with wild-type adults to test for the germline transmission of the *tpcn2* mutation (Figure 5.2Bii). Eventually, two germline transmitted *tpcn2* mutant alleles were identified in the $F_1$ from two different heterozygous females (Figure 5.2Biii). One of the mutant alleles was identified to be an 8-bp deletion via Sanger sequencing (Figure 5.2D). This was predicted to lead to a frameshift mutation at amino acid (aa) position 228 of TPC2, which would generate a premature stop codon in the protein coding region, and in this way it would lead to a loss of TPC2 function. Such a mutation was subsequently named *tpcn2^{dhkzla}* according to the ZFIN zebrafish nomenclature guideline (http://zfin.org). The heterozygous female carrying the *tpcn2^{dhkzla}* allele was then outcrossed with wild-type males to generate $F_2$ heterozygotes (Figure 5.2Biv), after which a number of the male and female $F_2$ heterozygotes were further incrossed to generate a combination of homozygotes, heterozygotes and wild-type $F_3$ fish (Figure 5.2Bv). The *tpcn2^{dhkzla}* mutation was again confirmed in the $F_3$ generation: (1) at the DNA level using PCR and Sanger sequencing analysis; (2) at the RNA level using RT-PCR (Figure 5.2Ei,Eii); and (3) at the protein level by whole-mount immunohistochemistry (Kelu et al., 2017). The *tpcn2^{dhkzla}* mutants were subsequently shown to have a defect in myotomal patterning and sarcomere formation, as well as defects in Ca$^{2+}$ signalling in the developing SMCs and PMNs (Kelu et al., 2017, 2018).

### 5.3.3 Morpholino Oligonucleotide Technology versus CRISPR/Cas9 Gene-Editing

Despite the fact that MOs have contributed greatly to the identification of hundreds of genes that are crucial for development, as well as to the elucidation of gene function, their use has recently been severely criticized due to their potential off-target effects (Eisen and Smith, 2008; Gerety and Wilkinson, 2011; Robu et al., 2007), as well as their failure to phenocopy the corresponding mutants (Kok et al., 2015). This led to the research community moving towards the use of permanent gene knock out techniques such as CRISPR/Cas9 gene-editing. However, reports now indicate that CRISPR/Cas9 might also be affected by off-targeting effects (Kuscu et al., 2014; Tsai and Joung, 2016). Indeed, it was recently suggested that the phenotypic discrepancies observed between some morphants and their corresponding mutants, might be due to the presence of genetic compensation in the mutants (Rossi et al., 2015). Thus, at least some of the differences observed between the morphants and the corresponding mutants might not just be attributable to the off-target effects of MOs; they might also be a result of the poor characterization of the mutants (Kok et al., 2015). However, with the appropriate controls, MOs can still be considered to be a reliable and valuable tool (Blum et al., 2015; Schulte-Merker and Stainier, 2014; Stainier et al., 2015, 2017). In addition, by using a combination of complementary transient-knock down (with MOs) and permanent-knock out (via CRISPR/Cas9), it is possible to obtain comprehensive data for a more thorough, comparable analysis.

### 5.3.4 Using a Pharmacological Approach to Inhibit TPC Action

In addition to the genetic manipulation of TPC2, two-pore channels have also been attenuated and inhibited pharmacologically in zebrafish (Kelu et al., 2015, 2017). *Trans*-ned-19 is an NAADP receptor antagonist (Naylor et al., 2009), whereas bafilomycin A1 is a vacuolar type $H^+$ ATPase inhibitor (Bowman et al., 1988; Yoshimori et al., 1991). Although neither of these inhibitors is specific for TPC2, they do help to establish the contribution of NAADP and acidic stores to the differentiation and onset of function of SMCs and PMNs in the zebrafish trunk. By the end of epiboly (i.e., ~10 hpf), zebrafish embryos, like other teleost embryos, are somewhat impermeable to drugs due to the formation of the enveloping layer (i.e., an embryonic periderm), which completely encloses the developing blastoderm and acts as an ionic and osmotic barrier (Bruce, 2016; Collazzo et al., 1994; Keller and Trinkaus, 1987). Thus, to treat embryos at ~17–18 hpf or older with pharmacological agents, the terminal tip of the tail (i.e., ~100 µm) can be excised just before the start of the drug treatment to ensure that they can penetrate and diffuse into the muscle precursor tissue of the trunk (Brennan et al., 2005; Cheung et al., 2011; Liu and Westerfield, 1990). The exposed tail cells do heal relatively quickly forming an injury-response blastema; for example, in adult zebrafish it is reported that within 1–3 h following amputation of the caudal (tail) fin, a thin epidermis migrates to cover the wound, and then over the following 12–18 h additional epidermal layers accumulate (Azevedo et al., 2011; Poss et al., 2003). However, the experiments conducted with bafilomycin A1 or *trans*-ned-19 were relatively short-term such that embryos were treated with the drugs at ~17 hpf and data were either collected immediately or else within ~8 h of the start of treatment. In this way, bafilomycin

A1 and *trans*-ned-19 were shown to have a dose-dependent effect on SMC development, with bafilomycin A1 being used at concentrations ranging between 100 nM and 5 μM, and *trans*-ned-19 being used at concentrations ranging between 50 μM and 500 μM (Kelu et al., 2015, 2017). Stock solutions of bafilomycin A1 and *trans*-ned-19 were prepared in DMSO and then diluted in Danieau's solution just prior to incubation with embryos. *Trans*-ned-19 has a tendency to precipitate in aqueous solution at high concentration, but heating the drug to 65°C for 5 min (and then allowing it to cool to ~28°C) just before it was used to treat embryos helped to resolve this issue (Kelu et al., 2017). In addition, tail-excised embryos were treated with Danieau's solution containing DMSO as negative controls.

## 5.4   READ-OUT: CA²⁺ SIGNALLING, MORPHOLOGY AND MOTILITY

Three different types of experiments were conducted to determine the effect of TPC2 knock down, knock out and inhibition on SMC and/or PMN differentiation. These were: (1) monitoring the release of $Ca^{2+}$ from intracellular stores in the SMCs and PMNs using bioluminescence- and fluorescence-based $Ca^{2+}$ detection techniques; (2) investigating the morphology of the SMCs via immunolabelling; and (3) examining the motility of embryos. These are discussed in detail in the following sections.

### 5.4.1   MONITORING CA²⁺ RELEASE FROM INTRACELLULAR STORES

The $Ca^{2+}$ signals generated in the SMCs were monitored using a transgenic line of zebrafish that expresses apoaequorin, the protein portion of the bioluminescent $Ca^{2+}$ reporter complex aequorin, specifically in the skeletal muscles. The $Ca^{2+}$ signals were then confirmed with the fluorescent $Ca^{2+}$ reporter, calcium green-1 dextran (Cheung et al., 2011).

The transgenic line of zebrafish was generated by injecting an *apoaequorin* (*aeq*) construct into 1-cell stage (i.e., newly fertilized) embryos. The construct was driven by an *α-actin* promoter, to target the *aeq* gene to the skeletal muscles (Higashijima et al., 1997). In addition, the construct contained an *EGFP* marker. This was regulated by an internal ribosome entry site sequence, which allowed for the *aeq* and *EGFP* genes to both be translated from a single mRNA (Fahrenkrug et al., 1999; Jang et al., 1988; Wang et al., 2000). In this way, *aeq* transgenic fish could be readily identified due to the EGFP fluorescence in the skeletal muscles (Cheung et al., 2011) such that the expression and localization of EGFP accurately reflected the expression and localization of apoaequorin protein. When first preparing the transgenic line of fish, the construct was microinjected into embryos at the 1-cell stage and these were then grown up to adulthood (~3 months post-fertilization; Kimmel et al., 1995). Any individuals that developed with EGFP fluorescence in the trunk were considered to be potential transgenic founder ($F_0$) fish. As only one founder fish was identified from all the candidates injected with the plasmid, this was outcrossed with a wild-type fish to generate the $F_1$ transgenic line. $F_1$ fish that expressed EGFP were then incrossed to establish the $F_2$ generation, which could then be used for experimentation (Cheung et al., 2011).

Once the transgenic lines were established, the trunk $Ca^{2+}$ signals were characterized. Transgenic individuals were incubated with the apoaequorin co-factor, *f*-coelenterazine to reconstitute active holo-*f*-aequorin (Shimomura, 1991; Shimomura and Johnson, 1975, 1978). Various coelenterazine incubation protocols were tested but the optimal method proved to be incubation of embryos with 50 μM coelenterazine from ~1.25 hpf (i.e., the 8-cell stage) until ~16.5 hpf (i.e., the 16-somite stage) at which time $Ca^{2+}$ imaging was initiated (Cheung et al., 2011). As coelenterazine itself generates luminescence due to a reaction with free radicals (Shimomura and Teranishi, 2000), embryos were washed with Danieau's solution to remove the excess co-factor just prior to the start of $Ca^{2+}$ measurements.

Aequorin-generated luminescence data were acquired with either a custom-designed luminescence imaging microscope (LIM) system, to provide both temporal and spatial $Ca^{2+}$ signalling information, or (more commonly) a photomultiplier tube-based system, to provide temporal luminescence detection information alone (Miller et al., 1994; Webb et al., 2010). Using aequorin-based luminescence imaging, two distinct $Ca^{2+}$ signalling periods (SP) were identified in the developing trunk SMCs (Cheung et al., 2011). The first, named SP1, occurred for 2 h between ~17.5 hpf and ~19.5 hpf. This confirmed a previous report showing an increased frequency of $Ca^{2+}$ signals between ~17.5 hpf and 22 hpf when zebrafish embryos were loaded with the fluorescent $Ca^{2+}$ reporter, Oregon Green BAPTA 488 dextran (Brennan et al., 2005). The SP1 was followed by a quiet period (QP) with little-to-no $Ca^{2+}$ signals, which lasted ~3.5 h (i.e., from ~19.5 hpf to ~22.5 hpf), after which a second series of $Ca^{2+}$ signals (called SP2) began. SP2 persisted from ~22.5 hpf until at least 30 hpf when data acquisition was concluded. This aequorin-based luminescence measurement method was the primary read-out used to determine the effect of TPC2 knock down, knock out and pharmacological inhibition on the SMC-generated $Ca^{2+}$ signals. Once the main $Ca^{2+}$ measurements were completed, Triton X-100 was added to the embryo bathing medium. This detergent permeabilizes the plasma membrane and exposes any unspent cytoplasmic aequorin to extracellular $Ca^{2+}$ in the medium (Cheung et al., 2011). This was especially important in cases when the $Ca^{2+}$ signals were completely inhibited (e.g., following injection of *TPCN2*-MO + *p53*-MO, or following incubation with *trans*-ned-19), as it demonstrated whether the lack of luminescence observed might be due to the $Ca^{2+}$ signals being actively inhibited by the treatment or if it was simply due to an overall lack of active aequorin remaining in embryos due to factors such as the failed reconstitution of apoaequorin with coelenterazine to form active holo-aequorin (Cheung et al., 2011).

Aequorin-based imaging demonstrated that embryos injected with standard control-MO or *p53*-MO alone still generated SP1 and SP2 $Ca^{2+}$ signals with a distinct QP between the two (Kelu et al., 2015). When embryos were injected with *TPCN2*-MO-T or *TPCN2*-MO-S, however, the SP1 and SP2 were completely abolished, but when *TPCN2*-MO-T and *tpcn2* mRNA were co-injected into embryos, a partial rescue of the muscle-generated $Ca^{2+}$ signals was observed (Kelu et al., 2015, 2017). The SP1 and SP2 $Ca^{2+}$ signals were also rescued when embryos that had been injected with *TPCN2*-MO-T were bathed in the membrane-permeable D-*myo*-Ins(1,4,5)P$_3$ hexakis(butyrloxy-methyl) ester (IP$_3$/BM), whereas the SP2 signals alone were rescued when *TPCN2*-MO-T-injected embryos were bathed with the RyR agonist, caffeine (Kelu et al., 2017).

Aequorin-based experiments are ideal for identifying $Ca^{2+}$ signals generated by intact zebrafish embryos over the long periods of time that are required for developmental events; this method is non-disturbing and allows for continual visualization of $Ca^{2+}$ signalling events from fertilization to >30 hpf (Webb and Miller, 2003, 2007; Webb et al., 2010). One disadvantage of this method, however, is that it only generates two-dimensional and relatively low-resolution $Ca^{2+}$ information (Cheung et al., 2006, 2011; Yuen et al., 2013). Thus, after using the aequorin-based approach to establish the location and time that $Ca^{2+}$ transients arose in the developing skeletal musculature, the signals were then examined at higher spatial resolution by loading embryos with the fluorescent $Ca^{2+}$ reporter, calcium green-1 dextran and using high-resolution laser scanning confocal microscopy. This method allowed the subcellular identification of $Ca^{2+}$ signals in the SMCs of normally developing embryos between ~17 hpf and ~24 hpf (Cheung et al., 2011). Furthermore, this imaging technique would be very useful for investigating at high resolution the effect of TPC2 knock down, knock out and inhibition on the SMC-generated $Ca^{2+}$ signals.

The $Ca^{2+}$ signals generated in the PMNs were monitored using the SAIGFF213A;UAS:GCaMP7a double-transgenic line of fish, which expresses GCaMP7a strongly in the caudal primary motor neurons (Muto et al., 2011). GCaMPs are calmodulin-based fluorescent genetically encoded $Ca^{2+}$ indicators (GECI), which have been used to image $Ca^{2+}$ signals generated in cells in culture, tissues and freely moving organisms (Helassa et al., 2016). GCaMP7a was developed specifically to show the $Ca^{2+}$ signals associated with neuronal activity in the zebrafish (Muto et al., 2013). The SAIGFF213A;UAS:GCaMP7a line of fish was generated by crossing the Gal4:SAIGFF213A and UAS:GCaMP7a transgenic lines (both obtained from Koichi Kawakami, NIG, Japan). Time-lapse laser scanning confocal microscopy was then used to image the $Ca^{2+}$ transients generated by the PMNs. We showed that disruption of TPC2 function (by knock down, knock out or pharmacological inhibition) resulted in a loss of both the normal ipsilateral correlation and contralateral anti-correlation of the $Ca^{2+}$ signalling in the CaPs (Kelu et al., 2018), which was first reported by Muto et al. (2011). There was also a reduction in the frequency and amplitude of the $Ca^{2+}$ transients recorded from the CaPs, and a concomitant increase in the duration of the CaP $Ca^{2+}$ transients (Kelu et al., 2018).

In summary, TPC2 knock down, knock out or pharmacological inhibition was demonstrated to inhibit the $Ca^{2+}$ signals generated in the SMCs and disrupt the $Ca^{2+}$ signals generated in the PMNs in living zebrafish embryos (Kelu et al., 2017; 2018). In addition, the rescue of normal SMC and PMN $Ca^{2+}$ signalling was achieved by co-injection of the *TPCN2*-MO-T with a *tpcn2* mRNA or incubation of *TPCN2*-MO-T injected embryos with $IP_3$/BM (Kelu et al., 2017; 2018).

### 5.4.2   DETERMINING THE EFFECT OF TPC2 KNOCK DOWN, KNOCK OUT OR INHIBITION ON SMC MORPHOLOGY

To determine the morphology of the SMCs following TPC2 knock down, knock out or inhibition, the MHC and F-actin, two of the main proteins in skeletal muscle, were visualized via immunolabelling with the F59 antibody (Devoto et al.,

1996; described in Section 5.2), and incubation with fluorescent-phalloidin (Wulf et al., 1979) respectively. Embryos were initially whole-mount immunolabelled using the methodology described in Section 5.2, after which they were incubated with fluorescent-phalloidin for 3 h in the dark. After washing to remove the excess phalloidin, embryos were either placed in grooves made in agarose or else were mounted under AF1 mountant (as described in Section 5.2) prior to visualization via confocal microscopy. In another series of experiments embryos were immunolabelled (using standard methods) with an anti-prox1 primary antibody, which labels the SMC nuclei (Roy et al., 2001). Following confocal microscopy, the images acquired were analyzed and various parameters of the fluorescently labelled myotome were measured. These included determination of the number of SMCs, the width of the myotome, the shape of the somites (determined by measuring the angle between the bilaterally paired blocks), the width of myofibers and the ratio between the length of the myofiber and length of the somite (Kelu et al., 2017). TPCN2 knock down (with *TPCN2*-MO-T alone, *TPCN2*-MO-S alone or with *TPCN2*-MO-T plus *TPCN2*-MO-S), *TPCN2* knock out (in *tpcn2* heterozygous or homozygous mutants) or TPC2 inhibition (with bafilomycin A1 or *trans*-ned-19) all demonstrated that the number of SMCs, myotome width and myofiber width were significantly lower, whereas the somite angle and myofiber:somite ratio were significantly greater than the controls (untreated and standard control-MO or *p53*-MO injected embryos; Kelu et al., 2017). Furthermore, the effect of *TPCN2* knock down or pharmacological inhibition could be rescued either by co-injection of the *TPCN2*-MO-T with *tpcn2* mRNA or treatment of *TPCN2*-MO-T-injected embryos with IP$_3$/BM (Kelu et al., 2017).

### 5.4.3  DETERMINING THE EFFECT OF TPC2 KNOCK DOWN ON EMBRYO MOTILITY

Zebrafish embryos are reported to demonstrate three sequential motor behaviours during development. The first motile behaviour is called spontaneous coiling and this starts at ~17 hpf. This is followed by a touch-evoked response at ~21 hpf and then organized swimming, which begins at ~27 hpf (Kimmel et al., 1995; Saint-Amant and Drapeau, 1998). The effect of TPC2 knock down on the spontaneous coiling behaviour was determined by video microscopy, whereas the touch-evoked response was determined by gently touching the embryos on the head twice and recording their response (i.e., if they moved or not). The data showed that when compared with the various control groups (i.e., the untreated, standard control-MO injected and *p53*-MO injected embryos), none of the embryos injected with *TPCN2*-MO-T (plus *p53*-MO) exhibited spontaneous coiling behaviour and only a small percentage responded to touch. In contrast, when embryos were injected with *TPCN2*-MO-T (plus *p53*-MO) and *tpcn2* mRNA, there was partial rescue of both the spontaneous coiling and touch-evoked behaviours (Kelu et al., 2017).

### 5.5  CONCLUSIONS

Over the last few years, we have accumulated evidence for a role for TPC2 in the neuromuscular development in zebrafish embryos. This has been achieved via the use of *TPCN2* knock down, *TPCN2* knock out and pharmacological inhibition of

TPCs, both in intact zebrafish and in SMCs and PMNs isolated from fish, together with different read-out techniques, including temporal and/or spatial $Ca^{2+}$ measurements using luminescent or fluorescent GECIs (i.e., apoaequorin and GCaMP7a, respectively), morphological analysis and motility studies. However, this is by no means the end of the story. It is important to determine: (1) if there is a link between TPC2-dependent $Ca^{2+}$ signalling in the PMNs and that in the SMCs; and (2) what the signalling pathway or pathways might be and what the downstream targets are in these two cell types. In addition, it would be interesting to determine if TPC1 and TPC3, which are reported to be expressed in endosomes (Calcraft et al., 2009), are also expressed in zebrafish embryos, and if so, then how they might play a role in developmental processes. Gaining a better understanding of the function of TPCs and their endogenous agonist(s) might reveal new opportunities for therapeutic intervention with respect to treating diseases such as Ebola virus disease, metabolic disorders such as fatty liver disease, and cancer.

## 5.6  PROTOCOLS FOR IMMUNOLABELLING EXPERIMENTS

### 5.6.1  Whole-Mount Dual-Immunolabelling TPC2 and the Myosin Heavy Chain in Zebrafish Embryos at 24 hpf

#### 5.6.1.1  Equipment

- Zebrafish embryos at 24 hpf (AB wild-type).
- MS-222 (ethyl 3 aminobenzoate methanesulfonate; e.g., A5040, Sigma-Aldrich Corp., St Louis, MO, USA).
- Paraformaldehyde (e.g., 16% solution, 15710, Electron Microscopy Sciences, Hatfield, PA, USA).
- PBS (phosphate-buffered solution; 137 mM NaCl, 2.68 mM KCl, 16 mM $Na_2HPO_4$, 4 mM $NaH_2PO_4.2H_2O$, pH 7.3).
- Triton X-100 (e.g., T8787, Sigma-Aldrich Corp.).
- DMSO (dimethyl sulphoxide; e.g., D2650; Sigma-Aldrich Corp.).
- Goat serum (e.g., 16210-064, Gibco, Invitrogen Corp., Eugene, OR, USA).
- BSA (bovine serum albumin; e.g., A7906, Sigma-Aldrich Corp.).
- 2137A TPC2 antibody (raised in rabbit, custom-made by Covalab UK Ltd., Cambridge, UK).
- F59 IgG1 myosin heavy chain antibody (Developmental Studies Hybridoma Bank, Iowa City, IA, USA).
- Atto 647 (STED/GSD) goat anti-rabbit IgG (e.g., 15048, Active Motif).
- Alexa Fluor 488 F(ab')2 goat anti-mouse IgG (H+L) (e.g., A11070, Molecular Probes Inc., Invitrogen).
- AF1 mountant (Citifluor Ltd., Leicester, UK).
- Milli-Q water.
- Bench top centrifuge.
- Tweezers (fine or super-fine points, No. 0 or 5; e.g., Regine, Switzerland).
- Gilson pipetmen (P10, P100 and P1000) and associated tips.
- Confocal microscope equipped with a 63× objective lens and suitable for 633 nm excitation and 669 nm detection, and 488 nm excitation and 519 nm detection to capture the Atto 647 and Alexa Fluor 488 fluorescence, respectively.

## 5.6.1.2  Step-by-Step Protocol

1. Dechorionate embryos manually with tweezers.
2. Anaesthetize embryos briefly with 0.02% MS-222 and then fix them with PBS (pH 7.3) containing 4% paraformaldehyde for 4–6 h at room temperature (or overnight at 4°C).
3. Wash embryos with PBS for 3 × 10 min.
4. Wash embryos with PBS containing 0.1% triton X-100 (PBT) – 3 × 10 min.
5. Incubate embryos with PBS containing 0.1% triton X-100 + 1% DMSO (PBDT) – 1 h.
6. Incubate embryos with blocking buffer (PBDT containing 10% goat serum + 1% BSA) – 2 h
7. Incubate some embryos with anti-TPC2 antibody (diluted 1:10 in blocking buffer) – overnight at 4°C. A few embryos should be incubated with blocking buffer alone. These are the secondary antibody controls.
8. Wash embryos with wash buffer (PBDT containing 1% goat serum + 0.1% BSA) – 5 × 10 min.
9. Incubate embryos with F59 IgG1 myosin heavy chain antibody (diluted 1:10 in blocking buffer) – overnight at 4°C. The localization pattern of the F59 antibody in zebrafish SMCs is well-established (Devoto et al., 1996), and so there is no need to prepare secondary antibody controls for this primary antibody.
10. Wash embryos with wash buffer – 5 × 10 min.

**All the subsequent steps should be conducted in the dark**

11. Prepare the first secondary antibody solution, Atto 647N-tagged goat anti-rabbit IgG (diluted 1:200 with blocking solution), then centrifuge at 13,000 rpm for 5 min just prior to use.
12. Incubate embryos with Atto 647N-tagged goat anti-rabbit IgG overnight at 4°C.
13. Wash embryos with wash buffer – 5 × 10 min.
14. Prepare a second secondary antibody solution, Alexa Fluor 488 goat anti-mouse IgG (H+L) antibody (diluted 1:200 with blocking solution), then centrifuge at 13,000 rpm for 5 min just prior to use.
15. Incubate embryos with Alexa Fluor 488 goat anti-mouse IgG overnight at 4°C.
16. Wash with PBDT for 3 × 10 min.
17. Wash with PBT for 3 × 10 min.
18. Wash with PBS for 1 × 10 min.
19. Rinse briefly with Milli-Q water.
20. Excise and discard the head and yolk of the dual-immunolabelled embryos.
21. Mount the remaining trunk region under AF1 mountant.
22. Store at 4°C pending imaging with a confocal microscope.

**Note**: This protocol can also be used to whole-mount immunolabel the SMC nuclei (using an anti-prox1 antibody, e.g., 11-002, AngioBio, San Diego, CA, USA, at 1:500 dilution), or whole-mount label F-actin (e.g., using Alexa Fluor 568-conjugated phalloidin, A12380, Molecular Probes Inc., Invitrogen, at 1:50 dilution), where embryos are incubated with the latter for 3 h at room temperature in the dark just prior to the final washes and specimen mounting (Steps 16–22 above; Kelu et al., 2017).

### 5.6.2 Preparation of Zebrafish Primary Muscle Cell Cultures

#### 5.6.2.1 Equipment

- Zebrafish embryos at 17 hpf (AB wild-type).
- Bleach solution (e.g., >6.25% sodium hypochlorite solution, Clorox Company, Oakland, CA, USA).
- Ethanol (e.g., >95% solution, 64-17-5, Anaqua Chemicals Supply, Inc., Houston, USA).
- Danieau's solution (17.4 mM NaCl, 0.21 mM KCl, 0.12 mM $MgSO_4\cdot7H_2O$, 0.18 mM $Ca(NO_3)_2\cdot4H_2O$ and 1.5 mM HEPES; pH 7.2). Autoclave to sterilize.
- Micro-dissection scissors (e.g., 14003, World Precision Instruments, FL, USA).
- Tweezers (see Section 5.6.1.1).
- Custom ATV solution (5.5 mM D-glucose, 5.4 mM KCl, 136.8 mM NaCl, 5.5 mM $Na_2CO_3$ and 0.05% trypsin [with EDTA; e.g., 15400-054, Gibco, Invitrogen Corp., Eugene, OR, USA]) with 2% penicillin-streptomycin (e.g., 15140-122, Gibco, Invitrogen Corp., Eugene, OR, USA).
- PBS (see Section 5.6.1.1).
- Muscle culture medium (50% Leibovitz's L-15 [e.g., 11415-064, Gibco, Invitrogen Corp.], 48% 0.1× Ringer's solution [116 mM NaCl, 2.9 mM KCl, 1.8 mM $CaCl_2\cdot2H_2O$, 5 mM HEPES], 1% fetal bovine serum [e.g., 12657029, Gibco, Invitrogen Corp.] and 1% penicillin-streptomycin [Gibco, Invitrogen Corp.]).
- Glass coverslips (e.g., 0117530, Precision cover glasses No. 1.5H, Paul Marienfeld GmbH & Co. KG).
- 4-well plates (e.g., 167063, Nunc Nunclon Δ Surface 4-well plate, Thermo Fisher Scientific, Geel, Belgium).
- Eppendorf tubes (1.5 ml).

#### 5.6.2.2 Step-by-Step Protocol

1. Sterilize embryos (in their intact chorions) by washing: first with ~0.07% bleach solution, second with ~75% ethanol, and third with sterile Danieau's solution, each for 30 seconds. Maintain the washed embryos in sterile Danieau's solution.
2. Clean the micro-dissection scissors and tweezers in ~75% ethanol prior to use.
3. Dechorionate ~10 sterile embryos manually with tweezers. Dissect and discard the head and the yolk sac from the embryos using the micro-dissection scissors, leaving the majority of the trunk region (i.e., from the somite 1 to somite 16) for subsequent enzymatic digestion. Try to remove as much of the attaching yolk sac as possible using the tweezers.

4. Transfer the dissected trunks to an Eppendorf tube in 500 µl custom ATV solution (containing 2% penicillin-streptomycin) and incubate for 15–30 min at room temperature (i.e., ~23°C). Briefly tap the Eppendorf tube containing the custom ATV solution and trunks to facilitate cell dissociation. Do not disturb the tube after 5 min.
5. Remove most of the custom ATV solution without disturbing the trypsinized trunk tissue at the bottom of the Eppendorf tube. Suspend the trypsinized trunk tissue in PBS and triturate to facilitate cell dissociation further.
6. To remove any further residual custom ATV solution, centrifuge at 1,000 rpm for 5 min at room temperature and then discard the supernatant.
7. Re-suspend the cell pellet in muscle culture medium (to a volume of ~100 µL/ dissected trunk).
8. Pipette ~200 µL dissociated cells onto each glass coverslip in a 4-well plate and incubate for 1 h at room temperature.
9. Add ~300 µL muscle culture medium to each well. Culture cells for either 24 h or 48 h at ~28°C.

### 5.6.3   DUAL IMMUNOLABELING OF TPC2 AND THE MYOSIN HEAVY CHAIN IN ZEBRAFISH CULTURED MUSCLE CELLS

#### 5.6.3.1   Equipment
- Paraformaldehyde (see Section 5.6.1.1).
- Triton X-100 (see Section 5.6.1.1).
- Goat serum (see Section 5.6.1.1).
- BSA (see Section 5.6.1.1).
- 2137A TPC2 antibody (see Section 5.6.1.1).
- F59 IgG1 myosin heavy chain antibody (see Section 5.6.1.1).
- Atto 647N goat anti-rabbit antibody (see Section 5.6.1.1).
- Alexa Fluor 488 goat anti-mouse antibody (see Section 5.6.1.1).
- ProLong Gold antifade reagent containing DAPI (e.g., P36931, Molecular Probes, Invitrogen Corp.).
- Milli-Q water.
- Bench top centrifuge.
- Gilson pipetmen (P10, P100 and P1000) and associated tips.
- Confocal microscope (as described in Section 5.6.1.1; but with the additional capability to capture DAPI fluorescence, i.e., 358 nm excitation and 641 nm emission).

#### 5.6.3.2   Step-by-Step Protocol
1. Briefly wash the 24-h- and 48-h-cultured cells with PBS. Fix the cells with PBS containing 4% paraformaldehyde for 15 min at room temperature.
2. Wash fixed cells with PBS – 3 × 5 min.
3. Permeabilize cells with PBS containing 0.1% triton X-100 (PBT) – 10 min.
4. Incubate cells with blocking buffer (PBT containing 10% goat serum + 1% BSA) – 30 min.

5. Incubate cells with anti-TPC2 antibody (diluted 1:10 with blocking buffer) – 1 h at room temperature. At least one of the coverslips containing cells should be incubated with blocking buffer alone as the secondary antibody control.
6. Wash cells with wash buffer (PBT containing 1% goat serum and 0.1% BSA) – 3 × 5 min.
7. Incubate cells with the F59 antibody (diluted 1:10 with blocking buffer) – 1 h at room temperature.
8. Wash cells with wash buffer – 3 × 5 min.

## All the subsequent steps should be conducted in the dark

9. Prepare the Atto 647N-tagged goat anti-rabbit IgG as described in step 11 of Section 5.6.1.2.
10. Incubate cells with the Atto 647N-tagged goat anti-rabbit IgG – 1 h at room temperature.
11. Wash cells with wash buffer – 3 × 5 min.
12. Prepare the Alexa Fluor 488 goat anti-mouse IgG (H+L) antibody as described in step 14 of Section 5.6.1.2.
13. Incubate cells with the Alexa Fluor 488 goat anti-mouse IgG (H+L) antibody – 1 h at room temperature.
14. Wash cells with PBT – 3 × 5 min.
15. Wash cells with PBS – 3 × 5 min.
16. Rinse briefly with Milli-Q water.
17. Mount the labelled cells under Prolong Gold antifade reagent containing DAPI overnight at room temperature.
18. Store at 4°C pending imaging with a confocal microscope.

**Note**: The same protocol can be used to immunolabel muscle cells in culture with antibodies to the RyR (with the 34C anti-RyR antibody, e.g., R129, Sigma-Aldrich, at 1:500 dilution), $IP_3$ receptor type I (e.g., 407145, Calbiochem, Merck KGaA, Darmstadt, Germany, at 1:10 dilution), $IP_3$ receptor type II (e.g., I7654, Sigma-Aldrich, at 1:10 dilution), $IP_3$ receptor type III (e.g., I7529, Sigma-Aldrich, at 1:250 dilution) or the lysosomes (with an anti-LAMP1 antibody, e.g., ab24170, Abcam, Cambridge, UK, at 1:100 dilution; Kelu et al., 2015, 2017).

## ACKNOWLEDGEMENTS

We acknowledge funding support from Hong Kong Research Grants Council (RGC) General Research Fund awards 16101714, 16100115 and 16100719, the ANR/RGC joint research scheme award A-HKUST601/13 and the Hong Kong Innovation and Technology Commission (ITCPD/17-9).

## REFERENCES

Aarhus, R., Dickey, D.M., Graeff, R.M., Gee, K.R., Walseth, T.F., and Lee, H.C. (1996). Activation and inactivation of $Ca^{2+}$ release by $NAADP^+$. *J. Biol. Chem.* *271*(15), 8513–8516.

Aley, P.K., Mikolajczyk, A.M., Munz, B., Churchill, G.C., Galione, A., and Berger, F. (2010). Nicotinic acid adenine dinucleotide phosphate regulates skeletal muscle differentiation via action at two-pore channels. *Proc. Natl. Acad. Sci. U.S.A. 107*(46), 19927–19932.

Ambrosio, A.L., Boyle, J.A., Aradi, A.E., Christian, K.A., and Di Pietro, S.M. (2016). TPC2 controls pigmentation by regulating melanosome pH and size. *Proc. Natl. Acad. Sci. U.S.A. 113*(20), 5622–5627.

Arredouani, A., Ruas, M., Collins, S.C., Parkesh, R., Clough, F., Pillinger, T., Coltart, G., Rietdorf, K., Royle, A., Johnson, P., et al. (2015). Nicotinic acid adenine dinucleotide phosphate (NAADP) and endolysosomal two-pore channels modulate membrane excitability and stimulus-secretion coupling in mouse pancreatic β cells. *J. Biol. Chem. 290*(35), 21376–21392.

Attili, S., and Hughes, S.M. (2014). Anaesthetic tricaine acts preferentially on neural voltage-gasyed sodium channels and fails to block directly evoked muscle contraction. *PLoS One 9*(8), e103751. doi: 10.1371/journal.pone.0103751.

Azevedo, A.S., Bartholomäus, G., Jacinto, A., Weidinger, G., and Saúde, L. (2011). The regenerative capacity of the zebrafish caudal fin is not affected by repeated amputations. *PLoS One 6*(7), e22820. doi: 10.1371/journal.pone.0022820.

Berg, I., Potter, B.V.L., Mayr, G.W., and Guse, A.H. (2000). Nicotinic acid adenine dinucleotide phosphate (NAADP+) is an essential regulator of T-lymphocyte $Ca^{2+}$ signalling. *J. Cell Biol. 150*(3), 581–588.

Bestman, J.E., and Cline, H.T. (2013). Morpholino studies in *Xenopus* brain development. *Methods Mol. Biol. Brain Dev. 1082*, 155–171.

Bill, B.R., Petzold, A.M., Clark, K.J., Schimmenti, L.A., and Ekker, S.C. (2009). A primer for morpholino use in zebrafish. *Zebrafish 6*(1), 69–77.

Blum, M., De Robertis, E.M., Wallingford, J.B., and Niehrs, C. (2015). Morpholinos: Antisense and sensibility. *Dev. Cell 35*(2), 145–149.

Bowman, E.J., Siebers, A., and Altendorf, K. (1988). Bafilomycins: A class of inhibitors of membrane ATPases from microorganisms, animal cells, and plant cells. *Proc. Natl., Acad., Sci. U.S.A. 85*(21), 7972–7976.

Brailoiu, E., Churamani, D., Pandey, V., Brailoiu, G.C., Tuluc, F., Patel, S., and Dun, N.J. (2006). Messenger-specific role for nicotinic acid adenine dinucleotide phosphate in neuronal differentiation. *J. Biol. Chem. 281*(23), 15923–15928.

Brailoiu, E., Hoard, J.L., Filipeanu, C.M., Brailoiu, G.C., Dun, S.L., Patel, S., and Dun, N.J. (2005). Nicotinic acid adenine dinucleotide phosphate potentiates neurite outgrowth. *J. Biol. Chem. 280*(7), 5646–5650.

Brennan, C., Mangoli, M., Dyer, C.E.F., and Ashworth, R. (2005). Acetylcholine and calcium signaling regulates muscle fiber formation in the zebrafish embryo. *J. Cell Sci. 118*(22), 5181–5190.

Bruce, A.E.E. (2016). Zebrafish epiboly: Spreading thin over the yolk. *Dev. Dynam. 245*(3), 244–258.

Burry, R.W. (2011). Controls for immunochemistry: An update. *J. Histochem. Cytochem. 59*(1), 6–12.

Calcraft, P.J., Arredouani, A., Ruas, M., Pan, Z., Cheng, X., Hao, X., Tang, J., Rietdorf, K., Teboul, L., Chuang, K.T., et al. (2009). NAADP mobilizes calcium from acidic organelles through two-pore channels. *Nature 459*(7246), 596–600.

Cancela, J.M., Churchill, G.C., and Galione, A. (1999). Coordination of agonist-induced $Ca^{2+}$-signalling patterns by NAADP in pancreatic acinar cells. *Nature 398*(6722), 74–76.

Capel, R.A., Bolton, E.L., Lin, W.K., Aston, D., Wang, Y., Liu, W., Wang, X., Burton, R.-A.B., Bloor-Young, D., Shade, K.T., et al. (2015). Two-pore channels (TPC2s) and nicotinic acid adenine dinucleotide phosphate (NAADP) at lysosomal-sarcoplasmic reticular junctions contribute to acute and chronic β-adrenoceptor signaling in the heart. *J. Biol. Chem. 290*(50), 30087–30098.

Capriotti, K., and Capriotti, J.A. (2012). Dimethyl sulfoxide: History, chemistry, and clinical utility in dermatology. *J. Clin. Aesth. Dermatol. 5*(9), 24–26.

Carroni, M., and Saibil, H.R. (2016). Cryo electron microscopy to determine the structure of macromolecular complexes. *Methods 95*, 78–85.

Chang, N., Sun, C., Gao, L., Zhu, D., Xu, X., Zhu, X., Xiong, J.W., and Xi, J.J. (2013). Genome editing with RNA-guided Cas9 nuclease in zebrafish embryos. *Cell Res. 23*(4), 465–472.

Cheung, C.Y., Webb, S.E., Love, D.R., and Miller, A.L. (2011). Visualization, characterization and modulation of calcium signaling during the development of slow muscle cells in intact zebrafish embryos. *Int. J. Dev. Biol. 55*(2), 153–174.

Cheung, C.Y., Webb, S.E., Meng, A., and Miller, A.L. (2006). Transient expression of apoaequorin in zebrafish embryos: Extending the ability to image calcium transients during later stages of development. *Int. J. Dev. Biol. 50*(6), 561–569.

Chu, V.T., Weber, T., Wefers, B., Wurst, W., Sander, S., Rajewsky, K., and Kühn, R. (2015). Increasing the efficiency of homology-directed repair for CRISPR-Cas9-induced precise gene editing in mammalian cells. *Nat. Biotechnol. 33*(5), 543–548.

Churchill, G.C., Okada, Y., Thomas, J.M., Genazzani, A.A., Patel, S., and Galione, A. (2002). NAADP mobilizes $Ca^{2+}$ from reserve granules, lysosome-related organelles, in sea urchin eggs. *Cell 111*(5), 703–708.

Collazzo, A., Bolker, J.A., and Keller, R. (1994). A phylogenetic perspective on teleost gastrulation. *Am. Nat. 144*(1), 133–152.

Cong, L., Ran, F.A., Cox, D., Lin, S., Barretto, R., Habib, N., Hsu, P.D., Wu, X., Jiang, W., Marraffini, L.A., and Zhang, F. (2013). Multiplex genome engineering using CRISPR/Cas systems. *Science 339*(6121), 819–823.

de Ménorval, M.-A., Mir, L.M., Fernández, M.L., and Reigada, R. (2012). Effects of dimethyl sulfoxide in cholesterol-containing lipid membranes: A comparative study of experiments *in silico* and with cells. *PLoS One 7*(7), e41733. doi: 10.1371/journal.pone.0041733.

Devoto, S.H., Melançon, E., Eisen, J.S., and Westerfield, M. (1996). Identification of separate slow and fast muscle precursor cells *in vivo*, prior to somite formation. *Development 122*(11), 3371–3380.

Doudna, J.A., and Charpentier, E. (2014). The new frontier of genome engineering with CRISPR-Cas9. *Science 346*(6213), 1258096. doi: 10.1126/science.1258096.

Eisen, J.S., and Smith, J.C. (2008). Controlling morpholino experiments: Don't stop making antisense. *Development 135*(10), 1735–1743.

Ekker, S.C., and Larson, J.D. (2001). Morphant technology in model developmental systems. *Genesis 30*(3), 89–93.

Ezeani, M., and Omabe, M. (2016). A new perspective of lysosomal cation channel-dependent homeostasis in Alzheimer's disease. *Mol. Neurobiol. 53*(3), 1672–1678.

Fahrenkrug, S.C., Clark, K.J., Dahlquist, M.O., and Hackett Jr, P.B. (1999). Dicistronic gene expression in developing zebrafish. *Mar. Biotechnol. 1*(6), 552–561.

Fameli, N., Ogunbayo, O.A., van Breemen, C., and Evans, A.M. (2014). Cytoplasmic nanojunctions between lysosomes and sarcoplasmic reticulum are required for specific calcium signaling. *F1000Res. 3*, 93. doi: 10.12688/f1000research.3720.1.

Flanagan-Steet, H., Fox, M.A., Meyer, D., and Sanes, J.R. (2005). Neuromuscular synapses can form *in vivo* by incorporation of initially aneural post-synaptic specializations. *Development 132*(20), 4471–4481.

Galione, A., Evans, A.M., Ma, J., Parrington, J., Arredouani, A., Cheng, X., and Zhu, M.X. (2009). The acid test: The discovery of two-pore channels (TPCs) as NAADP-gated endolysosomal $Ca^{2+}$ release channels. *Pflug. Arch. Eur. J. Physio.* doi: 10.1007/s00424-009-0682-y.

García-Rúa, V., Feijóo-Bandín, S., Rodríguez-Penas, D., Mosquera-Leal, A., Abu-Assi, E., Beiras, A., María Seoane, L., Lear, P., Parrington, J., Portolés, M., et al. (2016). Endolysosomal two-pore channels regulate autophagy in cardiomyocytes. *J. Physiol. (Lond.) 594*(11), 3061–3077.

Genazzani, A.A., and Galione, A. (1996). Nicotinic acid-adenine dinucleotide phosphate mobilizes Ca$^{2+}$ from a thapsigargin-insensitive pool. *Biochem. J. 315*(3), 721–725.

Gerety, S.S., and Wilkinson, D.G. (2011). Morpholino artifacts provide pitfalls and reveal a novel role for pro-apoptotic genes in hindbrain boundary development. *Dev. Biol. 350*(2), 279–289.

Grimm, C., Holdt, L.M., Chen, C.C., Hassan, S., Müller, C., Jörs, S., Cuny, H., Kissing, S., Schröder, B., Butz, E., et al. (2014). High susceptibility to fatty liver disease in two-pore channel 2-deficient mice. *Nat. Commun. 5*,4699. doi: 10.1038/ncomms5699.

Helassa, N., Podor, B., Fine, A., and Török, K. (2016). Design and mechanistic insight into ultrafast calcium indicators for monitoring intracellular calcium dynamics. *Sci. Rep. 6*, 38276. doi: 10.1038/srep38276.

Hell, S.W., and Wichmann, J. (1994). Breaking the diffraction resolution limit by stimulated emission: Stimulated-emission-depletion fluorescence microscopy. *Opt. Lett. 19*(11), 780–782.

Higashijima, S., Okamoto, H., Ueno, N., Hotta, Y., and Eguchi, G. (1997). High-frequency generation of transgenic zebrafish which reliably express GFP in whole muscles or the whole body by using promoters of zebrafish origin. *Dev. Biol. 192*(2), 289–299.

Hirata, H., Watanabe, T., Hatakeyama, J., Sprague, S.M., Saint-Amant, L., Nagashima, A., Cui, W.W., Zhou, W., and Kuwada, J.Y. (2007). Zebrafish *relatively relaxed* mutants have a ryanodine receptor defect, show slow swimming and provide a model of multi-minicore disease. *Development 134*(15), 2771–2781.

Hockney, L.N., Kilpatrick, B.S., Eden, E.R., Lin-Moshier, Y., Brailoiu, G.C., Brailoiu, E., Futter, C.E., Schapira, A.H., Marchant, J.S., and Patel, S. (2015). Dysregulation of lyso-somal morphology by pathogenic LRRK2 is corrected by TPC2 inhibition. *J. Cell Sci. 128*(2), 232–238.

Hong, N., Li, M., Yuan, Y., Wang, T., Yi, M., Xu, H., Zeng, H., Song, J., and Hong, Y. (2016). Dnd is a critical specifier of primordial germ cells in the medaka fish. *Stem Cell Rep. 6*(3), 411–421.

Hsu, P.D., Lander, E.S., and Zhang, F. (2014). Development and applications of CRISPR-Cas9 for genome engineering. *Cell 157*(6), 1262–1278.

Hwang, W.Y., Fu, Y., Reyon, D., Maeder, M.L., Kaini, P., Sander, J.D., Joung, J.K., Peterson, R.T., and Yeh, J.R. (2013). Heritable and precise zebrafish genome editing using a CRISPR-Cas system. *PLoS One 8*(7), e68708.

Irion, U., Krauss, J., and Nüsslein-Volhard, C. (2014). Precise and efficient genome editing in zebrafish using the CRISPR/Cas9 system. *Development 141*(24), 4827–4830.

Ishino, Y., Shinagawa, H., Makino, K., Amemura, M., and Nakata, A. (1987). Nucleotide sequence of the *iap* gene, responsible for alkaline phosphatase isozyme conversion in *Escherichia coli*, and identification of the gene product. *J. Bacteriol. 169*(12), 5429–5433.

Jahidin, A.H., Stewart, T.A., Thompson, E.W., Roberts-Thomson, S.J., and Monteith, G.R. (2016). Differential effects of two-pore channel protein 1 and 2 silencing in MDA-MB-468 breast cancer cells. *Biochem. Biophys. Res. Commun. 477*(4), 731–736.

Jang, S.K., Kräusslich, H.G., Nicklin, M.J., Duke, G.M., Palmenberg, A.C., and Wimmer, E. (1988). A segment of the 5′ nontranslated region of encephalomyocarditis virus RNA directs internal entry of ribosomes during *in vitro* translation. *J. Virol. 62*(8), 2636–2643.

Jao, L.E., Wente, S.R., and Chen, W. (2013). Efficient multiplex biallelic zebrafish genome editing using a CRISPR nuclease system. *Proc. Natl. Acad. Sci. U.S.A. 110*(34), 13904–13909.

Jinek, M., Chylinski, K., Fonfara, I., Hauer, M., Doudna, J.A., and Charpentier, E. (2012). A programmable dual-RNA-guided DNA endonuclease in adaptive bacterial immunity. *Science 337*(6096), 816–821.

Jinek, M., East, A., Cheng, A., Lin, S., Ma, E., and Doudna, J. (2013). RNA-programmed genome editing in human cells. *eLIFE*. doi: 10.7554/eLife.00471.001.

Keller, R.E., and Trinkaus, J.P. (1987). Rearrangement of enveloping layer cells without disruption of the epithelial permeability barrier as a factor in *Fundulus* epiboly. *Dev. Biol. 120*(1), 12–24.

Kelu, J.J., Chan, H.L.H., Webb, S.E., Cheng, A.H.H., Ruas, M., Parrington, J., Galione, A., and Miller, A.L. (2015). Two-pore channel 2 activity is required for slow muscle cell-generated $Ca^{2+}$ signaling during myogenesis in intact zebrafish. *Int. J. Dev. Biol. 59*(7–9), 313–325.

Kelu, J.J., Webb, S.E., Galione, A., and Miller, A.L. (2018). TPC2-mediated $Ca^{2+}$ signaling is required for the establishment of synchronized activity in developing zebrafish primary motor neurons. *Dev. Biol. 438*(1), 57–68.

Kelu, J.J., Webb, S.E., Galione, A., and Miller, A.L. (2019). Characterization of ADP-ribosyl cyclase 1-like (ARC1-like) activity and NAADP signaling during slow muscle development in zebrafish embryos. *Dev. Biol. 445*(2), 211–225.

Kelu, J.J., Webb, S.E., Parrington, J., Galione, A., and Miller, A.L. (2017). $Ca^{2+}$ release via two-pore channel type 2 (TPC2) is required for slow muscle cell myofibrillogenesis and myotomal patterning in intact zebrafish embryos. *Dev. Biol. 425*(2), 109–129.

Kimmel, C.B., Ballard, W.W., Kimmel, S.R., Ullmann, B., and Schilling, T.F. (1995). Stages of embryonic development of the zebrafish. *Dev. Dynam. 203*(3), 253–310.

Kimura, Y., Hisano, Y., Kawahara, A., and Higashijima, S. (2014). Efficient generation of knock-in transgenic zebrafish carrying reporter/driver genes by CRISPR/Cas9-mediated genome engineering. *Sci. Rep. 4*, 6545. doi: 10.1038/srep06545.

Kinnear, N.P., Boittin, F.X., Thomas, J.M., Galione, A., and Evans, A.M. (2004). Lysosome-sarcoplasmic reticulum junctions: A trigger zone for calcium signalling by nicotinic acid adenine dinucleotide phosphate and endothelin-1. *J. Biol. Chem. 279*(52), 54319–54326.

Kok, F.O., Shin, M., Ni, C.W., Gupta, A., Grosse, A.S., van Impel, A., Kirchmaier, B.C., Peterson-Maduro, J., Kourkoulis, G., Male, I., et al. (2015). Reverse genetic screening reveals poor correlation between morpholino-induced and mutant phenotypes in zebrafish. *Dev. Cell 32*(1), 97–108.

Komor, A.C., Badran, A.H., and Liu, D.R. (2017). CRISPR-based technologies for the manipulation of eukaryotic genomes. *Cell 168*(1–2), 20–36.

Kuscu, C., Arslan, S., Singh, R., Thorpe, J., and Adli, M. (2014). Genome-wide analysis reveals characteristics of off-target sites bound by the Cas9 endonuclease. *Nat. Biotechnol. 32*(7), 677–683.

Lawson, N.D., and Wolfe, S.A. (2011). Forward and reverse genetic approaches for the analysis of vertebrate development in the zebrafish. *Dev. Cell 21*(1), 48–64.

Lear, P.V., González-Touceda, D., Porteiro Couto, B., Viaño, P., Guymer, V., Remzova, E., Tunn, R., Chalasani, A., García-Caballero, T., Hargreaves, I.P., et al. (2015). Absence of intracellular ion channels TPC1 and TPC2 leads to mature-onset obesity in male mice, due to impaired lipid availability for thermogenesis in brown adipose tissue. *Endocrinol. 156*(3), 975–986.

Lee, H.C., and Aarhus, R. (1995). A derivative of NADP mobilizes calcium stores insensitive to inositol trisphosphate and cyclic ADP-ribose. *J. Biol. Chem. 270*(5), 2152–2157.

Li, M., Zhao, L., Page-McCaw, P.S., and Chen, W. (2016). Zebrafish genome engineering using the CRISPR-Cas9 system. *Trends Genet. 32*(12), 815–827.

Liu, D.W.C., and Westerfield, M. (1990). The formation of terminal fields in the absence of competitive interactions among primary motoneurons in the zebrafish. *J. Neurosci. 10*(12), 3947–3959.

López, J.J., Dionisio, N., Berna-Erro, A., Galán, C., Salido, G.M., and Rosado, J.A. (2012). Two-pore channel 2 (TPC2) modulates store-operated Ca$^{2+}$ entry. *Biochim. Biophys. Acta* *1823*(10), 1976–1983.

Makarova, K.S., Aravind, L., Grishin, N.V., Rogozin, I.B., and Koonin, E.V. (2002). A DNA repair system specific for thermophilic Archaea and bacteria predicted by genomic context analysis. *Nucleic Acids Res.* *30*(2), 482–496.

Marchant, J.S., and Patel, S. (2015). Two-pore channels at the intersection of endolysosomal membrane traffic. *Biochem. Soc. Trans.* *43*(3), 434–441.

Maruyama, T., Dougan, S.K., Truttmann, M.C., Bilate, A.M., Ingram, J.R., and Ploegh, H.L. (2015). Increasing the efficiency of precise genome editing with CRISPR-Cas9 by inhibition of nonhomologous end joining. *Nat. Biotechnol.* *33*(5), 538–542.

Meyer, L., Wildanger, D., Medda, R., Punge, A., Rizzoli, S.O., Donnert, G., and Hell, S.W. (2008). Dual-color STED microscopy at 30-nm focal plane resolution. *Small* *4*(8), 1095–1100.

Miller, A.L., Karplus, E., and Jaffe, L.F. (1994). Use of aequorin for [Ca$^{2+}$]i imaging. In: *Methods in Cell Biology, Volume 40: A Practical Guide to the Study of Ca$^{2+}$ in Living Cells*, R. Nuccitelli, ed. (Academic Press, Inc., San Diego, CA), pp. 305–338.

Missinato, M.A., Saydmohammed, M., Zuppo, D.A., Rao, K.S., Opie, G.W., Kühn, B., and Tsang, M. (2018). Dusp6 attenuates Ras/MAPK signalling to limit zebrafish heart regeneration. *Development* *145*(5), dev157206. doi: 10.1242/dev.157206.

Mojica, F.J., Díez-Villaseñor, C., Soria, E., and Juez, G. (2000). Biological significance of a family of regularly spaced repeats in the genomes of Archaea, Bacteria and mitochondria. *Mol. Microbiol.* *36*(1), 244–246.

Morgan, A.J., Davis, L.C., Wagner, S.K.T.Y., Lewis, A.M., Parrington, J., Churchill, G.C., and Galione, A. (2013). Bidirectional Ca$^{2+}$ signalling occurs between the endoplasmic reticulum and acidic organelles. *J. Cell Biol.* *200*(6), 789–805.

Morgan, A.J., Platt, F.M., Lloyd-Evans, E., and Galione, A. (2011). Molecular mechanisms of endolysosomal Ca$^{2+}$ signalling in health and disease. *Biochem. J.* *439*(3), 349–374.

Muto, A., Ohkura, M., Abe, G., Nakai, J., and Kawakami, K. (2013). Real-time visualization of neuronal activity during perception. *Curr. Biol.* *23*(4), 307–311.

Muto, A., Ohkura, M., Kotani, T., Higashijima, S.I., Nakai, J., and Kawakami, K. (2011). Genetic visualization with an improved GCaMP calcium indicator reveals spatiotemporal activation of the spinal motor neurons in zebrafish. *Proc. Natl. Acad. Sci. U.S.A.* *108*(13), 5425–5430.

Naito, Y., Hino, K., Bono, H., and Ui-Tei, K. (2015). CRISPRdirect: Software for designing CRISPR/Cas guide RNA with reduced off-target sites. *Bioinformatics* *31*(7), 1120–1123.

Nasevicius, A., and Ekker, S.C. (2000). Effective targeted gene 'knockdown' in zebrafish. *Nat. Genet.* *26*(2), 216–220.

Naylor, E., Arredouani, A., Vasudevan, S.R., Lewis, A.M., Parkesh, R., Mizote, A., Rosen, D., Thomas, J.M., Izumi, M., Ganesan, A., et al. (2009). Identification of a chemical probe for NAADP by virtual screening. *Nat. Chem. Biol.* *5*(4), 220–226.

Nguyen, O.N.P., Grimm, C., Schneider, L.S., Chao, Y.K., Atzberger, C., Bartel, K., Watermann, A., Ulrich, M., Mayr, D., Wahl-Schott, C., et al. (2017). Two-pore channel function is crucial for the migration of invasive cancer cells. *Cancer Res.* *77*(6), 1427–1438.

Nishimune, H., Badawi, Y., Mori, S., and Shigemoto, K. (2016). Dual-color STED microscopy reveals a sandwich structure of Bassoon and Piccolo in active zones of adult and aged mice. *Sci. Rep.* *6*, 27935. doi: 10.1038/srep27935.

Norris, A., and Streit, A. (2014). Morpholinos: Studying gene function in the chick. *Methods* *66*(3), 454–465.

Notch, E.G., Shaw, J.R., Coutermarsh, B.A., Dzioba, M., and Stanton, B.A. (2011). Morpholino gene knockdown in adult *Fundulus heteroclitus*: Role of SGK1 in seawater acclimation. *PLoS One* *6*(12), e29462. doi: 10.1371/journal.pone.0029462.

Notomi, T., Ezura, Y., and Noda, M. (2012). Identification of two-pore channel 2 as a novel regulator of osteoclastogenesis. *J. Biol. Chem. 287*(42), 35057–35064.

Oulhen, N., Onorato, T.M., Ramos, I., and Wessel, G.M. (2014). Dysferlin is essential for endocytosis in the sea star oocyte. *Dev. Biol. 388*(1), 94–102.

Park, K.H., Kim, K.N., Park, D.R., Jang, K.Y., and Kim, U.H. (2015). Role of nicotinic acid adenine dinucleotide phosphate (NAADP) in keratinocyte differentiation. *J. Invest. Dermatol. 135*(6), 1692–1694.

Parrington, J., and Tunn, R. (2014). $Ca^{2+}$ signals, NAADP and two-pore channels: Role in cellular differentiation. *Acta Physiol. (Oxford.) 211*(2), 285–296.

Patel, S., Churchill, G.C., and Galione, A. (2001). Coordination of $Ca^{2+}$ signalling by NAADP. *Trends Biochem. Sci. 26*(8), 482–489.

Pineda, R.H., Svoboda, K.R., Wright, M.A., Taylor, A.D., Novak, A.E., Gamse, J.T., Eisen, J.S., and Ribera, A.B. (2006). Knockdown of Nav1.6a $Na^+$ channels affects zebrafish motoneuron development. *Development 133*(19), 3827–3836.

Pipalia, T.G., Koth, J., Roy, S.D., Hammond, C.L., Kawakami, K., and Hughes, S.M. (2016). Cellular dynamics of regeneration reveals role of two distinct Pax7 stem cell populations in larval zebrafish muscle repair. *Dis. Models Mech. 9*(6), 671–684.

Poss, K.D., Keating, M.T., and Nechiporuk, A. (2003). Tales of regeneration in zebrafish. *Dev. Dynam. 226*(2), 202–210.

Rivero-Ríos, P., Fernández, B., Madero-Pérez, J., Lozano, M.R., and Hilfiker, S. (2016). Two-pore channels and Parkinson's disease: Where's the link? *Messenger (LA) 5*(1–2), 67–75.

Robu, M.E., Larson, J.D., Nasevicius, A., Beiraghi, S., Brenner, C., Farber, S.A., and Ekker, S.C. (2007). p53 activation by knockdown technologies. *PLOS Genet. 3*(5), e78. doi: 10.1371/journal.pgen.0030078.

Rossi, A., Kontarakis, Z., Gerri, C., Nolte, H., Hölper, S., Krüger, M., and Stainier, D.Y. (2015). Genetic compensation induced by deleterious mutations but not gene knock-downs. *Nature 524*(7564), 230–233.

Roy, S., Wolff, C., and Ingham, P.W. (2001). The *u-boot* mutation identifies a Hedgehog-regulated myogenic switch for fiber-type diversification in the zebrafish embryo. *Genes Dev. 15*(12), 1563–1576.

Saint-Amant, L., and Drapeau, P. (1998). Time course of the development of motor behaviors in the zebrafish embryo. *J. Neurobiol. 37*(4), 622–632.

Saito, S., Hamanaka, G., Kawai, N., Furukawa, R., Gojobori, J., Tominaga, M., Kaneko, H., and Satta, Y. (2017). Characterization of TRPA channels in the starfish *Patiria pectinifera*: Involvement of thermally activated TRPA1 in thermotaxis in marine planktonic larvae. *Sci. Rep. 7*(1), 2173. doi: 10.1038/s41598-017-02171-8.

Sakurai, Y., Kolokoltsov, A.A., Chen, C.C., Tidwell, M.W., Bauta, W.E., Klugbauer, N., Grimm, C., Wahl-Schott, C., Biel, M., and Davey, R.A. (2015). Ebola virus. Two-pore channels control Ebola virus host cell entry and are drug targets for disease treatment. *Science 347*(6225), 995–998.

Santella, L., Kyozuka, K., Genazzani, A.A., De Riso, L., and Carafoli, E. (2000). Nicotinic acid adenine dinucleotide phosphate-induced $Ca^{2+}$ release. *J. Biol. Chem. 275*(12), 8301–8306.

Schulte-Merker, S., and Stainier, D.Y. (2014). Out with the old, in with the new: Reassessing morpholino knockdowns in light of genome editing technology. *Development 141*(16), 3103–3104.

Shi, J., Bi, P., Pei, J., Li, H., Grishin, N.V., Bassel-Duby, R., Chen, E.H., and Olson, E.N. (2017). Requirement of the fusogenic micropeptide myomixer for muscle formation in zebrafish. *Proc. Natl. Acad. Sci. U.S.A. 114*(45), 11950–11955.

Shimomura, O. (1991). Preparation and handling of aequorin solutions for the measurement of cellular $Ca^{2+}$. *Cell Calcium 12*(9), 635–643.

Shimomura, O., and Johnson, F.H. (1975). Regeneration of the photoprotein aequorin. *Nature 256*(5514), 236–238.

Shimomura, O., and Johnson, F.H. (1978). Peroxidized coelenterazine, the active group in the photoprotein aequorin. *Proc. Natl. Acad. Sci. U.S.A.* 75(6), 2611–2615.

Shimomura, O., and Teranishi, K. (2000). Light-emitters involved in the luminescence of coelenterazine. *Luminescence* 15(1), 51–58.

Siddall, L.S., Barcroft, L.C., and Watson, A.J. (2002). Targeting gene expression in the pre-implantation mouse using morpholino antisense oligonucleotides. *Mol. Reprod. Dev.* 63(4), 413–421.

Singh, V., Braddick, D., and Dhar, P.K. (2017). Exploring the potential of genome editing CRISPR-Cas9 technology. *Gene 599*, 1–18.

Stainier, D.Y., Kontarakis, Z., and Rossi, A. (2015). Making sense of anti-sense data. *Dev. Cell 32*(1), 7–8.

Stainier, D.Y., Raz, E., Lawson, N.D., Ekker, S.C., Burdine, R.D., Eisen, J.S., Ingham, P.W., Schulte-Merker, S., Yelon, D., Weinstein, B.M., et al. (2017). Guidelines for morpholino use in zebrafish. *PLoS Genet. 13*(10), e1007000. doi: 10.1371/journal.pgen.1007000.

Storer, N.Y., and Zon, L.I. (2010). Zebrafish models of p53 functions. *Cold Spring Harb. Perspect. Biol. 2*(8), a001123. doi: 10.1101/cshperspect.a001123.

Summerton, J., and Weller, D. (1997). Morpholino antisense oligomers: Design, preparation, and properties. *Antisense Nucleic Acid Drug Dev. 7*(3), 187–195.

Topic Popovic, N., Strunjak-Perovic, I., Coz-Rakovac, R., Barisic, J., Jadan, M., Persin Berakovic, A., and Sauerborn Klobucar, R. (2012). Tricaine methane-sulfonate (MS-222) application in fish anaesthesia. *J. Appl. Ichthyol. 28*(4), 553–564.

Trevarrow, B., Marks, D.L., and Kimmel, C.B. (1990). Organization of hindbrain segments in the zebrafish embryo. *Neuron 4*(5), 669–679.

Tsai, S.Q., and Joung, J.K. (2016). Defining and improving the genome-wide specificities of CRISPR-Cas9 nucleases. *Nat. Rev. Genet. 17*(5), 300–312.

Tugba Durlu-Kandilci, N., Ruas, M., Chuang, K.T., Brading, A., Parrington, J., and Galione, A. (2010). TPC2 proteins mediate nicotinic acid adenine dinucleotide phosphate (NAADP)- and agonist-evoked contractions of smooth muscle. *J. Biol. Chem. 285*(32), 24925–24932.

Varshney, G.K., Pei, W., LaFave, M.C., Idol, J., Xu, L., Gallardo, V., Carrington, B., Bishop, K., Jones, M., Li, M., et al. (2015a). High-throughput gene targeting and phenotyping in zebrafish using CRISPR/Cas9. *Genome Res. 25*(7), 1030–1042.

Varshney, G.K., Sood, R., and Burgess, S.M. (2015b). Understanding and editing the zebrafish genome. *Adv. Genet. 92*, 1–52.

Wang, X., Wan, H., Korzh, V., and Gong, Z. (2000). Use of an IRES bicistronic construct to trace expression of exogenously introduced mRNA in zebrafish embryos. *BioTechniques 29*(814–816), 818, 820.

Webb, S.E., and Miller, A.L. (2003). Calcium signaling during embryonic development. *Nat. Rev. Mol. Cell Biol. 4*(7), 539–552.

Webb, S.E., and Miller, A.L. (2007). $Ca^{2+}$ signaling and early embryonic patterning during zebrafish development. *Clin. Exp. Pharmacol. Physiol. 34*(9), 897–904.

Webb, S.E., Rogers, K.L., Karplus, E., and Miller, A.L. (2010). The use of aequorins to record and visualize $Ca^{2+}$ dynamics: From subcellular microdomains to whole organisms. In: *Methods in Cell Biology, Volume 99: Calcium in Living Cells*, M. Whitaker, ed. (Academic Press, Inc., San Diego, CA), pp. 263–300.

Willig, K.I., Harke, B., Medda, R., and Hell, S. (2007). STED microscopy with continuous wave beams. *Nat. Methods 4*(11), 915–918.

Wulf, E., Deboben, A., Bautz, F.A., Faulstich, H., and Wieland, T. (1979). Fluorescent phal-lotoxin, a tool for the visualization of cellular actin. *Proc. Natl. Acad. Sci. U.S.A. 76*(9), 4498–4502.

Yoshimori, T., Yamamoto, A., Moriyama, Y., Futai, M., and Tashiro, Y. (1991). Bafilomycin A1, a specific inhibitor of vacuolar-type $H^+$-ATPase inhibits acidification and protein degradation in lysosomes of cultured cells. *J. Biol. Chem.* *266*(26), 17707–17712.

Yuen, M.Y.F., Webb, S.E., Chan, C.M., Thisse, B., Thisse, C., and Miller, A.L. (2013). Characterization of $Ca^{2+}$ signaling in the external yolk syncytial layer during the late blastula and early gastrula periods of zebrafish development. *Biochim. Biophys. Acta* *1833*(7), 1641–1656.

Zhang, Z.H., Lu, Y.Y., and Yue, J. (2013). Two pore channel 2 differentially modulates neural differentiation of mouse embryonic stem cells. *PLoS One.* doi: 10.1371/journal.pone.0066077.

Zhu, M.X., Ma, J., Parrington, J., Calcraft, P.J., Galione, A., and Evans, A.M. (2010). Calcium signaling via two-pore channels: Local or global, that is the question. *Am. J. Physiol. Cell Physiol.* *298*(3), C430–C441.

# 6 Functional Study of Lysosomal Nutrient Transporters

*Xavier Leray, Corinne Sagné, and Bruno Gasnier*

## CONTENTS

## 6.1   INTRODUCTION

Lysosomal hydrolysis of materials internalized by endocytosis and phagocytosis or sequestered by autophagy releases a wide variety of metabolites which are exported from the lysosomal lumen by specific transporters for reuse. This chapter focuses on the functional study of these transporters. Detecting and quantifying their transport activity poses several challenges. First, like any organellar transport protein, the intracellular localization limits their tractability. Second, they usually have low substrate affinity, in the millimolar range. This results in high background and poor signal to noise ratio compared to high-affinity plasma membrane transporters. Finally, the translocation of molecule or ion through transporters is very slow (10 to $10^3$ cycles per second) as it requires structural transitions that alternately expose the substrate binding site to either side of the membrane. This alternating-access mechanism is several orders of magnitude slower than the electrodiffusion of ions through channels ($10^6$ to $10^8$ ions per second). Therefore, detecting the activity of transporters requires much higher membrane densities than ion channels.

   Several approaches have been developed to overcome these technical bottlenecks. One efficient strategy consists of misrouting the transporter of interest to the cell surface by identifying in its sequence, and mutating, one or several motifs responsible for its delivery to lysosomes. Mutant proteins lacking such motifs are usually delivered by default to the plasma membrane. This approach, first applied to the lysosomal cystine transporter, cystinosin (Kalatzis et al., 2001), replaces the poorly tractable lysosomal export by a classical cellular influx. Lowering the extracellular pH mimics the lysosomal lumen acidity and generally activates the misrouted transporter (Figure 6.1).

   This whole-cell approach offers several advantages. First, the transport activity can be measured with a limited number of cells, ranging from a few 100,000 cultured cells per well for biochemical techniques to a single cell in electrophysiological assays, thus bypassing the need to purify lysosomes from tissues or large amounts of cultured cells. Second, the large internal volume of a cell maintains uptake at its initial velocity for a long period, allowing to amplify the transport signal over time. In contrast, uptake into, or efflux from, lysosomes or membrane vesicles reaches a plateau within a few minutes, resulting in low signals. Finally, a wide diversity of techniques ranging from radiotracer assays to electrophysiological or fluorescent recording can be easily applied to whole cells to monitor transport activities at the plasma membrane (Figure 6.1).

   However, some potential pitfalls may be encountered with the ectopic expression of a lysosomal transporter at the plasma membrane. The distinct lipid composition and

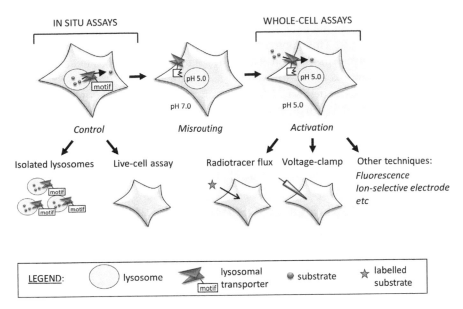

**FIGURE 6.1**   Overview of the methods used to study the activity of lysosomal transporters. Lysosomal metabolite transport can be measured in the native membrane using radiotracer flux assays with isolated lysosomes. It can also be indirectly assessed within live cells by monitoring a cellular response correlating with lysosomal accumulation of small molecules (see Figure 6.2). Alternately, recombinant lysosomal transporters can be redirected to the cell surface by mutation of their sorting motif(s). In this whole-cell configuration, topologically equivalent to inside-out lysosomes, lysosomal transporters can be studied by techniques routinely applied to plasma membrane transporters using radiotracers, electrophysiological recording, fluorescent reporters, etc. Lowering the extracellular pH to mimic the lysosomal lumen acidity activates the misrouted transporter.

the lack of interacting proteins (for instance, an unidentified beta subunit) may alter transport properties in the whole-cell assay. The lysosomal transporter may also be processed, and regulated, by lysosomal proteases in its native environment (Savalas et al., 2011). Recapitulating this processing in a whole-cell assay may prove difficult.

It is thus important to study lysosomal transporters as well in their native membrane (Figure 6.1). A classical approach used in early biochemical studies consists in isolating lysosomes or lysosomal membrane vesicles and measuring transmembrane fluxes with radiotracers (Gahl et al., 1982; Mancini et al., 1989; Pisoni and Thoene, 1991). A step-by-step protocol to measure lysosomal amino acid exchange ('countertransport' assay) in subcellular fractions is described in the next section.

Ideally, it would be useful to monitor lysosomal transport within live cells rather than in vitro, as subcellular fractionation might lose regulations by cytosolic factors. Although genetically encoded sensors have been developed for amino acids and sugars (Okumoto et al., 2012), their application to lysosomes and endosomes remains challenging. A way to circumvent this bottleneck consists of monitoring a biological response that directly depends on the activity of a specific lysosomal transporter to provide a proxy for its activity. We recently developed an approach exploiting the cellular distribution of the transcription factor EB (TFEB), a master gene for lyso-somal biogenesis (Sardiello et al., 2009), as a proxy for lysosomal accumulation of specific compounds. This approach could characterize lysosomal transporters for amino acids in live cells (Verdon et al., 2017). It might be extended to any lysosomal transporter if there is a way to overload its substrate(s) in lysosomes, for instance through the endocytic pathway. More generally, any cell response tightly correlated to lysosomal accumulation of specific compounds could be exploited to monitor cog-nate transporter(s). The TFEB-based assay described below should thus be taken as a guiding example among diverse options.

Depending on the specificity of the techniques covered in this chapter, we will provide step-by-step protocols or general guidelines.

## 6.2 IN SITU ASSAYS OF LYSOSOMAL TRANSPORTERS

### 6.2.1 RADIOTRACER ASSAYS WITH ISOLATED LYSOSOMES

#### 6.2.1.1 General Considerations

Radiotracer flux assays have been extensively used in the 1980s and 1990s to char-acterize small-molecule transport activities in isolated lysosomes or lysosomal membrane vesicles (Pisoni and Thoene, 1991). This technique consists in isolating a lysosomal fraction from cultured cells or tissues and incubating it with a radioactive compound. Membranes are then quickly separated from the incubation medium, and washed by filtration or centrifugation. The accumulated radioactivity is measured by scintillation counting. This method is straightforward and highly sensitive.

The homogenization step prior to subcellular fractionation is critical with cultured cells because disruption of isolated cells requires shearing forces at smaller scale than ground tissue. Several methods exist which use shearing forces and/or pressure differences between inside and outside of the cell to break the plasma membrane. These methods may require specific equipment (French press; Parr cell disruption bomb; BioNeb droplet low-pressure nebulizer) or may not (Potter-Elvehjem or Douce homogenizer; syringe/needle). The former methods are easier to scale up. Whatever method is chosen, it is essential to define in preliminary experiments the conditions that give the highest yield of cell breakage while preserving lysosome integrity. Cell breakage is easily monitored by comparing samples before and after homogenization under a microscope. Broken cells appear as nuclei without cytoplasm. Staining with a membrane-impermeant dye facilitates detection of remaining intact cells.

Lysosomal integrity is assessed by measuring the activity of an acidic hydrolase with and without Triton X-100 in an aliquot of homogenate. Without Triton X-100, the membrane-impermeant substrate cannot reach hydrolases contained in intact lysosomes. Adding the non-ionic detergent solubilizes cell membranes but keeps enzymes in native state, thus releasing 'latent' enzymatic activity from intact lyso-somes (hence the name 'latency assay'). Lysosomal integrity is expressed as the ratio of activity protected by a membrane over the total activity:

$$\frac{(\text{Activity}_{+\text{TX100}} - \text{Activity}_{-\text{TX100}})}{\text{Activity}_{-\text{TX100}}}$$

It is recommended to find homogenization conditions that give integrity values higher than 50%.

The level of lysosome purification needed depends on the selectivity of the transport assay. As lysosomal integrity decreases across purification steps, a trade-off should be found between purity on one hand, and yield and integrity on the other hand. A transport activity highly specific for lysosomes or availability of a specific inhibitor discriminating the lysosomal signal from contaminating organelles enables to assay the transporter in crude fractions with a maximal yield and integrity. In contrast, substrates transported into diverse cell compartments (mitochondria, contaminating plasma membrane vesicles, etc.), such as amino acids, require highly purified lysosomes prepared either by classical differential and isopycnic centrifugation (Chapel et al., 2013) or by fast immuno-isolation methods (Abu-Remaileh et al., 2017; Xiong et al., 2019) (see also Chapter 9). The former technique is easy to scale up, however its duration and the mechanical stress during ultracentrifugation tend to harm lysosomal integrity. The latter technique provides highly purified fractions with minimal lysosomal breakage, but its cost is high and its scale limited. In the case of amino acids, the counter-transport assay provides a simple way to satisfy both constraints as it allows lysosomal selectivity without extensive purification.

### 6.2.1.2 Principle and Experimental Design of the Counter-Transport Assay

The counter-transport assay has been used in the 1980s to biochemically identify lysosomal amino acid transport pathways in crude subcellular fractions (Pisoni and Thoene, 1991). In this assay, partially purified lysosomes are selectively loaded with the amino acid of interest using an ester precursor prior to transport measurements. The ester passively diffuses into all compartments. In lysosomes, it is cleaved by acidic hydrolases, leading to specific amino acid build-up in this compartment (Reeves, 1979). After this loading step, there are two options to assay the cognate amino acid transporter. If lysosomes were treated with a radiolabelled ester, they are next diluted and incubated in the presence of ATP to monitor the decay of lysosomal radioactivity over time – see Cang et al. (2013) for a recent example. ATP usually stimulates this decay through $H^+$ coupling with the vacuolar-type $H^+$-ATPase. This export assay is directly relevant to the physiological activity. However, radioactive esters are not commercially available and, although preparing a methyl ester from radiolabelled amino acids is straightforward (Cang et al., 2013; Reeves, 1979), modifying radiolabelled compounds is often not permitted by radiation safety committees.

An alternate approach, the counter-transport assay, consists in artificially loading lysosomes using an unlabelled ester and measuring an exchange reaction between the unlabelled, internal amino acid and the radioactive, externally added amino acid. Owing to a hallmark property of transporters known as 'trans-stimulation', the internal amino acid can drive uptake ('counter-transport') of the radiotracer into lysosomes over its external concentration, even though the transporter would export its substrates under physiological conditions. This effect results from the alternating-access mechanism of membrane transporters. Under standard conditions, these proteins randomly cycle through the whole set of structural and ligand occupancy states to catalyze a net flux. However, if the substrate is abundant on one side of the membrane such as in artificially loaded lysosomes, adding another substrate or a tracer to the other side will shift the transport cycle from a net flux to a ping-pong-like shuttle between inward-open and outward-open substrate-bound states. The preloaded internal amino acid thus drives the external radiotracer into the lysosome.

In practice, the loading step should be optimized individually for each ester as the permeation and hydrolysis rates vary with the amino acid and alcohol moieties. A simple approach consists in treating subcellular fractions with increased ester concentrations at 25°C or 37°C and measuring lysosomal integrity over time using a latency assay. Amino acid accumulation at exceeding level causes osmotic stress and lysosomal ruptures. The highest ester concentration fully preserving lysosomal integrity is used for counter-transport measurements. With some amino acids, such as glutamine, classical methyl esters proved inefficient in our hands. Using esters made with more hydrophobic alcohols circumvented this bottleneck (Verdon et al., 2017).

Amino acids can accumulate into mitochondria and other contaminating organelles, which may lead to a high non-specific signal for some amino acids, such as alanine or valine (Verdon et al., 2017). Assigning the trans-stimulated (ester-dependent) component of uptake to lysosomes should thus be confirmed by another criterion. A simple approach consists in selectively rupturing lysosomes at the end of the uptake period to release their internal radioactivity. Glycine methyl ester (GME) (Goldman and Kaplan, 1973), L-leucyl-L-leucine methyl ester (LLOMe) (Thiele and Lipsky, 1990) or glycyl-L-phenylalanine 2-naphthylamide (GPN) (Berg et al., 1994) are commonly used for this purpose. GME and GPN promote osmotic rupture through fast cleavage in lysosomes (by cathepsin C for GPN), whereas LLOMe is converted by cathepsin C into short polyleucine chains which transiently permeabilize the lysosomal membrane (Repnik et al., 2017).

On the downside, it is worth noting that the counter-transport assay probes a partial reaction of the lysosomal transporter rather than the full transport cycle operating in the cell. Some important functional aspects may be missed. For instance, the $K_M$ for substrates on the luminal side, which is relevant for lysosomal export, cannot be determined in contrast with whole-cell approaches.

### 6.2.1.3 Detailed Protocol: Glutamine Counter-Transport in HeLa Cell Lysosomes

We provide here an example of amino acid counter-transport protocol used to characterize the lysosomal transporter for glutamine and asparagine SNAT7 (Verdon et al., 2017). Quantities are given to test up to four experimental conditions measured in triplicate at a single time point. If more conditions must be tested it is preferable to run separate experiments rather than scaling up the number of cells because lysosomal integrity decreases with lengthier cell fractionation. Alternately, cell homogenization can be done with a Parr cell disruption bomb or a BioNeb nebulizer to scale up the protocol without lengthening the homogenization step.

The day before the experiment:

(i)   Check that a minimal number of $25 \times 10^6$ HeLa cells will be available the next day.

(ii)     Prepare the material: tubes; syringe; needle; pipette tips, cut obliquely to minimize lysosomal breakage during pipetting.

Prepare 10 mL of lysosome isolation buffer: 250 mM sucrose, 10 mM triethanolamine, 10 mM acetic acid, 1 mM EDTA, adjusted to pH 7.4 with NaOH.

To minimize degradation of cell constituents, cell disruption and subcellular fractionation should be performed in a cold room with pre-chilled material and buffer.

The next day:

(iii)    Add protease inhibitor cocktail (Halt Protease Inhibitor Cocktail 100×, Thermo Fischer Scientific) and 5 mM ATP-$Mg^{2+}$ (from a stock solution adjusted to pH 7.4) to the isolation buffer.

(iv)     Harvest cells by trypsinization and count them. Collect the medium containing $25 \times 10^6$ cells in a 50-mL conical tube. Centrifuge at $200 \times g$ for 10 min and wash the cells once with 50 mL phosphate buffer saline (PBS). Centrifuge again and discard the supernatant.

(v)      Resuspend the cell pellet in 1.1 mL isolation buffer. Transfer the cell suspension into the cold room and allow it to cool down on ice. Keep the material at 4°C in all subsequent steps except mentioned otherwise.

(vi)     Break the cells by 50 passages through a 27 Gauge, ¾ inch-length syringe needle, being careful to avoid generating air bubbles. Centrifuge the suspension at $750 \times g$ for 10 min to pellet unbroken cells and cell debris. Remove the post-nuclear supernatant (carefully avoid taking the pellet). Resuspend the pellet in 1.1 mL isolation buffer. Centrifuge again at $750 \times g$ for 10 min. Pool the two post-nuclear supernatants. Centrifuge at $1,500 \times g$ for 15 min. At this step, the pellet should be small and barely visible.

(vii)    Centrifuge the supernatant at $20,000 \times g$ for 15 min. The supernatant should now appear clear. Resuspend the pellet in 75 µL isolation buffer. Adjust the final volume to 125 µL.

(viii)   Mix 100 µL of the lysosome-enriched fraction with 11 µL of a 37.5 mM stock solution of L-glutamine tert-butyl ester (final concentration 3.7 mM). Incubate for 15 min at 25°C to artificially load lysosomes with L-glutamine. Transfer the glutamine-loaded lysosomes into four tubes (4 × 25 µL). Centrifuge at $20,000 \times g$ for 15 min at 4°C. Discard the supernatants.

If the experiment aims to compare lysosomes with and without internal glutamine, treat only half of the lysosome-enriched fraction with the tert-butyl ester.

The next step should be done in a room dedicated to the use of radiolabelled compounds according to local radiation safety guidelines.

(ix)     Resuspend each slightly yellow pellet in 400 µL isolation buffer supplemented with L-[$^3$H]glutamine (4 µCi, 200 nM), ATP-$Mg^{2+}$ and any drug to be tested. For each tested condition, split the 400-µL mix into 50-µL aliquots transferred into seven hemolysis tubes kept on ice. One tube is directly filtered (see below) without incubation to determine the radioactivity background. The other six tubes are incubated for 30 min at 37°C. Three mixes are filtered just after this incubation to determine in triplicate the level of L-[³H]glutamine accumulated into all organelles (after subtracting the background level averaged across the four tested conditions). The remaining mixes are supplemented with 10 mM GME and incubated further for 10 min to selectively release radioactivity from lysosomes. These samples provide the level of accumulation into non-lysosomal organelles in triplicate.

For filtration, samples are diluted with 3 mL ice-cold PBS and filtered under vacuum onto a 0.45-µm pore nitrocellulose membrane (HAWP02500; Millipore). The membrane is immediately washed three times with chilled PBS. The radioactivity retained on filters is determined by scintillation counting.

Lysosomal [³H] glutamine counter-transport is determined for each tested condition by subtracting the GME-resistant signal from the signal measured in untreated samples. As mentioned, up to four conditions (28 filtrations) can be tested from $25 \times 10^6$ HeLa cells with this protocol.

## 6.2.2 USING THE TRANSCRIPTION FACTOR TFEB AS A PROXY FOR LYSOSOMAL EXPORT IN LIVE CELLS

### 6.2.2.1 Principle

To screen for potential lysosomal amino acid transporters, we developed a novel assay using the distribution of the transcription factor EB (TFEB) as a proxy to detect lysosomal amino acid overload in live cells (Verdon et al., 2017). Lysosomes can be artificially overloaded with specific amino acids within live cells using the same ester precursors as those used in vitro for the counter-transport assay. Inside cells, cytosolic esterases cleave the ester group, thus limiting access to intracellular organelles. However, if the ester concentration is high enough, some intact molecules enter into the lysosomes to accumulate the corresponding amino acid in their lumen. This lysosomal accumulation can be detected by taking advantage of a transcriptional feedback loop which adapts lysosomal biogenesis to cell degradative needs (Sardiello et al., 2009).

Lysosomal biogenesis is indeed orchestrated by TFEB and other members of the MiT-TFE family of basic helix-loop-helix leucine-zipper transcription factors (Puertollano et al., 2018). Under healthy, nutrient-replete conditions, TFEB is maintained in a phosphorylated form by mTORC1 and other kinases, leading to its retention in the cytoplasm (Martina et al., 2012; Roczniak-Ferguson et al., 2012; Settembre et al., 2012). When undegraded macromolecules or small molecules accumulate in lysosomes, TFEB is dephosphorylated, leading to its translocation to the nucleus to upregulate lysosomal genes (Puertollano et al., 2018; Sardiello et al., 2009). The distribution or the phosphorylation state of MiT-TFE family transcription factors thus offers a simple way to detect lysosomal overload with specific amino acids and the rescue of this overload by cognate lysosomal transporters (Figure 6.2).

This approach may be used to detect lysosomal accumulation of any compound, not just amino acids. For instance, endocytosis of cleavable polymer precursors might be considered to release, and accumulate, other types of compound in the lysosomal lumen.

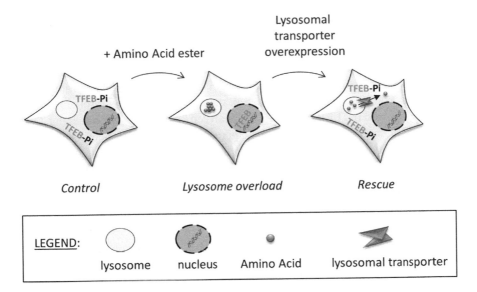

**FIGURE 6.2** Principle of the TFEB-based assay of lysosomal amino acid transporters in live cells. In untreated cells, the transcription factor TFEB is phosphorylated and retained in the cytoplasm (left scheme). Treatment with a membrane-permeant ester precursor induces artificial overload of lysosomes with the corresponding amino acid. This triggers TFEB dephosphorylation and its translocation to the nucleus to activate lysosomal genes (centre). Overexpression of the cognate lysosomal exporter mitigates this lysosomal overload, thus rescuing TFEB nuclear translocation (right).

## 6.2.2.2  Technical Considerations

As with subcellular fractions, each amino acid ester should be individually tested in a dose-response curve, starting with the simple methyl ester and extending to other alcohol derivatives if necessary. An additional complexity with live cells compared with cell fractions arises from the competition between ester cleavage in the cytoplasm and ester entry in intact form into lysosomes. High ester concentrations favour the latter process. The distribution of TFEB is a good readout to perform these preliminary experiments. TFEB distribution can be assessed either by expressing a tagged recombinant construct or by analyzing the endogenous protein with an antibody. Ester treatments inducing ~30% nuclear translocation provide a good starting point to detect with good sensitivity both decreases and increases in lysosomal overload upon transporter expression. Optimal working concentrations for 11 amino acid esters applied for 2 h to HeLa cells are provided in our study of the transporter SNAT7 (Verdon et al., 2017).

Another technical aspect to consider is the method used to express recombinant proteins. Lipofection should be avoided because endocytosis of DNA/lipofectant complexes induces a long-lasting lysosomal stress, resulting in a strong nuclear translocation of TFEB even 72 h after transfection. In contrast, electroporation promotes DNA entry through transient holes in the plasma membrane. Although nuclear translocation of TFEB also occurs on the first day, this effect fully reverses after 48 h if no other lysosomal stress (ester treatment) is delivered. Another advantage of electroporation over lipofection is the lower level of expression, yielding better lysosomal targeting of the recombinant transporter.

This approach can efficiently deorphanize putative lysosomal transporters and it does not require prior identification of lysosomal sorting motifs. Moreover, a small number of cells ($10^6$ per transporter) is enough to test ~15 amino acids in two weeks with the protocol described in the next section. This throughput can be greatly improved if TFEB distribution is analyzed by high-content screening. On the downside, it should be noted that this approach probes steady-state levels of lysosomal accumulation rather than dynamic fluxes. The ester treatment and the TFEB response are too slow to monitor the dynamics of lysosomal import or export.

### 6.2.2.3   Example of Protocol

The following protocol can be easily implemented in diverse cell lines.

(i)  On day 1, HeLa cells are transiently transfected by electroporation with two plasmids, one encoding a TFEB construct tagged with a fluorescent protein (for instance mRFP) and another encoding the candidate transporter. Electroporated cells are plated on glass coverslips into 24-well plates.

   If no specific antibody is available, the candidate transporter should be tagged with an epitope or another fluorescent protein (for instance EGFP). For negative control, this construct is replaced by a well-targeted, inactive lysosomal protein – for instance the P334R mutant of human sialin (Morin et al., 2004) – to exclude the possibility that overexpression of a lysosomal membrane protein *per se* might impact TFEB phosphorylation.

   Seed approximately 20,000 cells per well to keep confluency below 60% after 2 days of culture. At higher confluency, lower cell spreading would hinder TFEB analysis.

(ii)  On day 3, cells are incubated for 2 h with the tested amino acid ester(s) at their optimal concentration (see above) in a culture medium supplemented with 10% fetal calf serum and 25 mM HEPES pH 7.4. Cells are then washed twice with PBS supplemented with 0.1 mM $Ca^{2+}$ and 0.1 mM $Mg^{2+}$ and fixed with 4% paraformaldehyde.

   As amino acid esters are often purchased as hydrochloride salts and used at high concentration, the pH of stock solutions (for instance 500× in PBS) should be adjusted to pH 7.4 to avoid acidifying the culture medium.

(iii)  Coverslips are washed and mounted in a medium supplemented with DAPI to label cell nuclei.

(iv)  Cells are then imaged and scored under an epifluorescence microscope at low magnification (10× or 20×). Select a field showing transporter-expressing cells in the green fluorescence channel. Shift to the red channel to observe TFEB and classify its distribution in each cell into three categories: 'cytoplasmic', i.e. TFEB signal is higher in the cytoplasm, the nucleus appearing in black; 'nuclear', i.e. the intensity is higher in the nucleus than in the cytoplasm; and 'mixed', i.e. TFEB signal is similar in the two compartments.

It should be noted that TFEB distribution usually varies across cells from a given field. To get reliable averages of the whole population, observe the following precautions: (a) examine at least five different fields per coverslip and score a minimum of 50 cells per condition; (b) avoid scoring neighbouring cells as they may represent daughter cells from the same transfected cell; scoring daughter cells may induce biases; (c) it is better to have this scoring step done by an independent observer in a blind manner.

## 6.3   WHOLE-CELL APPROACHES TO STUDY LYSOSOMAL TRANSPORTERS: GENERAL CONSIDERATIONS

### 6.3.1   OVERVIEW AND ADVANTAGES

As mentioned earlier, whole-cell assays of lysosomal transporters provide direct access to their transport activity by replacing the poorly tractable lysosomal export by a topologically equivalent cellular influx. This influx is measured at low extracellular pH to mimic the acidic lysosomal lumen (Figure 6.1). These whole-cell assays require much fewer cells than those with isolated lysosomes since a single 24-multiwell plate or, in some techniques, a single cell is sufficient to provide valuable information. Moreover, they are less labour intensive, and their signal to noise ratio is higher than those with isolated lysosomes.

In principle, the ectopic expression of a lysosomal transporter at the plasma membrane might alter its transport properties. Although this risk should be kept in mind, whole-cell assays of several transporters proved to be remarkably consistent with earlier studies in isolated lysosomes (Jézégou et al., 2012; Kalatzis et al., 2001; Morin et al., 2004).

For lysosomal transporters associated with genetic diseases, another advantage of whole-cell approaches is that the impact of pathogenic mutations on the transport activity, on one hand, and on the delivery to lysosomes, on the other hand, can be analysed distinctly, in contrast with isolated lysosome studies. See, for instance, Kalatzis et al. (2004) for cystinosis and Morin et al. (2004) and Wreden et al. (2005) for Salla disease.

### 6.3.2   MISROUTING LYSOSOMAL TRANSPORTERS TO THE CELL SURFACE

Resident membrane proteins are targeted to the lysosome from the *trans*-Golgi network either directly via the endosomes or indirectly by default routing to the plasma membrane followed by internalization into the endocytic pathway. In both cases, short sequence motifs present in their cytosolic domains are recognized by adaptor proteins that drive their incorporation into protein-coated vesicles which eventually uncoat and fuse with the target membrane (Braulke and Bonifacino, 2009). Mutation of key residues in these motifs impairs the recognition step, resulting in default delivery of the mutated protein to the plasma membrane.

Designing a whole-cell assay of a given transporter thus consists in identifying, and mutating, candidate sorting motifs in its primary sequence and assessing the impact of such mutations on its intracellular localization. Diverse classes of lysosomal sorting motifs have been described, including the tyrosine-based motifs YXXØ and NPXY, where X is any amino acid and Ø is a bulky amino acid, and the dileucine-based motifs [D/E]XXXL[L/I] and DXXLL (Braulke and Bonifacino, 2009). YXXØ, NPXY and [D/E]XXXL[L/I] motifs interact with heterotetrameric adaptor protein complexes (AP-1, AP-2 or AP-3), whereas DXXLL motives bind Golgi localized, γ-adaptin ear-containing, ARF-binding protein (GGA) components of the clathrin coat. The tyrosine residue and the pair of leucine/isoleucine are critical for these interactions. Mutating these residues to alanine or glycine is sufficient to disrupt recognition by the trafficking machinery. Lipid modification, phosphorylation or even unconventional sorting motifs can also affect intracellular sorting of lysosomal membrane proteins (Storch et al., 2004, 2007).

As adaptor proteins recognize their cargo in the cytosol, the number of motif candidates can be reduced by focusing on cytosolic domains of the transporter. These domains can be inferred from a homologous 3D structure or by predicting the membrane topology with sequence algorithms (for instance, TMHMM or TMpred). Another criterion to select mutations is the evolutionary conservation of putative motifs. However, this criterion should be used with caution as sorting signals may be species-specific even within mammals. Some lysosomal proteins have multiple, functionally redundant sorting signals. Therefore, candidate mutations should be combined if individual mutations fail to disrupt lysosomal localization.

The localization of mutant and wild-type constructs is characterized by transient expression in HeLa cells, or another type of well-spread cell, and fluorescence microscopy. Disruption of lysosomal targeting shifts the distribution from a punctate pattern overlapping with lysosomal/late-endosomal markers such as LAMP1 to a diffuse staining visible up to filopodia. Localization of the sorting mutant at the plasma membrane may be confirmed by surface biotinylation. This assay is also useful to compare surface levels of different constructs and interpret changes in transport activity in the whole-cell assay.

### 6.3.3 Choice of Expression System for Transport Measurement

As transport activities are usually low, it is better to maximize expression for transport studies. For mammalian cells, HEK293T, COS-1 or COS-7 are choice expression systems as they stably express the Simian Virus 40 (SV40) large T antigen, which amplifies transfected plasmids harbouring an SV40 replication origin. This replication origin is often not mentioned in plasmid maps, although it is embedded in the SV40 early promoter used to confer neomycin resistance. Plasmid replication in HEK293T and COS cells results in much higher expression levels than in standard cell lines, such as HeLa.

Another criterion to consider is the existence of endogenous transporters for the tested substrate. For instance, the activity of the lysosomal transporter PQLC2 (its sorting mutant L290A/L291A) gives a poor signal to noise ratio in mammalian cells because of the high endogenous uptake of cationic amino acids (Jézégou et al., 2012). One option with such an issue may be to inhibit the endogenous transporter(s) (CAT1 in this case). However, pharmacological tools are often not available, and the molecular identity of background uptake may be elusive. Therefore, another option is to shift to a highly different expression system. Expression in *Xenopus* oocytes is a popular alternative in the transporter field because these cells have low endogenous transport activities, and synthetic mRNA injection yields huge expression levels. Moreover, this expression system is well tractable for electrophysiological studies.

### 6.3.4  Expression in *Xenopus laevis* Oocytes

#### 6.3.4.1  Some Considerations

Stage V–VI oocytes from the African clawed frog, *Xenopus laevis*, are giant cells (1–1.3 mm diameter) that can express up to ~$10^{11}$ copies of polytopic membrane protein in their plasma membrane (Ruivo et al., 2012). Intracellular trafficking machineries are conserved between frogs and mammals; therefore, a sorting mutant identified in HeLa cells usually behaves similarly in *Xenopus* oocytes. These properties make oocytes a choice model to study recombinant lysosomal transporters by whole-cell approaches. If the transporter is electrogenic, its activity can be monitored in real time using two-electrode voltage-clamp (TEVC) analysis. However, unlike mammalian cell lines which are easily bought and cultured, the use of *Xenopus* oocytes requires careful handling and specific preparation steps.

There are two supply options. One option is to purchase oocytes from commercial vendors. Several companies supply either oocyte-containing ovaries or ready-to-use defolliculated oocytes (for instance: EcoCyte Bioscience or the European *Xenopus* Resource Centre). Alternately, if the animal facility can house *Xenopus* frogs, ovarian lobes can be collected from anaesthetized females through surgical laparotomy. The surgical procedure, recovery time between laparotomies and number of surgeries on a single animal must obtain the approval of local ethics committees. As these guidelines vary across countries, this aspect is not detailed here. Preparing ready-to-use oocytes from ovarian lobes is relatively easy, and it provides extra-fresh oocytes. It is thus the solution commonly used in most laboratories.

#### 6.3.4.2  Protocol: Preparation of Oocytes from *Xenopus* Ovarian Lobes

Two buffers are used:

- Modified Barth's solution (MBS): 88 mM NaCl, 1 mM KCl, 2.4 mM NaHCO$_3$, 0.82 mM MgSO$_4$, 0.33 mM Ca(NO$_3$)$_2$, 0.41 mM CaCl$_2$, 5 mM Hepes pH 7.4. This solution is used to maintain oocytes.
- Ca$^{2+}$-free oocyte Ringer solution (OR2-): 82.5 mM NaCl, 2.5 mM KCl, 1 mM MgCl$_2$, 5 mM Hepes pH 7.4. This solution is used for collagenase treatment. The absence of Ca$^{2+}$ is critical to preserve oocyte integrity during defolliculation because purified collagenase preparations often contain contaminating proteases activated by Ca$^{2+}$.

We usually prepare and autoclave 1 L of each buffer. They can be stored at 4°C up to one year. Ovarian lobes collected by laparotomy are maintained at 16–19°C in MBS supplemented with 50 µg/mL gentamicin. To prepare oocytes, we use the following protocol:

(i)   Equilibrate 200 mL MBS and 200 mL OR2- at room temperature.
(ii)  Transfer ovarian lobes into a 90-mm Petri dish containing OR2-. Add 40 mg of Type II collagenase (Gibco) to 10 mL of OR2- in a 15-mL tube (final concentration: 4 mg/mL).
(iii) Prepare a T25 flask containing 5 mL of OR2-. Tease apart the lobes into ~30 mm$^3$ pieces (3 × 3 × 3 mm, containing ~10–20 oocytes) using tweezers

or sharp scissors. As things progress, add the pieces to the T25 flask until reaching a total volume of 10 mL (5 mL of OR2- + 5 mL tissue). It is important to use small pieces to get a homogenous collagenase treatment. Keep the remaining lobes in a 50 mL conic tube with 50 mL fresh MBS at 16–19°C supplemented with 50 µg/mL gentamicin. They can be used up to one week.

(iv) Add the 10-mL collagenase solution to the T25 flask containing the ovary pieces (final volume: 20 mL; final collagenase concentration: 2 mg/mL). Incubate horizontally for 1–1.5 h at 20°C, 80 rpm in an orbital shaker. Check the dissociation efficiency after 1 h: if ovarian pieces are digested and individualized oocytes predominate, engage the next step. If many pieces remain, sample some oocytes with a transfer pipette and check whether they still possess their follicle under a microscope. Do not incubate more than 1.5 h. This step may be adjusted by decreasing the collagenase concentration to 1 mg/mL or by increasing the temperature up to 25°C.

(v) Transfer the defolliculated oocytes into a 15-mL tube. Complete the volume up to 14 mL with OR2-. Shake gently by rotating the tube 10 times back and forth. Discard the OR2- solution and repeat this step 5 times until the solution is clear (too much washing is better than not enough).

(vi) Replace the OR2- solution by MBS. Upon gentle shaking, small white sheets, alike ghosts, should be seen floating in the solution. It means that follicles are dissociating from oocytes, which is what you want. Repeat this step 6 times.

(vii) Transfer oocytes into a new Petri dish with MBS. Select with a transfer pipette those containing a nice white belt separating the two poles (one pole is light yellow, the other one is brown). These are the stage V–VI oocytes used for injection. To avoid harming oocytes, we use general purpose transfer pipettes (Samco) with a 6-mm diameter tip. Discard the other oocytes.

(viii) Maintain selected and non-defolliculated oocytes in MBS supplemented with 50 µg/mL gentamicin in an incubator at 16–19°C. They can be kept up to one week. The next morning, discard unhealthy defolliculated oocytes and replace the medium by fresh MBS with gentamicin.

### 6.3.4.3   Expression of the Transporter in *Xenopus* Oocytes

Transporter expression is achieved by nanoinjection of synthetic RNA into defolliculated oocytes. The transporter cDNA is sub-cloned into a plasmid downstream of a bacterial RNA Polymerase promoter and transcribed in vitro with the mMessage mMachine kit (Thermo Fisher Scientific). *Xenopus* expression vectors, such as the pTLN and pOX(+) plasmids (Lorenz et al., 1996; Takanaga et al., 2005), have been optimized by flanking the cDNA cloning site with the 5' and 3' untranslated regions (UTR) of *Xenopus* β-globin to increase cRNA stability and translation efficiency. The template is linearized at a restriction site downstream the 3' β-globin UTR and the poly-A sequence before in vitro transcription.

cRNA microinjection is performed using a glass pipette pulled to obtain µm-scaled tip and mounted on a nanoinjector (Nanoject 2, Drummond). The procedure to pull micropipettes is extensively described in the *Pipette Cookbook* from Sutter

Instrument. Here is an example of protocol with a P-97 puller (Sutter Instrument) hosting an FB255B heating filament (Sutter Instrument) and 3-000-203-G/X glass capillaries (Drummond):

$$\text{HEAT} = 520, \text{PULL} = 30, \text{VEL.} = 120, \text{TIME} = 200$$

This will generate a ~6 mm long, extremely narrow tip that must be processed before use. Fill the entire capillary with mineral oil (Sigma) and stick it horizontally with a tack adhesive under a microscope. With the help of scissors, break the tip 1 mm from the extremity. Mineral oil should be seen moving into the broken tip. Mount the capillary onto the nanoinjector and use it to inject cRNA according to the manufacturer's instructions.

High expression levels are obtained by injecting 50 ng cRNA per oocyte. As cRNA is stored in water at 1 mg/mL (it may precipitate in the injection pipette at higher concentration), the volume injected (50 nL) represents about 1/7 of the oocyte water-accessible volume. It is thus recommended to wait a few seconds after injection before pipette removal. Injection is usually performed into the (brown) animal pole, but in some cases optimal expression may be obtained by injecting into the (yellowish) vegetal pole. The expressed transporter first locates in the membrane near the injection site and ultimately spreads to the entire oocyte surface. The duration of expression should be optimized in preliminary experiments for each protein to obtain the highest protein level without affecting oocyte health. The optimal time may range from a single day to a few days depending on the protein. If the recombinant transporter is fused to a fluorescent protein, oocytes can be screened for expression under a fluorescence microscope to select the best cells for transport experiments. Oocytes may be categorized into 3 or 4 expression levels in this manner. The selected oocytes are maintained at 16–19°C in a 24-well plate filled with gentamicin-containing MBS. We usually put 5–10 oocytes per well to minimize potential losses, as enzyme leakage from one unhealthy oocyte may harm its neighbours.

## 6.4 WHOLE-CELL RADIOTRACER ASSAY OF LYSOSOMAL TRANSPORTERS

### 6.4.1 RADIOTRACER ASSAY IN MAMMALIAN CELLS

Transporters are transiently expressed in COS-7 or HEK293T cells in 24-well plates. The optimal incubation time after transfection depends on the transporter, transfection method (lipofection, electroporation), amount of plasmid, etc. It may vary from 24 h to 72 h. This parameter should be determined in preliminary experiments using Western blotting or, more roughly, fluorescence microscopy to assess expression level.

To assay uptake, cells are washed twice with 0.5 mL of isotonic medium buffered at neutral pH (for instance, NaCl 140 mM, $MgSO_4$ 1 mM, D-glucose 5 mM, MOPS 10 mM adjusted to pH 7.0 with NaOH). They are then incubated with 200 µL of the same medium buffered either at pH 7.0 (negative control) or at pH 5.0 with

10 mM MES(Na$^+$) supplemented with the radiolabelled compound (0.5 µCi/well). Lysosomal transporters are usually activated at pH 5.0, mimicking the acidity of the lysosomal lumen. COS-7 and HEK293T cells can tolerate pH 5.0 during 20 min without noticeable impact on cell viability.

To avoid competition with high-affinity endogenous transporters or receptors, we recommend diluting the radiotracer with cold molecules to saturate such high-affinity processes and favour detection of the low-affinity lysosomal transporter. An overall tracer concentration equivalent to 1/10 or 1/5 the $K_M$ for the lysosomal transporter will keep the lysosomal signal to noise ratio at its maximum value. If this $K_M$ is unknown, a concentration of 10 µM or 100 µM is a good starting point.

After incubating the plates at room temperature or 37°C, radiotracer uptake is stopped by two quick washes with 500 µL ice-cold isotonic buffer. Cells are then lysed with freshly prepared NaOH 0.1 N to release their radioactivity (lysis with detergent is less practical as it creates bubbles). Lysates are then transferred into vials suitable for liquid scintillation counting. Uptake is measured in triplicate for each condition to average analytical variability.

### 6.4.2 RADIOTRACER ASSAY IN *XENOPUS* OOCYTES

All steps are carried out in modified Barth's solution (MBS: see Section 6.3.4.2) buffered with 5 mM Hepes, MES, or Bis-Tris propane adjusted to the required pH with NaOH. Uptake is measured in 24-well plates at 20°C because *Xenopus* oocytes are damaged at temperatures above 22°C. Each tested condition is applied to a batch of 10 oocytes to average the high intercellular variability in expression level. If oocytes have been pre-selected for expression by fluorescence microscopy (see above), this number may be reduced to five (triplicate is not enough). Oocytes are first washed in 500 µL MBS buffered at neutral pH. They are then transferred into 200 µL MBS adjusted to the desired pH (5.0–8.5) supplemented with the radiotracer (0.5 µCi/well; total concentration 10 µM or 100 µM). After the chosen duration, uptake is stopped by washing each well 2–4 times with 2 mL ice-cold MBS. Oocytes are then individually collected and lysed in NaOH 0.1 N or SDS 10% before scintillation counting.

## 6.5 WHOLE-CELL ELECTROPHYSIOLOGICAL STUDY OF LYSOSOMAL TRANSPORTERS

### 6.5.1 OVERVIEW AND ADVANTAGES

Electrophysiological techniques are choice methods to study the activity of electrogenic transporters. This occurs when the transport cycle transfers at least one electric charge across the membrane, which may be carried by the translocated molecule or by coupling to inorganic ions; for instance, H$^+$ symport of a neutral or zwitterionic molecule as observed for the cystine transporter cystinosin (Ruivo et al., 2012). Electrical recording allows one to study these activities in real time. Moreover, a wide range of substrates can be tested as this approach is not limited by the availability and cost of radioactive compounds.

As electrogenic transporters (and some electroneutral transporters) are influenced by the electrical membrane potential, radiotracer measurements in biochemical assays can yield inconsistent results because the membrane potential is not controlled in these techniques. This may result in high variability of uptake signals. Moreover, compounds altering endogenous channels, and hence the membrane potential, may be wrongly identified as inhibitors or activators of the electrogenic transporter. Electrophysiological techniques avoid these traps as they allow strict control of the membrane potential. Concomitant current recording with a time resolution up to milliseconds can reveal sub-steps of the transport cycle in voltage jump experiments, providing access to the transport mechanism (Ruivo et al., 2012).

Patch-clamp recording of artificially enlarged lysosomes has been successfully used to study several lysosomal channels (Cang et al., 2014, 2015; Dong et al., 2010, 2008; Wang et al., 2012). However, it has not yet been applied to lysosomal transporters, presumably because these proteins are too slow and their currents too small for this technique (see Figure 2D in (Cang et al., 2015)). Electrophysiological recording of lysosomal transporters redirected to the plasma membrane with a high density provides a good alternative. Two techniques are commonly used depending on the expression system: two-electrode voltage-clamp (TEVC) of *Xenopus* oocytes and whole-cell patch-clamp (PC) of mammalian cells. These techniques have been extensively used to study plasma membrane channels and transporters. Choosing one or the other depends on the questions addressed and experimenter training. TEVC does not require specific skills but the cytosolic compartment cannot be controlled. On the other hand, PC provides control of both extracellular and intracellular compartments but takes more effort to master. When possible, combining both techniques is a good way to cross check results and possibly unveil peculiar functional properties.

### 6.5.2 VOLTAGE-CLAMP RECORDING IN *XENOPUS* OOCYTES

TEVC applied to *Xenopus* oocytes requires a specific amplifier able to quickly and consistently inject microampere currents to clamp the electrical membrane potential of these giant cells. Measurement of membrane potential (through the 'V' electrode) and positive or negative current injection (through the 'I' electrode) are achieved using two sharp micropipette electrodes impaled into the oocyte. In voltage-clamp setting, the amplitude of the injected current required to clamp the potential at a fixed value chosen by the experimenter depends on endogenous oocyte channels (background current) and on the activity of the expressed transporter. Changes in the injected current directly reflect in real time opposite current changes across the biological membrane. Activation of the transporter upon substrate application is thus directly reflected in the current channel of the amplifier with, by convention, negative currents when positive charges flow into the cell across the biological membrane.

#### 6.5.2.1 Making Recording Electrodes

In TEVC recording, oocytes expressing the lysosomal transporter targeted to the plasma membrane are impaled in a perfusion chamber using two electrodes made of borosilicate glass, filled with 3 M KCl and containing an Ag/AgCl filament. Making good TEVC electrodes is not straightforward and has been extensively detailed in the *Pipette Cookbook* from Sutter Instrument . Here is an example of a protocol with a P-97 puller hosting an FB255B heating filament (both from Sutter Instrument) and GC150TF-10 borosilicate glass capillaries (Harvard Apparatus):

$$HEAT = 564, PULL = /, VEL. = 60, TIME = 180$$

Although this protocol is a good starting point to get oocyte recording electrodes, it should be adapted depending on filament 'ageing', local humidity, room temperature, etc. RAMP parameters of filament heating are fine-tuned to compensate these variations.

The shape and diameter of the micropipette electrode's tip are critical. The diameter must be small enough to impale oocytes without altering membrane integrity, but large enough to keep electric resistance between 0.5 M$\Omega$ and 1.5 M$\Omega$. Voltage clamping of the large oocyte membrane may not be fast enough if the $I$ electrode resistance is higher than 1.5 M$\Omega$. The length of the tip must be long enough to facilitate impalement, but short enough to avoid proximity of the electrode tips within the oocyte as this would hinder clamping and generate artefacts. Putting a metal shield connected to the ground between the impaled micropipettes prevents their electrical coupling. These electrodes can be reused several times if their resistance stays below 1.5 M$\Omega$, indicating that the tip is not stuffy. If the tip is accidentally broken, resistance drops below 0.5 M$\Omega$ and the electrode should be discarded.

### 6.5.2.2 Recording Currents

An electrode is made of a silver filament coated with silver-chloride (AgCl) inserted into a glass micropipette. When a negative current is injected into the oocyte, electrons convert AgCl to silver atoms and chloride anions that diffuse inside the solution. Repeated measurements deplete chloride from electrodes and affect the quality of recordings. Electrodes must thus be properly coated with a thin layer of AgCl. This is achieved by dipping them into 5% active chlorine bleach for a few minutes prior to each experiment. Then, clean the electrode with distilled water and follow this step-by-step protocol:

(i) *Optional step*: If the recombinant transporter is fused to a fluorescent tag, sort well-expressing oocytes under a fluorescence microscope. This improves the reproducibility of recording across oocytes and avoids wasting time with negative or low-expressing oocytes.

(ii) Fill the two recording electrodes with 3 M KCl. If you face difficulties to fill the tip (presence of air bubbles), dip the electrode upside down into 3 M KCl to fill the tip by capillarity (GC150TF-10 capillaries contain a microfilament to help this step). Then, add more KCl through the micropipette base, insert the AgCl-coated silver filaments and mount the two electrodes on the TEVC system.

(iii) Transfer one oocyte with a Samco transfer pipette into a Petri dish filled with ND96 buffer (96 mM NaCl, 2 mM KCl, 1 mM $MgCl_2$, 1.8 mM $CaCl_2$, 5 mM Hepes adjusted to pH 7.4 with NaOH). Then deposit it into the perfusion chamber already containing ND96 solution. Some chambers have a small hole in the bottom to help position the oocyte. Make sure that the oocyte is not in contact with air as this will kill it by shear stress. If the cRNA has been injected into the animal pole, the oocyte should be oriented with this pole upside to facilitate perfusion of the transporter.

(iv) Position with micromanipulators the electrode tips near the oocyte surface. Just before impaling, reset the offset of each electrode to zero on the amplifier. Then, carefully impale the oocyte with each electrode until they indicate the native membrane potential (usually between −20 and −60 mV depending on oocyte batches). Sometimes, when oocytes lack elasticity, a gentle nudge to the micromanipulator axis facilitates impalement.

(v) Activate the flow of ND96. Perfusion facilitates oocyte stability. The flow of the reference (ND96) and test (for instance, ND96 + substrate) solutions should be similar to avoid mechanical artefacts when the solution is changed.

(vi) Test for membrane current stability by applying a voltage step protocol over time. An example is shown in Figure 6.3. Apply this protocol every 30 s. If currents are stable over at least 5 min, run the experiment (for instance, recording in the absence and presence of transporter substrate).

### 6.5.2.3  Experimental Tips

This section contains several tips that proved helpful to study lysosomal transporters with an oocyte TEVC system.

**Changes in ion composition and use of an agar–KCl bridge.** Experiments often require modifying the perfused medium. For instance, cationic substrates may be added to the solution as chloride salt. As lysosomal transporters usually possess low affinity for their substrates, this could significantly alter chloride concentrations. This will modify the half-cell potential of the Ag/AgCl reference ($V_{ref}$) electrode used in the bath to measure membrane voltage, thus altering voltage measurement and the clamp. This effect can be compensated by adding an identical amount of inactive small-molecule cation, for instance N-Methyl-D-glucamine chloride, to the control solution (i.e. that without substrate). This is possible only if a single concentration of substrate is tested, and if the inactive compound in the control solution does not affect the transporter activity. Otherwise, a common strategy to alter freely the ionic composition consists of adding an agar–KCl bridge to the perfusion chamber. This is a glass tube filled with 3 M KCl, 2% agar-agar matrix that connects the oocyte bath to a 3 M KCl well containing the $V_{ref}$ electrode. This bridge buffers changes in chloride concentration to keep the $V_{ref}$ half-cell potential at constant value. A bridge can be reused indefinitely if properly conserved in 3 M KCl solution between experiments.

**Use of acidic external solutions.** Lysosomal transporters are often coupled to proton export from the lysosome or kinetically activated when the lysosomal lumen, corresponding to the extracellular compartment in this assay, is acidic. Therefore, it is essential to measure transport currents in an acidic environment. We routinely use an ND96 buffered at pH 5.0 with 5 mM MES rather than Hepes. Oocytes survive for several hours at pH 5.0, but the background current first needs to be stabilized in this unusual environment. To reduce this stabilization period, oocytes may be

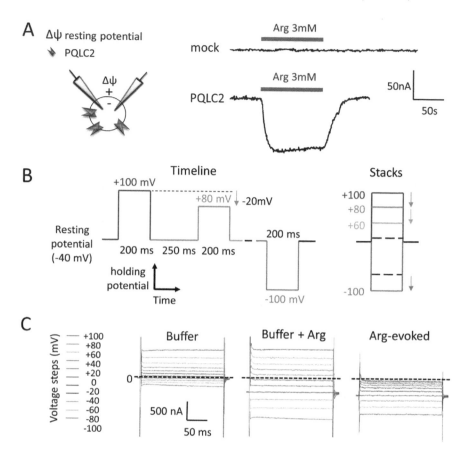

**FIGURE 6.3** Voltage-clamp analysis of lysosomal transporters in *Xenopus* oocytes. (A) Representative current traces of a water-injected oocyte ('mock') and an oocyte expressing the lysosomal transporter PQLC2 (mutant L290A/L291A) at the plasma membrane. Oocytes are clamped at −40 mV. Application of arginine at pH 5.0 induces an inward current in the PQLC2 oocyte, reflecting arginine influx through PQLC2. (B, C) Voltage jump protocol (B) and representative current traces (C) of a PQLC2 oocyte. Subtraction of the responses recorded in the presence and absence of arginine yields the arginine-evoked current carried by PQLC2. This current increases at hyperpolarizing (more negative) potentials. Unpublished data.

pre-incubated and impaled in this ND96 pH 5.0 buffer. In our hands, oocytes are damaged upon long incubations at a lower pH.

**Presence of internal nutrients.** The cytoplasm of *Xenopus* oocyte is rich in nutrients, including amino acids present at sub-mM to several mM levels (Bravo and Allende, 1976; Taylor et al., 1996). These levels may affect the behaviour of a recombinant transporter translocating such nutrients. This possibility should be considered when interpreting TEVC data. In some situations, for instance if the transporter of interest can be reversed, it may be possible to deplete these internal substrates by incubating oocytes for ≥1 hr in substrate-free medium before recording.

## 6.5.3   WHOLE-CELL PATCH-CLAMP RECORDING IN HEK293T CELLS

Like TEVC, PC study of misrouted lysosomal transporters essentially follows classical protocols used for plasma membrane transporters. In PC recording, a single Ag/AgCl electrode records membrane voltage and injects current to clamp the membrane potential at the chosen value. One of the main differences of whole-cell PC with TEVC in oocytes is that the cytosolic compartment of the cell is dialyzed with the medium in the micropipette. Therefore, the effect of cytosolic metabolites or cytosolic protein regulators can be studied by including them in the electrode solution. This dialysis also avoids accumulating substrates within the recorded cell, which might affect transport activity over time otherwise. Heterologous expression is usually done in HEK293T cells as protein is expressed to high levels and patch-clamping can be done efficiently in this cell line.

### 6.5.3.1   Cell Expression

HEK293T are grown and maintained in standard culture media (DMEM + GlutaMAX, 10% fetal calf serum, 1% Penicillin-Streptomycin; Gibco). We transfect them using Lipofectamine 2000 (Thermofisher) with plasmids like pEGFP-N vectors (now replaced by AcGFP1 vectors from Clontech) to fuse the protein of interest with a fluorescent tag and achieve good expression levels. Although facultative (and requiring preliminary experiments to assess its potential impact), the fluorescent tag facilitates detection of good-expressing cells for patching.

Recording requires a PC rig with a light stimulation system to screen for fluorescent cells. The optimal duration of expression is transporter-specific (see above) but could be as early as 24 h. On the day of experiment, check the expression level under a fluorescent microscope. Then, harvest by trypsinization and plate 150,000 transfected cells in a 35-mm culture dish containing glass coverslips coated with poly-D lysine. Cells must not contact each other, as gap-junction between neighbouring cells will prevent correct clamping and confound recordings. The use of glass coverslips will facilitate the transfer of a small quantity of cells in the perfusion chamber on the day of recording while keeping remaining cells in healthy conditions. A diamond cutter can split these coverslips into smaller pieces to increase the number of cells analyzed per batch. Wait at least 4 h to let cells adhere before running the experiment.

### 6.5.3.2   Electrode and Solutions

Cells are patched with electrodes made of borosilicate glass with a resistance between 3 M$\Omega$ and 5 M$\Omega$. Even more than TEVC electrodes, making good PC electrodes is not straightforward and is extensively detailed in the *Pipette Cookbook* from Sutter Instrument. Here is an example of a protocol with a P-97 puller hosting an FB255B heating filament and BF150-86-10 borosilicate glass capillaries (all from Sutter Instrument):

$$\text{HEAT} = 530, \ \text{PULL} = /, \ \text{VEL.} = 33, \ \text{DEL} = 1$$

The intrapipette solution composition varies depending on the property of the transporter (ion-coupling properties, etc.). Here is an example of classical intrapipette recipe: 130 mM KCl, 10 mM Hepes, 10 mM EGTA, 2 mM $CaCl_2$, 2 mM $MgCl_2$; pH adjusted with KOH and HCl. Osmolarity is usually around 295–305 mOsm and pH between 7.3 and 7.4 units. The extracellular solution is slightly more hypertonic (315–330 mOsm) to facilitate the seal between the electrode and the cell membrane. As mentioned for other assays, an acidic external buffer may be needed to activate the lysosomal transporter. Here is an example of composition: 140 mM NaCl, 5 mM KCl, 2 mM $CaCl_2$, 1 mM $MgCl_2$, 25 mM glucose, 20 mM MES, adjusted to pH 5.0 with NaOH and HCl.

### 6.5.3.3   Recording Currents

Before starting an experiment, make sure to coat the electrode filament with a thin layer of AgCl as described above. Then, follow this step-by-step protocol:

(i)   Take out transfected cells from the incubator and transfer one coverslip into a 35-mm culture dish containing PBS.

(ii)   Transfer the coverslip to the perfusion chamber of the patch-clamp rig already filled with external solution.

(iii)   Fill the electrode with internal solution. Prior dipping of the electrode's tip into this solution helps avoid stacking of air bubbles. Some capillaries contain a microfilament to facilitate this step. Then, mount the electrode on the holder and dip the tip into the solution. Check its resistance (3–5 M$\Omega$).

(iv)   At this point, HEK293T cells look like round, bright bubbles. If the recombinant transporter is fused to a fluorescent tag, look for a fluorescent cell with an even, bright membrane as these features usually correspond to healthy cells. Eventually, check that the cell adheres to the coverslip by gently shaking the PC chamber.

(v)   Position the perfusion system that will allow fast perfusion of the patched cell with compounds to test. Briefly activate the perfusion to make sure that the cell stays attached to the coverslip.

(vi)   Position the electrode near the cell, reset its offset to zero and patch the cell in whole-cell configuration.

   Optional stage: at this stage, if the seal is good, you may try to detach the cell from the coverslip by gently elevating the electrode with the micromanipulator. Although this is not critical, it might help stabilize the seal and increase the transport signal as the entire surface of the cell is perfused.

(vii)   Activate the fast perfusion system containing the external solution. The flow will facilitate membrane current stabilization and avoid artefacts when shifting solutions.

(viii)   Test for membrane current stability by applying a voltage step protocol over time (see Section 6.5.2 and 6.Figure 6.3) or a voltage ramp protocol as illustrated in Figure 6.4. Apply this protocol every 10 s three times. If membrane currents are stable, run the experiment.

### 6.5.3.4   Increasing the Transport Current Signal

Transport rate of small-molecule transporters is very low compared to channels that work orders of magnitude faster. Thus, it is critical to optimize every parameter to

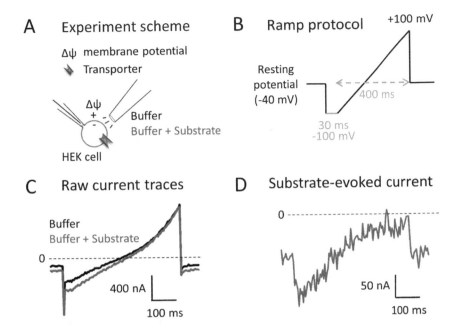

**A** Experiment scheme

Δψ membrane potential

Transporter

Δψ
+ −

Buffer
Buffer + Substrate

HEK cell

**B** Ramp protocol

+100 mV

Resting potential
(-40 mV)

400 ms

30 ms
-100 mV

**C** Raw current traces

Buffer
Buffer + Substrate

0

400 nA

100 ms

**D** Substrate-evoked current

0

50 nA

100 ms

**FIGURE 6.4** Whole-cell patch-clamp analysis of lysosomal transporters in HEK293T cells. Experiment scheme (A) and voltage ramp protocol (B) used to record the current response between −100 mV and +100 mV. Representative raw and subtracted current traces in a transfected HEK293T cell are shown in (C) and (D), respectively. Substrate application evokes an inward current at negative potentials.

facilitate detection of transport currents. An obvious one is to obtain a good expression level. Adding a fluorescent tag to the expressed protein allows one to focus on cells with the highest expression. Lowering the external pH may help increase the signal, as discussed above. HEK293T cells can survive for several hours at pH 5.0. Like with *Xenopus* oocytes, shifting the external pH from 7.0 to 5.0 alters endogenous membrane conductances that require time to stabilize. Incubating cells in pH 5.0 buffer before recording may shorten this step. Finally, the need to co-express an ancillary subunit or other interaction partners should be considered.

## 6.6 CONCLUSIONS

Detecting and characterizing the transport activity of lysosomal nutrient transporters poses several challenges due to their limited tractability, low substrate affinity and very slow transport rate compared to ion channels. Although classical radiotracer assays in isolated lysosomes remain a valuable approach, new methods have emerged to facilitate functional study of these proteins. Mutating lysosomal sorting motifs to redirect them to the plasma membrane allows the monitoring of their transport activity in mammalian cells or *Xenopus* oocytes using diverse techniques such as radiotracer assays and electrophysiological recording. Alternately, their activity can be indirectly assessed in lysosomes of live cells by taking advantage of adaptive cell responses to lysosomal overload. These responses, such as the nuclear translocation of the master gene for lysosomal biogenesis TFEB, provide a proxy to monitor lysosomal overload of specific compounds and its rescue by cognate lysosomal exporters.

## ACKNOWLEDGEMENTS

The related work in the Gasnier laboratory is supported by grants from the Agence Nationale de la Recherche (# ANR-18-CE11-0009-01) and the Cystinosis Research Foundation (# CRFS-2014-004).

## REFERENCES

Abu-Remaileh, M., Wyant, G.A., Kim, C., Laqtom, N.N., Abbasi, M., Chan, S.H., Freinkman, E., and Sabatini, D.M. (2017). Lysosomal metabolomics reveals V-ATPase and mTOR-dependent regulation of amino acid efflux from lysosomes. *Science 358*(6364), 807–813.

Berg, T.O., Strømhaug, P.E., Løvdal, T., Seglen, P.O., and Berg, T. (1994). Use of glycyl-l-phenylalanine 2-naphthylamide, a lysosome-disrupting cathepsin C substrate, to distinguish between lysosomes and prelysosomal endocytic vacuoles. *Biochem. J. 300*(1), 229–236.

Braulke, T., and Bonifacino, J.S. (2009). Sorting of lysosomal proteins. *Biochim. Biophys. Acta 1793*(4), 605–614.

Bravo, R., and Allende, J.E. (1976). Conditions affecting protein synthesis in amphibian oocytes. *Arch. Biochem. Biophys. 172*(2), 648–653.

Cang, C., Aranda, K., Seo, Y., Gasnier, B., and Ren, D. (2015). TMEM175 is an organelle K(+) channel regulating lysosomal function. *Cell 162*(5), 1101–1112.

Cang, C., Bekele, B., and Ren, D. (2014). The voltage-gated sodium channel TPC1 confers endolysosomal excitability. *Nat. Chem. Biol. 10*(6), 463–469.

Cang, C., Zhou, Y., Navarro, B., Seo, Y.J., Aranda, K., Shi, L., Battaglia-Hsu, S., Nissim, I., Clapham, D.E., and Ren, D. (2013). MTOR regulates lysosomal ATP-sensitive two-pore Na+ channels to adapt to metabolic state. *Cell 152*(4), 778–790.

Chapel, A., Kieffer-Jaquinod, S., Sagné, C., Verdon, Q., Ivaldi, C., Mellal, M., Thirion, J., Jadot, M., Bruley, C., Garin, J., et al. (2013). An extended proteome map of the lysosomal membrane reveals novel potential transporters. *Mol. Cell. Proteomics 12*(6), 1572–1588.

Dong, X., Shen, D., Wang, X., Dawson, T., Li, X., Zhang, Q., Cheng, X., Zhang, Y., Weisman, L.S., Delling, M., and Xu, H. (2010). PI(3,5)P(2) controls membrane trafficking by direct activation of mucolipin Ca(2+) release channels in the endolysosome. *Nat. Commun. 1*, 38.

Dong, X.P., Cheng, X., Mills, E., Delling, M., Wang, F., Kurz, T., and Xu, H. (2008). The type IV mucolipidosis-associated protein TRPML1 is an endolysosomal iron release channel. *Nature 455*(7215), 992–996.

Gahl, W.A., Bashan, N., Tietze, F., Bernardini, I., and Schulman, J.D. (1982). Cystine transport is defective in isolated leukocyte lysosomes from patients with cystinosis. *Science 217*(4566), 1263–1265.

Goldman, R., and Kaplan, A. (1973). Rupture of rat liver lysosomes mediated by L-amino acid esters. *Biochim. Biophys. Acta 318*(2), 205–216.

Jézégou, A., Llinares, E., Anne, C., Kieffer-Jaquinod, S., O'Regan, S., Aupetit, J., Chabli, A., Sagné, C., Debacker, C., Chadefaux-Vekemans, B., et al. (2012). Heptahelical protein PQLC2 is a lysosomal cationic amino acid exporter underlying the action of cysteamine in cystinosis therapy. *Proc. Natl. Acad. Sci. U. S. A. 109*(50), E3434–3443.

Kalatzis, V., Cherqui, S., Antignac, C., and Gasnier, B. (2001). Cystinosin, the protein defective in cystinosis, is a H(+)-driven lysosomal cystine transporter. *EMBO J. 20*(21), 5940–5949.

Kalatzis, V., Nevo, N., Cherqui, S., Gasnier, B., and Antignac, C. (2004). Molecular pathogenesis of cystinosis: Effect of CTNS mutations on the transport activity and subcellular localization of cystinosin. *Hum. Mol. Genet. 13*(13), 1361–1371.

Lorenz, C., Pusch, M., and Jentsch, T.J. (1996). Heteromultimeric CLC chloride channels with novel properties. *Proc. Natl. Acad. Sci. U. S. A. 93*(23), 13362–13366.

Mancini, G.M.S., De Jonge, H.R., Galjaard, H., and Verheijen, F.W. (1989). Characterization of a proton-driven carrier for sialic acid in the lysosomal membrane. Evidence for a group-specific transport system for acidic monosaccharides. *J. Biol. Chem. 264*(26), 15247–15254.

Martina, J.A., Chen, Y., Gucek, M., and Puertollano, R. (2012). MTORC1 functions as a transcriptional regulator of autophagy by preventing nuclear transport of TFEB. *Autophagy 8*(6), 903–914.

Morin, P., Sagne, C., and Gasnier, B. (2004). Functional characterization of wild-type and mutant human sialin. *EMBO J. 23*(23), 4560–4570.

Okumoto, S., Jones, A., and Mer, W.B. (2012). Quantitative imaging with fluorescent biosensors. *Annu. Rev. Plant Biol. 63*, 663–706.

Pisoni, R.L., and Thoene, J.G. (1991). The transport systems of mammalian lysosomes. *Biochim. Biophys. Acta 1071*(4), 351–373.

Puertollano, R., Ferguson, S.M., Brugarolas, J., and Ballabio, A. (2018). The complex relationship between TFEB transcription factor phosphorylation and subcellular localization. *EMBO J. 37*(11), 1–12.

Reeves, J. (1979). Accumulation of amino acids by lysosomes incubated with amino acid methyl esters. *J. Biol. Chem. 254*(18), 8914–8921.

Repnik, U., Distefano, M.B., Speth, M.T., Wui Ng, M.Y., Progida, C., Hoflack, B., Gruenberg, J., and Griffiths, G. (2017). L-leucyl-L-leucine methyl ester does not release cysteine cathepsins to the cytosol but inactivates them in transiently permeabilized lysosomes. *J. Cell Sci. 130*(18), 3124–3140.

Roczniak-Ferguson, A., Petit, C.S., Froehlich, F., Qian, S., Ky, J., Angarola, B., Walther, T.C., and Ferguson, S.M. (2012). The transcription factor TFEB links mTORC1 signaling to transcriptional control of lysosome homeostasis. *Sci. Signal. 5*(228), ra42.

Ruivo, R., Bellenchi, G.C.G.C., Chen, X., Zifarelli, G., Sagné, C., Debacker, C., Pusch, M., Supplisson, S., Gasnier, B., Sagneá, C., et al. (2012). Mechanism of proton/substrate coupling in the heptahelical lysosomal transporter cystinosin. *Proc. Natl. Acad. Sci. U. S. A. 109*(5), E210–E217.

Sardiello, M., Palmieri, M., di Ronza, A., Medina, D.L., Valenza, M., Gennarino, V.A., Di Malta, C., Donaudy, F., Embrione, V., Polishchuk, R.S., et al. (2009). A gene network regulating lysosomal biogenesis and function. *Science 325*(5939), 473–477.

Savalas, L.R.T.L.R.T., Gasnier, B., Damme, M., Lübke, T., Wrocklage, C., Debacker, C., Jézégou, A., Reinheckel, T., Hasilik, A., Saftig, P., et al. (2011). Disrupted in renal carcinoma 2 (DIRC2), a novel transporter of the lysosomal membrane, is proteolytically processed by cathepsin L. *Biochem. J. 439*(1), 113–128.

Settembre, C., Zoncu, R., Medina, D.L., Vetrini, F., Erdin, S., Erdin, S., Huynh, T., Ferron, M., Karsenty, G., Vellard, M.C., et al. (2012). A lysosome-to-nucleus signalling mechanism senses and regulates the lysosome via mTOR and TFEB. *EMBO J. 31*(5), 1095–1108.

Storch, S., Pohl, S., and Braulke, T. (2004). A dileucine motif and a cluster of acidic amino acids in the second cytoplasmic domain of the batten disease-related CLN3 protein are required for efficient lysosomal targeting. *J. Biol. Chem. 279*(51), 53625–53634.

Storch, S., Pohl, S., Quitsch, A., Falley, K., and Braulke, T. (2007). C-terminal prenylation of the CLN3 membrane glycoprotein is required for efficient endosomal sorting to lysosomes. *Traffic 8*(4), 431–444.

Takanaga, H., Mackenzie, B., Suzuki, Y., and Hediger, M.A. (2005). Identification of mammalian proline transporter SIT1 (SLC6A20) with characteristics of classical system imino. *J. Biol. Chem.* *280*(10), 8974–8984.

Taylor, P.M., Kaur, S., Mackenzie, B., and Peter, G.J. (1996). Amino-acid-dependent modulation of amino acid transport in Xenopus laevis oocytes. *J. Exp. Biol.* *199*(4), 923–931.

Thiele, D.L., and Lipsky, P.E. (1990). Mechanism of L-leucyl-L-leucine methyl ester-mediated killing of cytotoxic lymphocytes: Dependence on a lysosomal thiol protease, dipeptidyl peptidase I, that is enriched in these cells. *Proc. Natl. Acad. Sci. U. S. A.* *87*(1), 83–87.

Verdon, Q., Boonen, M., Ribes, C., Jadot, M., Gasnier, B., and Sagné, C. (2017). SNAT7 is the primary lysosomal glutamine exporter required for extracellular protein-dependent growth of cancer cells. *Proc. Natl. Acad. Sci. U. S. A.* *114*(18), E3602–E3611.

Wang, X., Zhang, X., Dong, X.P., Samie, M., Li, X., Cheng, X., Goschka, A., Shen, D., Zhou, Y., Harlow, J., et al. (2012). TPC proteins are phosphoinositide- activated sodium-selective ion channels in endosomes and lysosomes. *Cell* *151*(2), 372–383.

Wreden, C.C., Wlizla, M., and Reimer, R.J. (2005). Varied mechanisms underlie the free sialic acid storage disorders. *J. Biol. Chem.* *280*(2), 1408–1416.

Xiong, J., He, J., Xie, W.P., Hinojosa, E., Ambati, C.S.R., Putluri, N., Kim, H.E., Zhu, M.X., and Du, G. (2019). Rapid affinity purification of intracellular organelles using a twin strep tag. *J. Cell Sci.* *132*(24), jcs235390.

# 7 Lysosomal Vitamin B12 Trafficking

*Sean Froese and Matthias R. Baumgartner*

## CONTENTS

## 7.1 INTRODUCTION

Vitamin $B_{12}$ (cobalamin, Cbl) is required as cofactor for two essential human enzymes: cytosolic methionine synthase and mitochondrial methylmalonyl-CoA mutase. In order to reach these destination enzymes in the correct cofactor forms, Cbl must be taken up, modified and transported across the cell (Figure 7.1). Cellular entry of Cbl occurs through receptor mediated endocytosis, by which Cbl bound

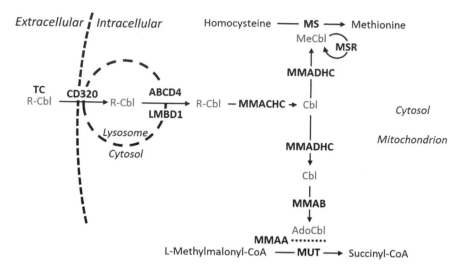

**FIGURE 7.1**   Intracellular cobalamin metabolism. Arrows depict enzymatic reactions or transport across membranes. Protein names are in bold. Cobalamin forms are in red. R-Cbl: cobalamin containing any upper-axial ligand. Cbl: cobalamin with no upper-axial ligand. Me-Cbl: methylcobalamin. Ado-Cbl: adenosylcobalamin. TC: transcobalamin. CD320: transcobalamin receptor. ABCD4: ATP-binding cassette subfamily D member 4. LBMD1: lipocalin-1 interacting membrane receptor domain containing 1. MMACHC: methylmalonic aciduria cblC-type with homocystinuria. MMADHC: methylmalonic aciduria cblD-type with homocystinuria. MS: methionine synthase. MSR: methionine synthase reductase. MMAB: methylmalonic aciduria type B. MMAA: methylmalonic aciduria type A. MUT: methylmalonyl-CoA mutase.

to the carrier protein transcobalamin is recognized by its nascent receptor CD320 (also known as the transcobalamin receptor, TCblR). Following progressive acidification in the transition from early- to late-endosomes, and finally lysosomes, the engulfed transcobalamin is degraded and Cbl is released. Free Cbl is then exported from the lysosome into the cytosol, where a series of metabolic steps results in the production of methyl-Cbl, the cofactor form for methionine synthase, or in transport into the mitochondria and the conversion to adenosyl-Cbl, the cofactor form for methylmalonyl-CoA mutase. Methionine synthase (E.C. 2.1.1.13), as part of the methionine cycle, is responsible for the production of methionine and ultimately S-adenosylmethionine. Methylmalonyl-CoA mutase (E.C. 5.4.99.2), a component of the propionate catabolic pathway for branched-chain amino acids, odd-chain fatty acids and the side chain of cholesterol, funnels catabolic intermediates into the tricarboxylic acid cycle.

The final production of the Cbl cofactor forms requires successful export of Cbl from the lysosome into the cytosol, but the exact mechanism through which this takes place is poorly understood. Based on genetic and experimental evidence, this export requires the concerted actions of two integral membrane proteins – ABCD4 and LMBD1. Cells from patients with inherited mutations in either *ABCD4* (Coelho et al., 2012) (which encodes ABCD4) or *LMBRD1* (Rutsch et al., 2009) (which encodes LMBD1) have been shown to accumulate free Cbl in their lysosomes (Coelho et al., 2012; Watkins and Rosenblatt, 1986), resulting in combined deficiency of methionine synthase and methylmalonyl-CoA mutase due to an inability to produce both the methyl-Cbl and adenosyl-Cbl cofactor forms. Although the explicit contribution to lysosomal Cbl export by both proteins has yet to be elucidated, it is tempting to rationalize their functions by comparison with their protein family members. LMBD1 (lipocalin membrane receptor domain containing protein 1) is so named due to its resemblance to the lipocalin membrane receptor (LIMR), which binds and internalizes lipocalins – small secreted proteins which bind protoporphin IX among other ligands (Dufour et al., 1990). With this in mind, a receptor–transporter role has been suggested for LMBD1 in Cbl transport (Rutsch et al., 2009). ABCD4 by contrast, is part of the ATP-binding cassette transporter subfamily D, whose closest members (ABCD1–3) are all located on peroxisomal membranes and function as importers (Contreras et al., 1994; Kamijo et al., 1990; Lombard-Platet et al., 1996; Mosser et al., 1994). This is suggestive of a direct transport function of Cbl for ABCD4. Unlike the other ABCD family members, ABCD4 lacks the N-terminal peroxisomal targeting motif (Lee et al., 2014) and is therefore not sorted towards the peroxisome. Singly over-expressed ABCD4 has been found in the endoplasmic reticulum (ER) (Kashiwayama et al., 2009) and autophagosomes (Fettelschoss et al., 2017), suggesting retention and degradation of mis-targeted or poorly folded protein. ABCD4 over-expressed in the presence of LMBD1, however, has been found to correctly localize to the lysosome (Fettelschoss et al., 2017; Kawaguchi et al., 2016), suggesting a targeting/chaperoning role of LMBD1 for ABCD4. This role is further supported by the fact that LMBD1 is heavily glycosylated (Rutsch et al., 2009), while ABCD4 appears not to be (Kashiwayama et al., 2009). Thus, the protective role of LMBD1 for ABCD4 may extend to their roles within the lysosome, as well as in transit. Although these putative roles have yet to be confirmed, the above data strongly suggests that ABCD4 and LMBD1 must physically interact to successfully carry out their physiological functions. This interaction has been shown in live cells (Fettelschoss et al., 2017) using a protocol detailed later in this chapter.

Following lysosomal release, Cbl is metabolized and chaperoned by the cytosolic protein MMACHC (Hannibal et al., 2009; Kim et al., 2008), which is targeted either to methionine synthase, together with its accessory protein methionine synthase reductase, or to the mitochondria, by the protein MMADHC (Coelho et al., 2008; Suormala et al., 2004). Methyl-Cbl, the cofactor form, is created on methionine synthase and maintained by methionine synthase reductase (Olteanu and Banerjee, 2001). Within the mitochondria, the protein MMAB is responsible for the formation of adenosyl-Cbl (Leal et al., 2003), which is delivered to methylmalonyl-CoA mutase in a reaction that is gated by the accessory protein MMAA (Padovani and Banerjee, 2009). Loss of function in any of the intermediate or final steps of Cbl cofactor synthesis, including impeded lysosomal Cbl release, disrupts the function of methionine synthase, methylmalonyl-CoA mutase, or both. With this in mind, assays measuring correct cofactor synthesis or of individual Cbl-dependent enzyme function can be exploited to determine indirectly the activity of the lysosomal Cbl enzymes. These "tricks" allow one to investigate the determinants of lysosomal export without having to know the specific components involved.

Here we present several protocols which may be used to indirectly measure the function of lysosomal vitamin $B_{12}$ trafficking. In the most straightforward approach, the first protocol measures the ability of cells to correctly produce the Cbl cofactor forms methyl- and adenosyl-Cbl following incubation with radio-labelled cyano-[$^{57}$Co]-Cbl. The second protocol, by contrast, follows the incorporation of [$^{14}$C]-propionate into acid precipitable proteins in intact cells. This assay is dependent on the correct function of adenosyl-Cbl bound methylmalonyl-CoA mutase, and is therefore indirectly dependent on proper lysosomal Cbl release. Both of these assays are very sensitive due to their use of radioactive material and have become routine assays in the diagnosis of intracellular Cbl disorders, including those affecting lysosomal function. Using primary or immortalized cells, they allow determination of lysosomal vitamin $B_{12}$ function without requiring detailed knowledge of the individual steps involved, and can succeed at the very low level at which the endogenous proteins are expressed. The third approach, by contrast, uses a flow-cytometer to measure Förster resonance energy transfer (FRET) between tagged over-expressed proteins of interest in live cells. This targeted approach provides a quantitative evaluation of physical interaction between any two lysosomal membrane proteins, including but not limited to proteins in the Cbl metabolic pathway.

In the coming sections, each of these approaches and their advantages will be discussed in turn, and detailed protocols suitable to perform these assays are provided.

## 7.2 COBALAMIN COFACTOR SYNTHESIS ASSAY

### 7.2.1 OVERVIEW AND ADVANTAGES

The cobalamin coenzyme synthesis assay monitors the uptake of radio-labelled, non-physiological cyano-([$^{57}$Co])-Cbl, and follows its intracellular conversion to hydroxo-Cbl and ultimately the cofactor forms adenosyl-Cbl and methyl-Cbl (Figure 7.2). It is therefore sensitive to the entire cellular metabolic Cbl pathway, including processing through the lysosomal compartment, and allows one to pinpoint the nature of the cellular defect of Cbl metabolism, regardless of its protein/organelle of nature. From the point of view of lysosomal investigation, this allows the researcher to assay any condition (e.g. small molecules, gene knock-out) that may result in alteration of lysosomal Cbl release. This method was originally described by Mahoney and Rosenberg (Mahoney and Rosenberg, 1971) and modified by Mellmen and colleagues (Mellman

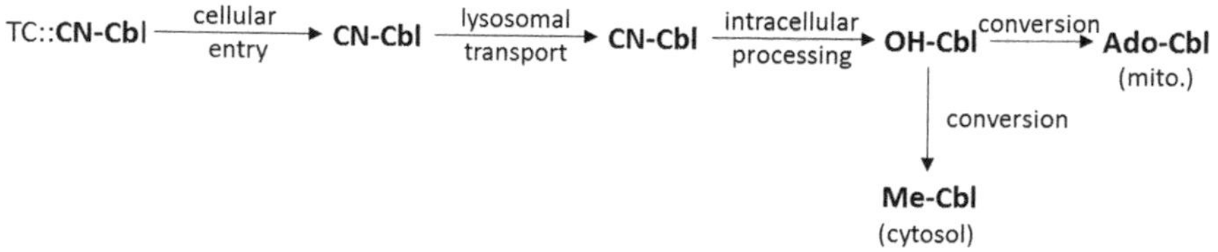

**FIGURE 7.2** Uptake, transport and modification of Cbl in the cobalamin cofactor synthesis assay. Radio-labelled cyano-Cbl (CN-Cbl) is provided to the cells bound to transcobalamin (TC). Cbl transported through the cells is modified to hydroxo-Cbl (OH-Cbl) and finally converted to the cofactor forms methyl-Cbl (Me-Cbl) and adenosyl-Cbl (Ado-Cbl).

et al., 1978). Here we present the updated method with our own modifications including the reagents and equipment used in our laboratory.

## 7.2.2 DETAILED PROTOCOL

### 7.2.2.1 Cell Preparation and Cyano-[57Co]-Cbl Incubation

Human adherent cells (e.g. fibroblasts, HEK293) with or without treatment (e.g. transfection, small molecule incubation) are cultured in T25cm$^2$ culture flasks (TPP) in routine culture medium consisting of Dulbecco's Modified Eagle's Medium (DMEM/F12 + GlutaMax™, Gibco) supplemented with 10% (v/v) foetal calf serum (FCS, Gibco) and 1% antibiotic-antimycotic mixture (penicillin 10,000 IU/mL, streptomycin 10,000 µg/mL, amphotericin B 25 µg/mL, Gibco). Concurrently, in the dark or under a red safelight (Dr. Fischer), cyano-[57Co]-Cbl (stock 10.5 µCi and 25 pg/mL, ICN Pharmaceuticals) is added to normal human serum (1 µL [57Co]-B$_{12}$ Tracer Stock/mL serum), covered with aluminium foil and pre-incubated for 30 min at 37°C to bind the labelled cobalamin to human transcobalamin. This serum is then added to DMEM/F12 + GlutaMax supplemented with 1% antibiotic-antimycotic (final concentration, 1:10 serum to medium) and filter-sterilized. Upon reaching 80–100% confluence, cells are first washed with 5 mL DMEM/F12 + GlutaMax to remove the FCS, then each flask is incubated with 2 mL of the filter-sterilized radio-labelled medium. Incubation takes place in a cell incubator at 37°C supplemented with 5% CO$_2$ for three days while covered in aluminium foil to prevent light exposure.

### 7.2.2.2 Total Counts Determination and Cobalamin Extraction

Following three days of incubation, the $^{57}$Co-labelled medium is removed under red safelight, cells are washed with phosphate-buffered saline (PBS, Ca$^{2+}$ and Mg$^{2+}$-free; Gibco) and then harvested using 0.25% Trypsin-EDTA (Gibco). Harvested cells are pelleted by centrifugation for 10 min at 350 × $g$ and resuspended in 5 mL PBS. A 1-mL aliquot of suspended cells is then transferred to microfuge tubes, pelleted by centrifugation (5 min at 350 × $g$) and put aside for determination of total radioactive counts measured by a gamma counter (see Section 7.3.4) as well as protein concentration determination, e.g. by the Lowry method (Lowry et al., 1951). The remaining 4 mL cell suspensions are centrifuged for 10 min at 350 × $g$, the supernatant removed and the pellet used for the extraction of cobalamins. In order to visualize the cobalamin peaks via high-performance liquid chromatography (HPLC, see Section 7.3.3), a 20 µl solution containing 1 mg/mL, each of adenosyl-Cbl, methyl-Cbl, cyano-Cbl and hydroxo-Cbl (all from Sigma-Aldrich; dissolved together in deionized water in the dark), is spiked into the cell pellet. Total cellular Cbl derivatives are then extracted from the cells by addition of 1 mL of 100% ethanol to the cell pellet. Resuspended cells are then incubated at 80°C for 10 min centrifuged at 350 × $g$ for 5 min and the supernatant transferred to a fresh tube. A further 1 mL of 100% ethanol is then added to the cell pellet and the procedure repeated in order to ensure all cobalamin derivatives have been recovered. Following the addition of both ethanol supernatants, the ethanol is removed by incubation at 80°C and flushing with nitrogen gas. When cooled to room temperature, the extracted cobalamins form a pellet which can be dissolved by the addition of 80 μL of 0.05 M phosphoric acid (titrated to pH 3.0 with concentrated ammonium hydroxide) which is then incubated at room temperature for 15 min with intermittent vortexing. Solubilized samples are transferred to a fresh microfuge tube and centrifuged for 5 min at 350 × $g$ to remove any undissolved materials. The final supernatant is then moved to a fresh microfuge tube and used for the next steps.

### 7.2.2.3   Separation of Radio-Labelled Cobalamins by HPLC

Cobalamin derivatives are separated by HPLC following a modified protocol first described by Jacobsen et al. (1982). For each sample, 40 μL is injected using a 50 μL glass syringe (Hamilton) at a flow-rate of 1 mL/min (Jasco PU-2089). Cobalamins are separated by a Lichrosorb RP-C8 column (Supelco) using a gradient of increasing concentration of 0.05 M phosphoric acid, pH 3.0 in 30% (v/v) acetonitrile (Buffer B). In this programme, over the first 15 min the concentration of Buffer B increases from 0% to 54% in the presence of 0.05 M phosphoric acid, pH 3.0 (Buffer A). Following this, a concentration of 54% Buffer B is maintained for a further 10 min (min 16–25), after which the concentration is increased to 100% Buffer B for 10 min (min 26–35). Fractions should be collected beginning 15 min after injection, with 48 fractions in total collected by changing the fraction every 22 seconds. Using this method, the expected retention times are: hydroxo-Cbl, 17–19 min (fractions: 6–12); cyano-Cbl, 18–20 min (fractions: 10–17); adenosyl-Cbl 26–29 min (fractions: 33–40); and methyl-Cbl 30–31 min (fractions: 42–45). These can be verified and refined by monitoring the retention of unlabelled cobalamins previously spiked into each sample by using a UV/Vis detector (Jasco UV-2070 Plus) at 254 nm.

### 7.2.2.4   Gamma Counting

Each fraction is moved to a gamma counter (e.g. LB2111, Berthold) which measures the gamma radiation emitted by the $^{57}$Co radionuclides. The total counts from the original input sample, as well from each fraction, should be subtracted from background counts taken from empty fractions to give corrected values. A histogram can then be created using the remaining counts per minute (cpm) values (Figure 7.3). If

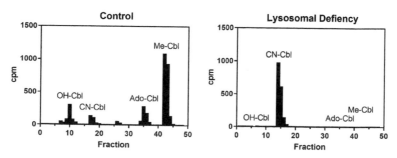

**FIGURE 7.3**   Histograms displaying radioactive counts of Cbl subtypes following separation by HPLC. Left panel: control fibroblasts (Control). In total, OH-Cb constitutes 14.7% of total radioactive counts, CN-Cbl: 7.6%, Ado-Cbl: 15.4%, Me-Cbl: 56.0%. Right panel: fibroblasts with dysfunctional LMBD (Lysosomal Deficiency). In total, OH-Cbl constitutes 1.8% of total radioactive counts, CN-Cbl: 94.8%, Ado-Cbl: 0.4%, Me-Cbl: 0.9%.

desired, the sum cpm in all fractions belonging to the same peak can be combined and compared against the sum total cpm of each sample, in order to determine the relative concentration of each cobalamin compound.

### 7.2.3 CONCLUSIONS

In all, this method allows evaluation of whether there is a block in the synthesis of the Cbl cofactor forms, and identification of where that block might be. In terms of lysosomal Cbl trafficking, it enables determination of the conditions under which Cbl is allowed or prevented to be released, visualized as conversion to hydroxo-, methyl- and adenosyl-Cbl, or a strong prevalence of cyano-Cbl, respectively.

## 7.3 [14C]-PROPIONATE INCORPORATION

### 7.3.1 OVERVIEW, ADVANTAGES AND CONSIDERATIONS

The [$^{14}$C]-propionate incorporation assay measures the amount of radio-labelled [$^{14}$C]-propionic acid that is incorporated into cellular macromolecules in intact cells. This assay utilizes the endogenous propionate catabolic pathway which feeds into the tricarboxylic acid (TCA) cycle, and makes use of the fact that TCA cycle intermediates are scavenged for the formation of various amino acids (Figure 7.4). This incorporation requires functional adenosyl-Cbl-dependent methylmalonyl-CoA mutase activity, and hence the successful intracellular metabolism of vitamin B$_{12}$. It

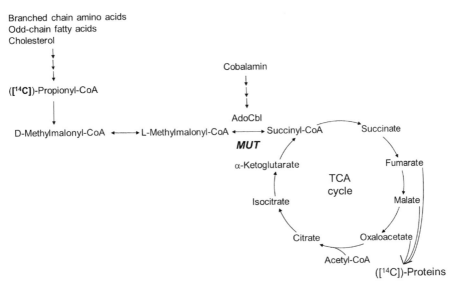

**FIGURE 7.4** Incorporation of $^{14}$C-propionyl-CoA into proteins through the propionic acid and tricarboxylic acid (TCA) metabolic pathways. Not depicted: conversion of [$^{14}$C]-propionate to [$^{14}$C]-propionyl-CoA, likely by acyl CoA synthetase. Arrows from fumarate, malate and oxaloacetate to proteins are for visualization; [$^{14}$C] may be incorporated into proteins from other TCA cycle intermediates.

is therefore used as a diagnostic assay for the establishment of intracellular cobala-min metabolism deficiency, as well as propionyl-CoA deficiency, or holocarboxylase synthetase deficiency. In the situation of a functional metabolic pathway, the addi-tion of radio-labelled propionate into cells results in the production of radio-labelled proteins (Figure 7.4). However, alterations in the function of any pathway step for the synthesis of adenosyl-Cbl, including lysosomal processing and release, results in a loss of TCA cycle intermediates arising from this pathway, and therefore decreased [$^{14}$C]-propionate incorporation into proteins. Additionally, the total incorporation is dependent on many variables (cell type, length of overnight incubation, media used), which means, among other things, that appropriate controls must be included each time this assay is performed. The methods presented here are an updated version of the original, first published by Willard et al. (1976).

## 7.3.2 Detailed Protocol

### 7.3.2.1 Cell Culture Conditions

In its capacity as a diagnostic assay, the [$^{14}$C]-propionate assay is routinely performed with cultured human skin fibroblasts from suspected patients and controls. However, like the Cbl cofactor synthesis assay, it is in principle compatible with any *in vitro* cultured mammalian cell line since it involves a metabolic pathway present in all mammalian cells.

Routine cell culture conditions as outlined in Section 7.2.2.1 should be used. Cells in T25cm$^2$ culture flasks in DMEM/F12 + GlutaMax™ supplemented with 10% FCS and 1x antibiotic-antimycotic are incubated at 37°C supplemented with 5% CO$_2$. We customarily prepare six flasks per experimental condition, three without and three with supplementation of 1 µg/mL hydroxo-Cbl (Sigma) to the media. Hydroxo-Cbl supplementation allows distinguishing between minor (or K$_m$) deficiencies and true blocks of pathway function for adenosyl-Cbl synthesis. Once cells are fully conflu-ent, the media should be aspirated and exchanged for 2 mL filter-sterilized assay medium containing Earle's Balanced Salt Solution (Gibco) supplemented with 5% FCS, 1.0 µCi/mL [$^{14}$C]-propionic acid (American radio-labelled chemicals, USA; catalog #ARC 0203A-50 µCi), 0.2 mM cold propionate (Sigma) and 1x antibiotic-antimycotic. Cells are incubated in this media overnight.

### 7.3.2.2 Cell Harvest and Trichloroacetic Acid (TCA) Extraction

The next day, for each flask the medium is removed and the cells are washed three times with PBS followed by detachment by the addition of 500 µL 0.25% Trypsin-EDTA. Once the cells are detached, the trypsin reaction is stopped by the addition of 1.5 mL stop solution (15% (v/v) FCS in PBS) and the cells are transferred to 10 mL conical tubes. The flasks are washed three more times with 2 mL of PBS each, adding each wash to the cell suspension in the conical tubes. The conical tubes are centrifuged at 200 × g for 10 min to sediment the cells. The supernatant is discarded, the cell pellet is washed with 3 mL of PBS and centrifugation is repeated, discarding the supernatant once more. The pellet is resuspended in 500 µL of 10% (w/v) TCA (Sigma) in PBS, vortexed well and incubated on ice for 10 min. Following incuba-tion, the sample is centrifuged at 200 × g, the supernatant is completely removed and the cell pellet is resuspended in 150 µL of 1 M NaOH.

### 7.3.2.3 Beta-Counting of Cell Homogenate

For each sample, 50 μL of resuspended cell pellet is added to Pico Prias (PerkinElmer) or equivalent vials containing 3 mL of scintillation cocktail (e.g. Optiphase Hisafe II; PerkinElmer). The rest of the cell homogenate can be stored at −20°C and used for determination of protein concentration, e.g. by the Lowry method. As controls, 50 μL of NaOH is added to 3 mL of scintillation cocktail (negative control), and 50 μL of $^{14}$C-propionate medium is added to 3 mL of scintillation cocktail (total input control). Close the vials, mix well and use a beta-counter (e.g. Tri-Carb C1900TR; PerkinElmer) to determine radioactive counts per minute (cpm) for each sample at least twice.

### 7.3.2.4 Results Calculation

Calculate the mean cpm of each sample vial, and subtract the mean cpm found in the negative control (background). This will provide the corrected cpm for each sample (see example below). To determine the amount of propionate (in pmols) per cpm, first calculate the corrected cpm for the total input control. Since the amount of total propionate ($^{14}$C-propionate + cold propionate ≈ 0.2 mM) in this sample is known, dividing the number of pmols propionate per 50 μL of medium by the corrected cpm of the total input control will provide the amount of propionate that corresponds to 1 cpm. This is shown in the following example:

- Determination of corrected cpm:
  - 221,416 cpm (total input) − 12 cpm (background) = 221,404 cpm (corrected)
- Determination of concentration (pmol) of propionate:
  - 0.0175 mM ($^{14}$C-propionate) + 0.1825 mM (cold propionate) = 0.200 mM (total propionate)
  - -corresponds to 200 μmol/L or 10,000 pmol/50 μL
- Determination of amount of propionate that corresponds to 1 cpm:
  - 10,000 pmol / 221,404 cpm = 0.045 pmol/cpm

With these values, the corrected cpm of each sample can be converted to the amount of incorporated propionate. By further relating the concentration of protein (in mg) per 50 μL sample, the amount of pmols propionate/mg of protein can finally be determined.

### 7.3.3 CONCLUSIONS

The $^{14}$C-propionate incorporation assay is a versatile technique which allows indirect determination of lysosomal Cbl release by utilizing a metabolic pathway which requires the adenosyl-Cbl cofactor form. By comparison to the cobalamin cofactor synthesis assay, the $^{14}$C-propionate incorporation assay requires less specialized equipment (e.g. no HPLC) and is therefore easier to perform, but, as an endpoint only assay, has the disadvantage that one cannot easily identify which aspect of the propionyl-CoA catabolic or adenosyl-Cbl synthesis pathway is dysfunctional when incorporation into proteins is low. Therefore, this assay is best used as a screening tool to identify conditions under which total synthesis is blocked, which can then be followed up by other assays to determine the nature of the block.

## 7.4   FLOW CYTOMETRY-BASED FRET

### 7.4.1   Overview and Advantages

In contrast to the previous assays illustrated in this chapter, which enable indirect evaluation of lysosomal function and do not require knowledge of the proteins involved, flow cytometry-based FRET instead allows evaluation of the physical interaction between two known proteins of interest, regardless of their contribution to overall function. This method can therefore be used on its own to map protein–protein interactions in a pathway or in a complex, or can be used in conjunction with a functional assay to determine the relative contribution of certain protein–protein interactions or their modulation to pathway function.

The use of FRET, which requires that the donor and acceptor chromophores tagged to the target proteins are extremely close to one another (~1–10 nm) in order to provide signal (Stryer and Haugland, 1967), ensures that only very specific inter-actions are measured. Utilization of a flow-cytometer to measure this FRET-signal enables (1) counting of a large number of cells, resulting in quantitative determination of the FRET-signal, as well as (2) the ability to monitor this interaction in live cells in real time. The combination of these advantages results in the ability to compare the strength of interactions between different proteins and conditions, and reliably identify under which conditions, or between which proteins, interaction is stronger or weaker. Flow cytometry-based FRET to detect protein–protein interactions has been successfully employed in HeLa, 293T and Jurkat cells to detect interactions at the plasma membrane, in synaptic vesicles and in the cytosol (Banning et al., 2010; Chan et al., 2001; He et al., 2003; Thyrock et al., 2010). However, these studies were based on cyan fluorescent protein and yellow fluorescent protein as the donor and acceptor chromophores, respectively, the universality of which may be limited by the availability of these chromophores and the requirement of a flow-cytometer possess-ing a 405-nm (violet) laser. We have developed a protocol which utilizes the combi-nation of green fluorescent protein (GFP) and a far-red fluorescent protein (fRFP) as the donor and acceptor chromophores, respectively. This combination is more widely available, and requires the flow-cytometer to instead possess a 488-nm (blue) laser – standard on even older models. Using the protocol outlined below, we have success-fully identified the interaction between the lysosomal membrane proteins LMBD1 and ABCD4, using human immortalized and primary fibroblasts, as well as HeLa cells, in both a FACSCalibur and a FACSAria III (BD Bioscience) flow-cytometer (Fettelschoss et al., 2017).

### 7.4.2   Experimental Considerations

DNA fragments incorporating the coding sequences of the genes of interest can be cloned in frame with N- or C-terminally tagged GFP and fRFP using established (e.g. pEGFP-N1, Clontech; pmKate2-N, Evrogen) or bespoke vectors. It is recom-mended that for each target protein, a GFP and an fRFP tagged construct be cre-ated because, in our experience, the nature of the protein-tag can have an effect on protein expression, even if the reasons for this are not necessarily clear. It is further important to keep in mind that GFP has severely diminished fluorescence intensity when in acidic compartments (Haupts et al., 1998), such as the lysosome, and that FRET will work poorly or not at all when fluorescent proteins are on opposite sides of the membrane. Therefore, it is recommended to use known protein structures or topologies to place the fluorescent tag on the protein terminus that is cytosolic for each target protein. In cases where protein topology is unknown, both the N- and C-termini should be separately tagged for each fluorescent protein. fRFP is recommended over shorter wavelength RFPs (e.g. DsRed or mCherry, Clontech) because the longer wavelength excitation spectrum of fRFP has essentially no overlap with the 488-nm laser, meaning very little background signal will arise from direct laser stimulation.

The choice of controls is particularly important in this assay, in order to ensure that true FRET positive signal is distinguishable from the background. Each chromophore-tagged target protein should be expressed separately and together to ensure FRET positive signal is only detectable in the presence of both proteins. Additionally, as negative control, a similarly localized (e.g. lysosomal membrane) but non-pathway-related chromophore-tagged protein can be expressed in the presence of the target proteins to prove FRET-signal specificity. Finally, when feasible, the creation of a fusion of the proteins of interest interspersed with the fluorescent tags (e.g. TargetA-GFP-TargetB-fRFP) can make an essential positive control, and can later be used for signal-gating in the flow-cytometer (see Section 7.4.3.2).

### 7.4.3 DETAILED PROTOCOL

#### 7.4.3.1 Cell Culture and Transfection

Following cloning of the target genes into the fluorescent tag containing vectors, appropriate cell types and transfection conditions should be selected. Cells should be grown under standard culture conditions, and when appropriate, can be handled as outlined in Section 7.2.2.1. Transfection efficiencies vary according to cell type and transfection protocol, so the best transfection method should be determined empirically in each situation. We have good experience with using $6-12 \times 10^6$ cells, within which we transfect 25 µg of plasmid for single transfections and 10–15 µg per plasmid for double transfections. We recommend transfection via lipofection for most immortalized cell lines (e.g. Lipofectamine 3000, Invitrogen), following manufacturer's instruction. For primary cell lines such as fibroblasts, efficiency can be increased by using electroporation (e.g. GENE PULSER® II, BioRad) (Burda et al., 2017). In the latter case, cells harvested from a T75 $cm^2$ flask (TPP) are resuspended in 0.3 mL DMSO-Medium (1.25% DMSO in DMEM/F12 + GlutaMax supplemented with 10% FCS and 1x antibiotic-antimycotic) and electroporated in a 0.4 cm gene-pulser cuvette (BioRad) using 260 V, 975 µF and 100 Ω. The electroporated cells are transferred into T25$cm^2$ culture flasks with 5 mL DMSO-Medium and placed into the incubator at 37°C and 5% $CO_2$ for 20–24 hours, after which the DMSO-Medium is replaced with DMEM/F12 + GlutaMax supplemented with 10% FCS and 1x antibiotic-antimycotic.

### 7.4.3.2 Flow Cytometry

To prepare the samples for flow cytometry, 36–72 hours after transfection, cells are harvested by trypsinization and pelleted at $250 \times g$ for 5 min. The cell pellet is washed with 5 mL HBSS, resuspended in 500–750 μL HBSS, transferred to flow-cytometry compatible tubes through a cell strainer snap cap (e.g. Corning #352235) and kept in the dark until measurement. This cell suspension, containing $0.5–3 \times 10^6$ cells, is added to the flow cell of the flow-cytometer and measured according to the manufacturer's instructions. Based on a FACSAriaIII (BD Bioscience), we suggest to excite GFP with the 488-nm laser and measure GFP fluorescence with a 540/30 filter and any occurring FRET-signal with a 695/40 filter. To confirm the presence of the fRFP-tagged protein, fRFP can be separately excited with a 561-nm laser and measured with a 610/20 filter (where available). Approximately 30,000 events for each sample should be collected and analyzed using appropriate software (e.g. FlowJo, BD Bioscience).

### 7.4.3.3 Controls and Gating

The example depicted in Figure 7.5 illustrates the use of appropriate controls to allow distinguishing non-specific from protein–protein interaction specific signal. Negative controls should include untransfected cells, singly transfected cells and cells co-transfected with a chromophore-tagged control protein known to be outside of the pathway of interest. An appropriate positive control may include a fused version of the target proteins. Using the untransfected cells, gates can be constructed to exclude background signal in both the GFP and FRET emission filters (Figure 7.5, first panel). These gates appear to look like cross-hairs. Using these gates, the percentage of cells present in the upper right-hand quadrant is representative of GFP and FRET positive cells. In the example in Figure 7.5 (grey values), it is clear that the percentage of cells in the positive control (28%) and following co-transfection of the target proteins (18%) is considerably higher than those in the negative controls (0–3%). However, where applicable, a stick-shaped gate can be drawn around the positive control, further delimiting the positive area. This extra gate enables exclusion of events in which extremely high GFP expression results in excitation of fRFP due to random association. This is depicted in the graphs

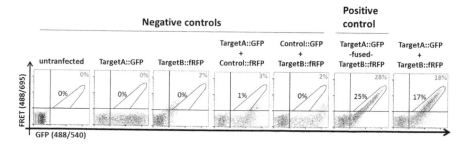

**FIGURE 7.5** An example of flow cytometry-based FRET including the appropriate controls. Detection of GFP emission is plotted on the X-axis against detection of FRET positive signal on the Y-axis.

TargetA::GFP + Control::fRFP and Control::GFP + TargetB::fRFP (Figure 7.5) as an increased FRET-signal at very high GFP levels. Within this new positive-gate (Figure 7.5, black values), the negative controls reach only a maximum of 1% positive signal, while co-transfection of the target proteins reaches 17% positive signal, thus increasing discrimination between the experimental condition and the controls. In this way, the amount of interaction in various experimental conditions, including co-transfection of various target proteins (e.g. TargetA + TargetB-Z) or co-transfection of the same target proteins in various conditions (e.g. mutant versions of TargetA or Target B, in the presence of small molecules, etc.), can be compared and quantified.

### 7.4.4 CONCLUSIONS

Flow cytometry-based FRET using cyan and yellow fluorescent proteins has been utilized for the identification of a number of protein–protein interactions in various cell types and organelles. The modification presented here enables extending this technique to GFP and fRFP-labelled proteins, increasing the utility of this technique. Since direct interaction of proteins is required for a host of processes, including lysosomal Cbl transport, this technique is of broad application.

## REFERENCES

Banning, C., Votteler, J., Hoffmann, D., Koppensteiner, H., Warmer, M., Reimer, R., Kirchhoff, F., Schubert, U., Hauber, J., and Schindler, M. (2010). A flow cytometry-based FRET assay to identify and analyse protein-protein interactions in living cells. *PLoS One 5*(2), e9344.

Burda, P., Suormala, T., Heuberger, D., Schafer, A., Fowler, B., Froese, D.S., and Baumgartner, M.R. (2017). Functional characterization of missense mutations in severe methylenetetrahydrofolate reductase deficiency using a human expression system. *J Inherit Metab Dis 40*(2), 297–306.

Chan, F.K., Siegel, R.M., Zacharias, D., Swofford, R., Holmes, K.L., Tsien, R.Y., and Lenardo, M.J. (2001). Fluorescence resonance energy transfer analysis of cell surface receptor interactions and signaling using spectral variants of the green fluorescent protein. *Cytometry 44*(4), 361–368.

Coelho, D., Kim, J.C., Miousse, I.R., Fung, S., du Moulin, M., Buers, I., Suormala, T., Burda, P., Frapolli, M., Stucki, M., et al. (2012). Mutations in ABCD4 cause a new inborn error of vitamin B12 metabolism. *Nat Genet 44*(10), 1152–1155.

Coelho, D., Suormala, T., Stucki, M., Lerner-Ellis, J.P., Rosenblatt, D.S., Newbold, R.F., Baumgartner, M.R., and Fowler, B. (2008). Gene identification for the cblD defect of vitamin B12 metabolism. *N Engl J Med 358*(14), 1454–1464.

Contreras, M., Mosser, J., Mandel, J.L., Aubourg, P., and Singh, I. (1994). The protein coded by the X-adrenoleukodystrophy gene is a peroxisomal integral membrane protein. *FEBS Lett 344*(2–3), 211–215.

Dufour, E., Marden, M.C., and Haertle, T. (1990). Beta-lactoglobulin binds retinol and protoporphyrin IX at two different binding sites. *FEBS Lett 277*(1–2), 223–226.

Fettelschoss, V., Burda, P., Sagne, C., Coelho, D., De Laet, C., Lutz, S., Suormala, T., Fowler, B., Pietrancosta, N., Gasnier, B., et al. (2017). Clinical or ATPase domain mutations in ABCD4 disrupt the interaction between the vitamin B12-trafficking proteins ABCD4 and LMBD1. *J Biol Chem 292*(28), 11980–11991.

Hannibal, L., Kim, J., Brasch, N.E., Wang, S., Rosenblatt, D.S., Banerjee, R., and Jacobsen, D.W. (2009). Processing of alkylcobalamins in mammalian cells: A role for the MMACHC (cblC) gene product. *Mol Genet Metab 97*(4), 260–266.

Haupts, U., Maiti, S., Schwille, P., and Webb, W.W. (1998). Dynamics of fluorescence fluctuations in green fluorescent protein observed by fluorescence correlation spectroscopy. *Proc Natl Acad Sci U S A 95*(23), 13573–13578.

He, L., Olson, D.P., Wu, X., Karpova, T.S., McNally, J.G., and Lipsky, P.E. (2003). A flow cytometric method to detect protein-protein interaction in living cells by directly visualizing donor fluorophore quenching during CFP-->YFP fluorescence resonance energy transfer (FRET). *Cytom A 55*(2), 71–85.

Jacobsen, D.W., Green, R., Quadros, E.V., and Montejano, Y.D. (1982). Rapid analysis of cobalamin coenzymes and related corrinoid analogs by high-performance liquid chromatography. *Anal Biochem 120*(2), 394–403.

Kamijo, K., Taketani, S., Yokota, S., Osumi, T., and Hashimoto, T. (1990). The 70-kDa peroxisomal membrane protein is a member of the Mdr (P-glycoprotein)-related ATP-binding protein superfamily. *J Biol Chem 265*(8), 4534–4540.

Kashiwayama, Y., Seki, M., Yasui, A., Murasaki, Y., Morita, M., Yamashita, Y., Sakaguchi, M., Tanaka, Y., and Imanaka, T. (2009). 70-kDa peroxisomal membrane protein related protein (P70R/ABCD4) localizes to endoplasmic reticulum not peroxisomes, and NH2-terminal hydrophobic property determines the subcellular localization of ABC subfamily D proteins. *Exp Cell Res 315*(2), 190–205.

Kawaguchi, K., Okamoto, T., Morita, M., and Imanaka, T. (2016). Translocation of the ABC transporter ABCD4 from the endoplasmic reticulum to lysosomes requires the escort protein LMBD1. *Sci Rep 6*, 30183.

Kim, J., Gherasim, C., and Banerjee, R. (2008). Decyanation of vitamin B12 by a trafficking chaperone. *Proc Natl Acad Sci U S A 105*(38), 14551–14554.

Leal, N.A., Park, S.D., Kima, P.E., and Bobik, T.A. (2003). Identification of the human and bovine ATP:Cob(I)alamin adenosyltransferase cDNAs based on complementation of a bacterial mutant. *J Biol Chem 278*(11), 9227–9234.

Lee, A., Asahina, K., Okamoto, T., Kawaguchi, K., Kostsin, D.G., Kashiwayama, Y., Takanashi, K., Yazaki, K., Imanaka, T., and Morita, M. (2014). Role of NH2-terminal hydrophobic motif in the subcellular localization of ATP-binding cassette protein subfamily D: Common features in eukaryotic organisms. *Biochem Biophys Res Commun 453*(3), 612–618.

Lombard-Platet, G., Savary, S., Sarde, C.O., Mandel, J.L., and Chimini, G. (1996). A close relative of the adrenoleukodystrophy (ALD) gene codes for a peroxisomal protein with a specific expression pattern. *Proc Natl Acad Sci U S A 93*(3), 1265–1269.

Lowry, O.H., Rosebrough, N.J., Farr, A.L., and Randall, R.J. (1951). Protein measurement with the Folin phenol reagent. *J Biol Chem 193*(1), 265–275.

Mahoney, M.J., and Rosenberg, L.E. (1971). Synthesis of cobalamin coenzymes by human cells in tissue culture. *J Lab Clin Med 78*(2), 302–308.

Mellman, I., Willard, H.F., and Rosenberg, L.E. (1978). Cobalamin binding and cobalamin-dependent enzyme activity in normal and mutant human fibroblasts. *J Clin Invest 62*(5), 952–960.

Mosser, J., Lutz, Y., Stoeckel, M.E., Sarde, C.O., Kretz, C., Douar, A.M., Lopez, J., Aubourg, P., and Mandel, J.L. (1994). The gene responsible for adrenoleukodystrophy encodes a peroxisomal membrane protein. *Hum Mol Genet 3*(2), 265–271.

Olteanu, H., and Banerjee, R. (2001). Human methionine synthase reductase, a soluble P-450 reductase-like dual flavoprotein, is sufficient for NADPH-dependent methionine synthase activation. *J Biol Chem 276*(38), 35558–35563.

Padovani, D., and Banerjee, R. (2009). A G-protein editor gates coenzyme B12 loading and is corrupted in methylmalonic aciduria. *Proc Natl Acad Sci U S A 106*(51), 21567–21572.

Rutsch, F., Gailus, S., Miousse, I.R., Suormala, T., Sagne, C., Toliat, M.R., Nurnberg, G., Wittkampf, T., Buers, I., Sharifi, A., et al. (2009). Identification of a putative lysosomal cobalamin exporter altered in the cblF defect of vitamin B12 metabolism. *Nat Genet 41*(2), 234–239.

Stryer, L., and Haugland, R.P. (1967). Energy transfer: A spectroscopic ruler. *Proc Natl Acad Sci U S A 58*(2), 719–726.

Suormala, T., Baumgartner, M.R., Coelho, D., Zavadakova, P., Kozich, V., Koch, H.G., Berghauser, M., Wraith, J.E., Burlina, A., Sewell, A., et al. (2004). The cblD defect causes either isolated or combined deficiency of methylcobalamin and adenosylcobalamin synthesis. *J Biol Chem 279*(41), 42742–42749.

Thyrock, A., Stehling, M., Waschbusch, D., and Barnekow, A. (2010). Characterizing the interaction between the Rab6 GTPase and Mint3 via flow cytometry based FRET analysis. *Biochem Biophys Res Commun 396*(3), 679–683.

Watkins, D., and Rosenblatt, D.S. (1986). Failure of lysosomal release of vitamin B12: A new complementation group causing methylmalonic aciduria (cblF). *Am J Hum Genet 39*(3), 404–408.

Willard, H.F., Ambani, L.M., Hart, A.C., Mahoney, M.J., and Rosenberg, L.E. (1976). Rapid prenatal and postnatal detection of inborn errors of propionate, methylmalonate, and cobalamin metabolism: A sensitive assay using cultured cells. *Hum Genet 34*(3), 277–283.

# 8 Detection of Lysosomal Membrane Permeabilization

*Anne-Marie Ellegaard, Line Groth-Pedersen, and Marja Jäättelä*

## CONTENTS

## 8.1  INTRODUCTION

### 8.1.1  LYSOSOME-DEPENDENT CELL DEATH

The concept of lysosome-dependent cell death was originally presented by Christian de Duve, a Belgian biochemist who received the Nobel Prize in 1974 for his discovery and characterization of lysosomes (de Duve, 1983). Today, lysosome-dependent cell death is defined as a form of regulated cell death that is initiated by lysosomal membrane permeabilization (LMP) in response to various perturbations of intracellular homeostasis, and executed by lysosomal hydrolases, especially cathepsins, with an optional involvement of caspases in the execution phase (Galluzzi et al., 2018). Lysosome-dependent cell death is evolutionarily conserved from yeast, roundworm and fruit fly to mammalian cells and tissues, and it contributes to numerous physiological processes (e.g. mammary involution) as well as degenerative, inflammatory and microbial diseases (Aits and Jäättelä, 2013; Appelqvist et al., 2013; Gómez-Sintes et al., 2016; Hafner Česen et al., 2012). In addition to the strictly lysosome-dependent cell death, LMP is a secondary event upon most other cell death subroutines (Vanden Berghe et al., 2010). Hence, studying whether LMP is the initial event or an amplifier of the cell death signal is important in deciphering the cell death pathway induced by a certain stimulus.

### 8.1.2  LYSOSOMES AND LYSOSOMAL HYDROLASES

Lysosomes are membrane-surrounded organelles that serve as sites for the degradation of cargo delivered to them through endocytosis, pinocytosis, phagocytosis or autophagy. To carry out their catabolic function, lysosomes contain over 60 hydrolases (proteases, lipases, sulfatases, glycosidases, nucleases, peptidases etc.) capable of degrading most cellular organelles and macromolecules (Xu and Ren, 2015). Cathepsin proteases are among the best-studied lysosomal hydrolases and their leakage to the cytosol is assumed to be essential for the cell death in most, if not all, lysosome-dependent cell death pathways. Depending on their catalytic site, cathepsins are divided into serine (e.g. cathepsin A), aspartic (e.g. cathepsin D) and cysteine (e.g. cathepsin B and L) proteases. Their concentrations can exceed 1 mM in the lysosomes and they have optimal activity in the acidic pH of the lysosomes (Turk et al., 2012). In spite of their acidic pH optima, some cathepsins retain their enzymatic activities for a short while or even gain new proteolytic activities after leaking to the cytosol (Prudova et al., 2016). Cytosolic cathepsin activity after LMP may be further assisted by the transient acidification of the cytosol upon concomitant leakage of $H^+$-ions from the lysosomes. Whereas the contribution of most cathepsins remains unknown, genetic studies have confirmed the role of cathepsin B (Foghsgaard et al., 2001; Guicciardi et al., 2000), cathepsin L (Fehrenbacher et al., 2004) and cathepsin D (Bidère et al., 2003) in the execution of lysosome-dependent cell death (reviewed in (Aits and Jäättelä, 2013)). Theoretically, the presence of a single cathepsin type (e.g. cathepsin D) in the cytosol is sufficient to kill the cell from inside (Roberg et al., 2002). Due to their highly redundant activities and concomitant leakage upon LMP, it is, however, difficult to pinpoint the cathepsins responsible for cell death.

The importance of individual cathepsins in this process is likely to depend on their relative expression levels in the model system studied. Furthermore, it should be noted that the role of other lysosomal hydrolases in lysosome-dependent cell death remains largely unstudied.

### 8.1.3 INDUCTION OF LYSOSOMAL MEMBRANE PERMEABILIZATION

Already in the 1970s, Christian de Duve initiated an intensive search for compounds that destabilize lysosomal membranes for the treatment of cancer. As a result, amines with long hydrophobic chains and high pK values were identified as lysosomotropic detergents with potential applications in cancer therapy (Firestone et al., 1979). One of the best-studied lysosomotropic detergents is L-leucyl-L-leucine methyl ester (LLOMe). It is endocytosed and first activated inside the lysosomes, where cathepsin C cleaves it to generate the active detergent that effectively permeabilizes the lysosomal membrane (Uchimoto et al., 1999). Due to the relatively low levels of cathepsin C in most cancer cells, LLOMe is not suitable for cancer therapy, whereas high cathepsin C levels in white blood cells has encouraged its development as a treatment for bone marrow transplantation-associated graft versus host disease (Charley et al., 1986). A recent report suggests, however, that LLOMe-induced cell death is not mediated by the leakage of active cathepsins but rather by the inactivation of cathepsins and subsequent loss of lysosomal function (Repnik et al., 2017).

The interest in lysosomotropic agents as potential anti-cancer drugs has revived recently due to the realization that many commonly used cationic amphiphilic drugs show cancer-specific toxicity (Ellegaard et al., 2013; Jahchan et al., 2013; Petersen et al., 2013; Shchors et al., 2015; Sukhai et al., 2013). Most cationic amphiphilic drugs accumulate in the lysosome, where they inhibit the conversion of sphingomyelin to ceramide by inhibiting acid sphingomyelinase (Kornhuber et al., 2010). The subsequent accumulation of sphingomyelin decreases the stability of the lysosomal limiting membrane and, hence, LMP is more likely to occur (Kirkegaard et al., 2010; Petersen et al., 2013).

In addition to lysosomotropic agents discussed above, a wide variety of other drugs and molecules are able to induce LMP (reviewed in (Aits and Jäättelä, 2013; Johansson et al., 2010)). Among these are classical apoptosis-inducers, such as tumour necrosis factor (TNF), tumour protein p53 (TP53) and the pro-apoptotic Bcl-2 family member Bax. While the exact molecular mechanisms responsible for the LMP are unknown, studies of TNF-induced LMP have revealed that it can occur either upstream, downstream or independent of caspase activation (Gyrd-Hansen et al., 2006; Taha et al., 2005), whereas DNA damage-activated TP53 can trigger LMP through direct interaction with lysosome-associated apoptosis-inducing protein containing the pleckstrin homology and FYVE domains on the lysosomal membrane (Li et al., 2007). Akin to the permeabilization of mitochondrial outer membrane in apoptosis, Bax has been suggested to induce LMP by forming pores in the lysosomal membrane (Bové et al., 2014; Feldstein et al., 2006; Guan et al., 2015; Karch et al., 2017). It should, however, be noted that LMP can occur independently of caspase activation, TP53 and Bax (Foghsgaard et al., 2001; Gyrd-Hansen et al., 2006).

Reactive oxygen species are among the few established mediators of LMP. They can be produced in the cell as by-products of mitochondrial respiration or lysosomal degradation of iron-containing proteins. In the presence of $H_2O_2$, lysosomal iron (II) can catalyse Fenton-type reactions leading to harmful oxygen radicals, which peroxidize the lysosomal membrane lipids and thereby destabilize the lysosomal limiting membrane (Kurz et al., 2008). Thus, iron chelators, like desferrioxamine, can protect cells from oxidative stress-induced LMP, but are without an effect in many other lysosome-dependent cell death models (Vanden Berghe et al., 2010).

### 8.1.4 CONSEQUENCES OF LYSOSOMAL MEMBRANE PERMEABILIZATION

Once the lysosomal membrane has been permeabilized, lysosomal contents spill out into the cytosol. Depending on its extent, LMP can trigger different types of cell death, a small leakage resulting in a regulated cell death programme with apoptotic or apoptosis-like features, and a major leak leading to necrosis characterized by an early permeabilization of the plasma membrane (Kågedal et al., 2001). Furthermore, it has recently become evident that LMP does not necessarily lead to cell death. Instead, lysosomes can recover their acidity or be removed by lysophagy (Aits et al., 2015a; Hung et al., 2013; Repnik et al., 2017).

As already mentioned, the cathepsin family of hydrolases plays an important role in the execution of cell death. In the cytosol, cathepsins can enhance the cell death signal by activating the apoptosis machinery thereby ensuring completion of the initiated cell death. Cathepsin D can directly cleave and activate caspase-8 (Conus et al., 2012), and multiple cathepsin family members can activate the pro-apoptotic Bcl-2 family member Bid and inactivate the anti-apoptotic Bcl-2 family members Bcl-2, Bcl-XL and Mcl-1 (Appelqvist et al., 2012; Cirman et al., 2004; Droga-Mazovec et al., 2008). This results in mitochondrial outer membrane permeabilization and consequential activation of the intrinsic apoptotic pathway. In the case of non-apoptotic lysosome-dependent cell death, the crucial cathepsin substrates are largely unknown (Aits and Jäättelä, 2013). Even though cathepsins participate in the execution of lysosome-dependent cell death, their inhibition merely delays cell death. Thus, more studies are needed to investigate the role of other lysosomal hydrolases, as well as $H^+$-ions and $Ca^{2+}$-ions in the cell death execution upon LMP (Gómez-Sintes et al., 2016; Loison et al., 2014).

All in all, LMP is an intricate cellular process. Whether it occurs or not, and its consequences to the cell, depend on the stimulus, the cell type and the cellular context. Thus, more research is needed in order to fully understand and potentially exploit this process.

## 8.2 EXPERIMENTAL DETECTION OF LYSOSOMAL MEMBRANE PERMEABILIZATION

### 8.2.1 INTRODUCTION

The study of LMP as a cell death initiator has been hampered by the lack of good methods to detect it. In recent years, more advanced and sensitive methods to study

LMP have emerged, of which only a handful are presented in this chapter. This development in methodology has provided us with a more nuanced view on this cellular phenomenon and its causes and effects.

The methods presented here address the stability of the lysosomal limiting membrane (Section 8.2.2), release of lysosomal contents (Section 8.2.3, Section 8.2.4 and Section 8.2.5) and the accumulation of cytosolic proteins on damaged lysosomes (Section 8.2.6). See Figure 8.1.

The examples of step-by-step protocols included below are meant as guides for the experimental procedures and should be modified and optimized according to the specific experimental setup. Also, none of the step-by-step protocols include treatment steps since this will vary greatly depending on the treatment type. The experimenter has to add this into the protocol at a suitable step for every experiment.

## 8.2.2 ACRIDINE ORANGE ASSAY

### 8.2.2.1 Introduction

The metachromatic weak base acridine orange (AO) accumulates in the lysosomes. The emission maximum of the compound's fluorescence depends on the concentration, pH and binding partners. It changes from 525 nm (green) at low concentration in the cytosol to 650 nm (red) at high concentration in acidic lysosomes. Consequently, staining cells with AO will result in green cells with red lysosomes (see Figure 8.1, Figure 8.2a). When residing in the lysosomes, AO can be photo-oxidized by blue light, which leads to destruction of the lysosomal membrane in a dramatic fashion resembling green explosions. Hence, the rates of the decrease of red fluorescence and increase of green fluorescence of AO over time are used as parameters for the stability of the lysosomal membrane.

AO localizes in the lysosomes due to trapping of the weakly basic molecules in the acid compartment upon protonation. Hence, decrease of red fluorescence of AO reflects a change in the surrounding pH due to a loss of the pH gradient of the lysosomes rather than the actual leakage of lysosomes. Therefore, the AO assay does not address the occurrence of LMP directly.

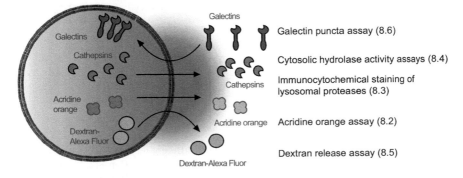

**FIGURE 8.1** Schematic overview of a lysosome with indications of the features measured in the methods presented here. In brackets: The section number corresponding to the method, see these for details.

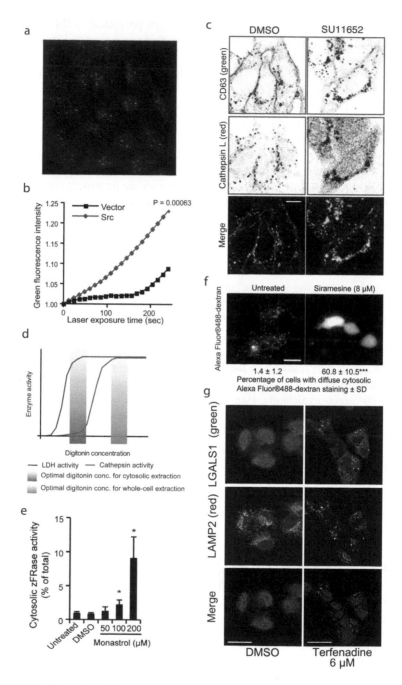

**FIGURE 8.2** Examples of results obtained with the different methods described. (a) U2OS cells stained with acridine orange (Petersen et al., 2010) (see Section 8.2.2). (b) graphical representation of the increase in green fluorescence as a measure for the membrane stabilities of two cell lines (vector and src) over time (Petersen et al., 2013) (see Section 8.2.2). (c) representative confocal images of HeLa-eGFP-CD63 cells treated for 8 h with DMSO or

**FIGURE 8.2 (CONTINUED)**

4 µM SU11652. Cathepsin L staining (red) is diffuse in drug-treated cells compared to control cells. e-GFP-CD63 (green) serves as a lysosomal marker (Ellegaard et al., 2013) (see Section 8.2.3). (d) schematic representation of the intervals of digitonin concentrations suitable for cytosolic (blue bar) and whole-cell (green bar) extractions based on measurements of cathepsin (red line) and LDH (blue line) activities at different digitonin concentrations (see Section 8.2.4). (e) graphical representation of cysteine cathepsin (zFRase) activity in MCF-7 cells left untreated or treated with DMSO or indicated concentrations of monastrol for 72 h. The activities in the cytosolic extracts are shown as a percentage of the activities in the corresponding total extracts (see Section 8.2.4) (Groth-Pedersen et al., 2012). (f) representative images of MCF-7 cells loaded with dextran-Alexa Fluor-488 and left untreated or treated with 8 µM siramesine for 20 h. The percentages of cells with diffuse cytosolic dextran-Alexa Fluor pattern as an indication of LMP were based on the quantification of at least 50 cells/condition (see Section 8.2.5) (Petersen et al., 2013). (g) representative confocal images of A549 cells treated with DMSO or 6 µM terfenadine for 24 h and stained for galectin-1 (LGALS1, green), LAMP-2 (red) and DNA (blue) (see Section 8.2.6) (Ellegaard et al., 2016).

## 8.2.2.2   Example of a Step-by-Step Protocol

This protocol applies to adherent cells but can easily be modified to cells in suspension, in which case the analysis is performed on a fluorescence-activated cell sorter (FACS). Depending on the treatment of interest, it can be added to the cells before or after loading with AO. If treatment is applied before AO loading, one must check that the loading of AO is not significantly affected by the treatment.

### 8.2.2.2.1   Materials and Equipment

Acridine orange, Hank's balanced salt solution (HBSS), fetal calf serum (FCS), fluorescence microscope with appropriate lamps/lasers and filters (see protocol for details), computational software for analysis.

### 8.2.2.2.2   Protocol

1. Grow cells of interest to sub-confluency.
2. Incubate the cells for 15 min at 37°C with 2 mg/mL acridine orange.
3. Wash cells in HBSS complemented with 3% FCS (concentration of FCS might vary with different cell types).
4. Expose the cells to 489 nm blue light in a fluorescence microscope (such as the Zeiss LSM LIVE DUO confocal system) while capturing micrographs of pre-defined sections of the cell sample every 0.5–12 s (this interval is cell type specific and should be determined in advance). The micrographs are captured in two channels defined by filters to capture the green (bandpass filter 495–555 nm) and red fluorescence (LP650 bandpass filter) of AO.
5. Analysis of decrease in green fluorescence and increase in red fluorescence of AO over time is done in suitable software (such as Zeiss LSM DUO software).

*Stability of the lysosomal membrane is visualized as a curve of increasing green fluorescence over time (see Figure 8.2b). The stability is measured relative to control cells in the same experiment.*

- The assay is easy to perform once the microscope and analysis software are set up.
- This assay addresses the lysosomal pH gradient rather than the occurrence of LMP.

*8.2.2.2.4   Limitations of This Method*
- AO fluoresces in a broad spectrum of red and green, rendering combination with other fluorescent markers almost impossible. Additionally, one has to consider if the compound of interest is fluorescent or the cells have a high autofluorescence and thereby might affect the measurements of changes in AO fluorescence.
- Furthermore, the computational analysis of the acquired micrographs can be rather substantial depending on the software.

## 8.2.3   Immunocytochemical Staining of Lysosomal Proteases

### 8.2.3.1   Introduction

One of the hallmarks of LMP is translocation of proteases such as cathepsins from the lysosomes to the cytosol. Here, the cathepsins have numerous targets, whose degradation is detrimental to the cell. Hence, the visualization of cathepsins in the cytosol is a way to determine that LMP has taken place. Different treatments induce different magnitudes of LMP and at different time points, which is why an exploration of the most optimal time point for the LMP detection is advised.

### 8.2.3.2   Example of a Step-by-Step Protocol

*8.2.3.2.1   Materials and Equipment*

Coverslips for cell culture, microscopy slides, methanol, 4% paraformaldehyde, phosphate-buffered saline with calcium and magnesium (PBS), 0.3% Triton X-100 in PBS with 1% FCS (buffer 1), 0.1% Triton X-100 in PBS with 0.25% FCS (buffer 2), 0.05% Tween-20 in PBS (buffer 3), Hoechst-33342 (or similar nuclear dye), primary and secondary antibodies (see description in the protocol), mounting medium, confocal fluorescent microscope with appropriate lasers/lamps and filters, preferably a computational software to analyze the micrographs.

*8.2.3.2.2   Protocol*
1. Grow the cells of interest on coverslips until approx. 70% confluency.
2. Wash the cells twice in PBS.
3. Fix the cells in ice-cold methanol for exactly 3 min or in 4% paraformaldehyde for 10 min at room temperature followed by incubation with 50 mM $NH_4Cl$ for 10 min.

*Which fixation method to use depends on the antibodies; some might require both to work optimally. If you work with fluorescent compounds, autofluorescing cells or genetically modified cells that express a fluorescent marker, this fluorescence can be abolished by fixing the cells in methanol. In contrast, if you are interested in keeping the fluorescent signal of a marker or compound in the cells, you should not fix the cells with methanol. In this case, be aware to choose secondary antibodies with fluorescent labels that are distinct from the fluorescence of your marker or compound in order to distinguish one from the other.*

4. Wash the cells twice in PBS.
5. Permeabilize the cells by incubating them in buffer 1 for 20 min.
6. Incubate the cells in buffer 1 containing 5% FCS and two primary antibodies for 1 h at room temperature or overnight at 4°C.

*The primary antibodies should recognize a lysosomal marker (such as LAMP-2) and a member of the cathepsin family (such as cathepsin B), respectively. The optimal concentration of the antibodies can vary greatly from 1:50 to 1:10,000, and this has to be determined beforehand.*

7. Wash the cells thrice in buffer 2.
8. Incubate the cells in buffer 2 containing 5% FCS and two secondary antibodies for 1 hour in the dark at room temperature.

*The secondary antibodies should recognize one of the primary antibodies each and be coupled to Alexa Fluor probes with different fluorescent labels, respectively. The optimal concentration of secondary antibodies from Molecular Probes is 1:1000.*

9. Wash the cells twice in buffer 3.
10. Incubate the cells with 5 μg/mL Hoechst-33342 for 2 min for visualization of the nucleus.

*Other nuclear dyes can be used as well or the nuclear staining can be omitted.*

11. Wash the cells twice in PBS.
12. Mount the coverslips on microscopy slides with a mounting medium (such as ProLong Gold Antifade from Molecular Probes) and let samples dry overnight in the dark at room temperature.
13. Store the slides in the dark at 4°C or −20°C.
14. Obtain confocal micrographs of the cells and analyze the percentage of cells with diffuse relative to dotty cathepsin staining.

*The lysosomal marker staining serves as a reference for the lysosomal compartment in cells with little or no cathepsin dots.*

### 8.2.3.2.3  Advantages of This Method

- This assay measures the presence of lysosomal cathepsins in the cytosol, which is a direct consequence of LMP.
- It is fairly easy to handle many samples simultaneously once the microscope settings and computational software for analysis have been set up.

### 8.2.3.2.4   *Limitations of This Method*

- The most prominent limitation of this assay is the large amount of cathepsins that needs to be released into the cytosol in order to visualize a diffuse staining pattern (Figure 8.2c). Minor volumes of leaked cathepsin will not be detectable with this assay. Thus, the threshold for the detection of LMP with this assay is rather high.
- The quality of immunocytochemical stainings always depends on the quality of the antibodies. For this assay, the specificity of the cathepsin antibody is paramount to the visualization of the diffuse pattern of cytosolic cathepsins.
- Addressing the presence of diffuse pattern of cytosolic cathepsin by computational analysis can be difficult. Alternatively, to analyze the micrographs manually is laborious and has to be blinded in order for the experimenter's bias to not influence the results.
- As mentioned in the step-by-step protocol, one has to consider if the detection of fluorescence from the immunocytochemically stained proteins can be disturbed by fluorescence from other sources, such as autofluorescence from the cells, fluorescence of a small molecule used in treatment or overexpression of a fluorescently labelled protein in the cells.

## 8.2.4   MEASUREMENT OF ACTIVITIES OF LYSOSOMAL HYDROLASES IN THE CYTOSOL

### 8.2.4.1   Introduction

A consequence of LMP is the release of lysosomal contents including soluble enzymes. The activity of these enzymes has an optimum at the acidic pH of the lysosomal lumen. However, some of them retain partial activity at neutral pH, which is found in the cytosol. This method measures the relative amount of this residual lysosomal enzyme activity present in the cytosol after LMP. Specifically, the measured activity of lysosomal enzymatic activity in a cytosolic extract is compared to the activity in a total cell extract.

The cytosolic and whole-cell extractions are performed with the cell membrane detergent digitonin. This compound binds cholesterol, which creates pores in the membranes (Geelen, 2005). Due to the lower level of cholesterol in the lysosomal membrane compared to the plasma membrane, low concentrations of digitonin permeabilize the plasma membrane while leaving the lysosomal membrane intact. This makes it possible to extract only the cytosolic contents from the cells, while high concentrations of digitonin permeabilize all cell membranes and allow for whole-cell extraction. Digitonin is very poorly dissolved in $H_2O$ and the exact concentration can differ between aliquots. Hence, for every new aliquot used, one has to determine the most optimal concentration of digitonin to use for the extractions. This is done in a pilot experiment where the activity of a soluble cytosolic enzyme (lactose dehydrogenase, LDH) serves as a marker for permeabilization of the plasma membrane and the activity of soluble lysosomal cysteine cathepsins serves as a measure for permeabilization of the lysosomal membrane. These enzyme activities are measured in extracts from cells incubated with a range of digitonin concentrations (see below for an example of a step-by-step protocol). In evaluating the results of this pilot experiment, one chooses a digitonin concentration for the cytosolic extraction that results in a high activity of LDH and none or very little activity of cathepsin. Additionally, a larger amount of digitonin is chosen for the whole-cell extraction where activities of both LDH and cathepsin are high. See Figure 8.2.d.

## 8.2.4.2   Example of a Step-by-Step Protocol

### 8.2.4.2.1   *Materials and Equipment*

Caspase reaction buffer (see Section 8.2.4.2.2), cathepsin reaction buffer (see Section 8.2.4.2.2), NAG reaction buffer (see Section 8.2.4.2.2), LDH activity assay (such as the Cytotoxicity Detection Kit from Sigma), digitonin extraction buffer (see Section 8.2.4.2.2), digitonin, Pefabloc, dithiothreitol (DTT), 1 M HCl, probes (see Section 8.2.4.2.4), black half-area 96-well plates, fluorescence plate reader, spectrophotometric plate reader.

### 8.2.4.2.2   *Before the First Experiment*

Prepare the digitonin extraction buffer and the enzyme reaction buffers as follows:

- Digitonin extraction buffer: Mix HEPES 20 mM, KCl 10 mM, $MgCl_2$ 1.5 mM, EDTA 1 mM, EGTA 1 mM and sucrose 250 mM in autoclaved MilliQ $H_2O$ up to 250 mL. Sterilize the filter and store at 4°C.
- Cathepsin reaction buffer: Mix Na-acetate 50 mM and EDTA 4 mM in MilliQ $H_2O$ up to 400 mL. Adjust the pH to 6.0 with 1 N NaOH and fill the bottle to 500 mL with MilliQ $H_2O$. Sterilize the filter and store at 4°C.
- N-acetyl-beta-D-glucosaminidase (NAG) reaction buffer: Dissolve 0.3 mg/mL 4-methylumbelliferyl N-acetyl-beta-D-glucosaminide in 0.2 M Na-citrate buffer at pH 4.5. Sterilize the filter and store at 4°C.
- Caspase reaction buffer: Mix HEPES 100 mM, DTT 5 mM, EDTA 0.5 mM and Chaps 0.1% in MilliQ $H_2O$ up to 300 mL. Adjust the pH to 7.5, add 20% glycerol and fill the bottle to 500 mL with MilliQ $H_2O$. Sterilize the filter and store at 4°C.

### 8.2.4.2.3   *Protocol for Determining the Optimal Digitonin Concentration*

1. Seed cells in 24-, 12- or 6-well plates to approx. 70% confluency.
2. Mix digitonin extraction buffer (200 µL/well for 24-well plate; 300 µL/well for 12-well plate; 400 µL/well for 6-well plate) with 0.5 mM Pefabloc and create a digitonin titration curve by adding 0, 5, 10, 15, 20, 25, 30, 50, 100, 200, 300, 500 µg/mL digitonin from the new aliquot.

*Digitonin needs to be heated up to 65°C and vortexed just prior to use in order to solubilize all precipitates.*

3. Place cells on ice.
4. Remove the growth medium from the wells one well at a time (maximum 8 wells at a time to prevent the cells from drying out).

5. Add extraction buffer to each well and treat the cells exactly 15 min on ice on a rocking table. Make sure that all wells are treated for the exact same amount of time.

*The incubation time needed might vary between cell lines.*

6. While treating with digitonin, place a 96-well plate on ice.
7. After exactly 15 min of digitonin treatment, transfer extracts (180 μL/well for 24-well plate; 280 μL/well for 12-well plate; 380 μL/well for 6-well plate) to the pre-cooled 96-well plate in the same order as you added the extraction buffer.
8. Keep extracts on ice.
9. Measure cathepsin and LDH activities as described in Section 8.2.4.2.4.
10. Based on the resulting data, choose a low concentration of digitonin for the cytosolic extraction (where LDH activity is high but cathepsin activity is low) and a high concentration of digitonin for the whole-cell extraction (where both the LDH activity and cathepsin activity are high) (see Figure 8.2d).

### 8.2.4.2.4    Protocol
*Extraction*
1. Seed cells in 24-, 12- or 6-well plates to approx. 70% confluency. Make two identical sets of samples (one for cytosolic extraction and one for whole-cell extraction).
2. Prepare the cytosolic and whole-cell extraction buffers: Mix digitonin extraction buffer (200 μL/well in 24-well plate; 300 μL/well in 12-well plate; 400 μL/well in 6-well plate) with 0.5 mM Pefabloc and low concentration (cytosolic extraction) or high concentration (whole-cell extraction) of digitonin as determined in the pilot experiment.

*Digitonin needs to be heated up to 65°C and vortexed just prior to use in order to solubilize all precipitates.*

3. Place cells on ice.
4. Remove the growth medium from the wells one well at a time (maximum 8 wells at a time to prevent the cells from drying out).
5. Add extraction buffer to each well and treat the cells exactly 15 min on ice on a rocking table. Make sure that all wells are treated for the exact same amount of time.

*The incubation time might vary between cell lines.*

6. While treating with digitonin, place a 96-well plate on ice.
7. After exactly 15 min of digitonin treatment, transfer extracts (180 μL/well for 24-well plate; 280 μL/well for 12-well plate; 380 μL/well for 6-well plate) to the pre-cooled 96-well plate in the same order as you added the extraction buffer.
8. Keep extracts on ice.

*Cysteine Cathepsin (zFRase) Activity Assay*
1. Mix cathepsin reaction buffer (50 µL/reaction) with 0.5 mM Pefabloc, 8 mM DTT and 50 µM of a fluorescent probe. For measurement of cysteine cathepsin activity (primarily cathepsin B and L) use benzyloxycarbonyl-Phe-Arg-aminotrifluoromethylcoumarin (z-FR-AFC; excitation: 395–400 nm and emission: 495–505 nm) or benzyloxycarbonyl-Phe-Arg-aminomethylcoumarin (z-FR-AMC; excitation: 360–380 nm and emission: 440–460 nm).
2. Transfer 50 µL/well extract to a pre-cooled, non-coated, black 96-well plate on ice.
3. Add 50 µL/well reaction buffer.
4. Incubate 3–5 min at room temperature.
5. Measure the emitted fluorescence in a fluorescence plate reader (such as VarioSkan Flash) every 40 s for 20 min.
6. Plot the time vs. fluorescence and calculate the Vmax from the linear part of the curve. Use these data to calculate the relative cysteine cathepsin activity later (see calculations and Figure 8.2e).

*Internal Standard for Cell Number (LDH assay)*
For some treatments, the level of LDH might be affected. In case this is suspected, one can use the BCA assay according to the manufacturer's protocol to normalize the enzyme activities to cell number.

1. Transfer 30 µL/well extract to a transparent 96-well plate.
2. Mix LDH Cytotoxicity Detection Kit reagents (LDH reaction mix) according to the manufacturer's protocol.
3. Add 30 µL/well of the LDH reaction mix to the plate with cell extracts.
4. Incubate 5–30 min at room temperature. A clear colour change from pale pink to dark red should be visible in some wells.
5. Stop the reaction with 20 µL/well 1 M HCl in the same order as you added the LDH reaction mix.
6. Measure the absorbance at 490 nm with a spectrophotometric plate reader (such as the VarioSkan Flash).

*Calculations*
1. Adjust the measured enzyme activity values with the LDH values for each well:

$$\text{Adjusted value} = \frac{\text{Cathepsin activity value}}{\text{LDH activity value}} \times 100\%$$

2. Calculate the percentage of released cathepsin activity in each well:

$$\text{Cathepsin release} = \frac{\text{Adjusted cytosolic activity}}{\text{Adjusted total activity}} \times 100\%$$

*Caspase Activity Assay*

For measurement of caspase activity, use the probe N-acetyl-Asp-Glu-Val-Asp-7-aminotrifluoromethylcoumarin (ac-DEVD-afc) and the caspase reaction buffer. Otherwise, follow the protocol for measuring cysteine cathepsin activity above. Excitation: 400 nm and emission: 505 nm.

*NAG Activity Assay*

For measuring NAG activity, use the NAG reaction buffer. No additional probe is needed; it is already in the buffer. Otherwise, follow the protocol for measuring cysteine cathepsin activity (Section 8.2.4.2.4). Excitation: 400 nm and emission: 505 nm.

### 8.2.4.2.5    Advantages of This Method

- Once you have the cytosolic and whole-cell extracts, you can measure the activities of several enzymes from the same extracts. This way, you can directly compare activity levels of cysteine cathepsins and NAG with activity levels of caspases. In a kinetic investigation of cell death, this is a way to address if LMP precedes caspase activity.

### 8.2.4.2.6    Limitations of This Method

- This is done on a population of cells and, thus, the result will be an average across the population. Accordingly, a minor release of enzymes in a subpopulation of the cells will be difficult to detect with this method.
- For treatments that alter the cholesterol composition of the cell membranes, this method cannot be used. In this case, you cannot rely on the assumption that the permeabilization of the plasma membrane and lysosomal membrane with digitonin is similar in treated and untreated cells.

## 8.2.5    RELEASE OF FLUORESCENTLY LABELLED DEXTRAN FROM THE LYSOSOMES

### 8.2.5.1    Introduction

When LMP happens, holes occur in the lysosomal membrane leading to release lysosomal contents. To visualize this process, lysosomes can be loaded with dextran molecules labelled with a fluorescent Alexa Fluor marker. The dextran is added extracellularly and will be taken up by the cells via endocytosis and transported to the lysosomes through vesicular transport. Here, the dextran-Alexa Fluor marker retains its structure and fluorescent activity, thus, enabling visualization of the lysosomes under a fluorescent microscope. Upon induction of LMP, dextran is released from the lysosomes into the cytosol (Figure 8.2f). Dextran comes in different sizes and the hole sizes induced in the lysosomal membranes by different stimuli can be assessed by comparing the releases of different sizes of dextran molecules.

### 8.2.5.2    Example of a Step-by-Step Protocol

#### 8.2.5.2.1    Materials and Equipment

Dextran labelled with Alexa Fluor (many sizes of dextran and many types of Alexa Fluor labels are available), PBS, HBSS, FCS, HEPES, fluorescence or confocal microscope.

## 8.2.5.2.2  Protocol

1. Seed cells in plates or chambers suitable for microscopy.
2. Incubate the cells with 75–200 µg/mL dextran-Alexa Fluor for 4–18 h.
3. Wash the cells in PBS and add fresh medium to the cells.
4. Leave the cells for 1–2 h to allow all the dextran-Alexa Fluor to be transported to the lysosomes.
5. Remove the medium and add a suitable microscopy buffer (such as HBSS + FCS + 25 mM HEPES).

*For live-imaging or other longer-term experiments, the cells might prefer clear medium + FCS + 25 mM HEPES.*

6. Acquire micrographs in a microscope of choice (fluorescence or confocal microscope).

*If desired, live imaging can be used to detect the dynamics of LMP if the inducing stimuli is added to the well in the microscope.*

## 8.2.5.2.3  Advantages of This Method

- The fluorescence of the Alexa Fluor label is stable in the hostile environment of the lysosomes. Additionally, the probe does not bleach significantly by repeated exposures to the light of the microscope. Hence, one can follow the dynamics of the lysosomal compartment including LMP events over time.
- With this method, LMP in every cell is evaluated, and thus, in case LMP only happens in a sub-population of the cells, this can be assessed.
- Loading the lysosomes with dextran-Alexa Fluor and visualizing the LMP in real-time interferes relatively little with the cells compared with other methods.
- If desired, fixation of the cells with 4% PFA will preserve the fluorescence of the Alexa Fluor label and hence other cellular features can be investigated alongside LMP in the cells by immunocytochemical stainings.

## 8.2.5.2.4  Limitations of This Method

- Due to the reliance on the fluorescence of the Alexa Fluor label in this method, one has to consider if any other fluorescence arising from autofluorescence of the cells, treatment with a fluorescent small molecule or overexpression of a fluorescently tagged protein might interfere with the detection of the Alexa Fluor. Luckily, dextran coupled to many different Alexa Fluor labels is available, which makes it possible to solve this issue.
- Acquisition and quantification of a large enough number of cells for statistically reliable results are time-consuming and laborious. This process is preferably automated to limit the workload and to avoid any investigator biases in the interpretation of the images.
- As with the method for *Immunocytochemical staining of lysosomal proteases* (Section 8.2.3), a major limitation to this method is the fact that one is looking at a reduction in punctate lysosomal staining and an appearance of

diffuse cytosolic staining. This requires the LMP to be of a certain magnitude to be detectable by microscopy. A limited release of dextran-Alexa Fluor could go undetected in this method.

### 8.2.6   DETECTION OF GALECTIN PUNCTA

#### 8.2.6.1   Introduction

When LMP occurs, not only are the lysosomal contents released to the cytosol, but the soluble cytosolic proteins also gain access to the inside of the lysosomes. Among these are the galectin family proteins, which bind with high affinity to beta-galactosides. These sugars are not present in the cytosol, but the glycocalyx on the inside of the lysosomal membrane is rich in beta-galactosides. Consequently, when LMP occurs, the galectins gain access to lysosomal lumen, bind to beta-galactosides and rapidly accumulate inside the lysosomes. As demonstrated in Figure 8.2g, by visualizing galectins, even small levels of LMP can be detected as a punctate pattern in the cells (Aits et al., 2015b). This can be done either by immunocytochemical stainings or overexpression of a fluorescently tagged galectin. Here, we will concentrate on the immunocytochemical staining of galectins, but overexpression of fluorescently tagged galectin is more suitable in some experimental settings such as large-scale screening.

#### 8.2.6.2   Example of a Step-by-Step Protocol

##### 8.2.6.2.1   Materials and Equipment

Coverslips specifically for cell culture, microscopy slides, 4% PFA, PBS, 0.3% Triton X-100 in PBS with 1% FCS (buffer 1), 0.1% Triton X-100 in PBS with 0.25% FCS (buffer 2), 0.05% Tween-20 in PBS (buffer 3), Hoechst-33342 (or similar nuclear dye), primary and secondary antibodies (see description in the protocol), mounting medium, confocal fluorescence microscope with appropriate lasers/lamps and filters, preferably a computational software to analyze the micrographs.

##### 8.2.6.2.2   Protocol

1. Grow cells of interest on coverslips until approx. 70% confluency.
2. Wash the cells twice in PBS.
3. Fix the cells in 4% paraformaldehyde for 10 min at room temperature followed by incubation with 50 mM $NH_4Cl$ for 10 min.
4. Wash the cells twice in PBS.
5. Permeabilize the cells by incubating them in buffer 1 for 20 min.
6. Incubate the cells in buffer 1 containing 5% FCS and primary antibodies for 1 h at room temperature or overnight at 4°C.

*The primary antibodies should recognize a galectin and a lysosomal marker (such as LAMP-2). The expression pattern of the members of the galectin family varies between tissues, and the stability of the formed puncta also varies between different galectins. In most cases we have seen staining for galectin-1 or -3 to be successful, however, we recommend that the most optimal galectin marker in the given experimental setup is determined beforehand. The optimal concentration of the antibodies can vary greatly from 1:50 to 1:10,000, and this has to be determined beforehand.*

7. Wash the cells thrice in buffer 2.
8. Incubate the cells in buffer 2 containing 5% FCS and secondary antibodies for 1 h in the dark at room temperature.

*The secondary antibodies should recognize one of the primary antibodies each and be coupled to Alexa Fluor probes with different fluorescent labels. The optimal concentration of the secondary antibodies from Molecular Probes is 1:1000.*

9. Wash the cells twice in buffer 3.
10. Incubate the cells with 5 μg/mL Hoechst-33342 for 2 min for visualization of the nucleus (other nuclear stains can be used as well).
11. Wash the cells twice in PBS.
12. Mount the coverslips on microscopy slides with a mounting medium (such as ProLong Gold Antifade from Molecular Probes) and let samples dry overnight in the dark at room temperature.
13. Store the slides in the dark at 4°C or −20°C.
14. Obtain confocal micrographs of the cells and analyze the percentage of cells positive for galectin puncta (a limit such as ≥3 puncta per cell is advised, however, depending on the experimental question to be answered, this limit can be adjusted up or down). The lysosomal marker serves as a reference. Hence, there should be a substantial overlap between the lysosomal marker and the galectin puncta.

### 8.2.6.2.3 Advantages of This Method

- The most prominent advantage of this method is its sensitivity. It can detect even a partial leakage of a single lysosome! The galectin mark remains in lysosomes for several hours allowing also the detection of lysosomes that have leaked and recovered. This makes it the most sensitive method that allows the studying of LMP at the single lysosome level, which has previously not been possible.
- Once the optimal conditions and antibodies have been identified, it is fairly easy to use this method for a relatively large number of samples in parallel. However, an automated process of acquisition and quantification of galectin positive cells is advised.
- For large experiments or screens, transient overexpression of fluorescently labelled galectin or the creation of a stable cell line overexpressing a fluorescently labelled galectin might ease the workload.
- This assay can be adapted to paraffin-embedded tissues and live cell imaging (Aits et al., 2015b).

### 8.2.6.2.4 Limitations of This Method

- The acquisition of the micrographs and quantification of galectin positive cells can be quite laborious. Preferably, these two steps should be done in an automated fashion to decrease workload and to avoid any biases.
- It is advised to add a positive control such as LLOMe. However, some cells lack cathepsin C activity, which is needed for converting LLOMe into a lysosomal detergent.

## 8.3  CONCLUSIONS

Development of reliable methods to detect LMP has revived the interest in lysosomal cell death. Subsequently, emerging genetic data has corroborated the role of cathepsins as evolutionarily conserved executors of cell death, and lysosomal leakage as a significant mediator of both physiological and pathological cell demise (Boya and Kroemer, 2008; Hafner Česen et al., 2012; Kirkegaard and Jäättelä, 2009; Kreuzaler and Watson, 2012; Yamashima and Oikawa, 2009). The addition of the highly sensitive galectin puncta assay to the tool kit may open an entirely new research on the possible role of nonlethal LMP, for example as a cause of inflammation and senescence in lysosomal storage disorders and other degenerative diseases.

## ACKNOWLEDGEMENTS

The related work in the Jäättelä laboratory is supported by grants from the European Research Council (AdG 340751), Danish National Research Foundation (DNRF125), Danish Cancer Society (R90-A5783 and R167-A11061), Novo Nordisk Foundation (NNF15OC0016914) and Independent Research Fund Denmark (DFF-7016-00360).

## REFERENCES

Aits, S., and Jäättelä, M. (2013). Lysosomal cell death at a glance. *J. Cell Sci. 126*(9), 1905–1912.

Aits, S., Jäättelä, M., and Nylandsted, J. (2015a). Methods for the quantification of lysosomal membrane permeabilization: A hallmark of lysosomal cell death. *Methods Cell Biol. 126*, 261–285.

Aits, S., Kricker, J., Liu, B., Ellegaard, A.M., Hämälistö, S., Tvingsholm, S., Corcelle-Termeau, E., Høgh, S., Farkas, T., Jonassen, A.H., et al. (2015b). Sensitive detection of lysosomal membrane permeabilization by lysosomal galectin puncta assay. *Autophagy 11*(8), 1408–1424.

Appelqvist, H., Sandin, L., Björnström, K., Saftig, P., Garner, B., Öllinger, K., and Kågedal, K. (2012). Sensitivity to lysosome-dependent cell death is directly regulated by lysosomal cholesterol content. *PLoS One 7*(11), e50262.

Appelqvist, H., Wäster, P., Kågedal, K., and Öllinger, K. (2013). The lysosome: From waste bag to potential therapeutic target. *J. Mol. Cell Biol. 5*(4), 214–226.

Bidère, N., Lorenzo, H.K., Carmona, S., Laforge, M., Harper, F., Dumont, C., and Senik, A. (2003). Cathepsin D triggers Bax activation, resulting in selective apoptosis-inducing factor (AIF) relocation in T lymphocytes entering the early commitment phase to apoptosis. *J. Biol. Chem. 278*(33), 31401–31411.

Bové, J., Martínez-Vicente, M., Dehay, B., Perier, C., Recasens, A., Bombrun, A., Antonsson, B., and Vila, M. (2014). BAX channel activity mediates lysosomal disruption linked to Parkinson disease. *Autophagy 10*(5), 889–900.

Boya, P., and Kroemer, G. (2008). Lysosomal membrane permeabilization in cell death. *Oncogene 27*(50), 6434–6451.

Charley, M., Thiele, D.L., Bennett, M., and Lipsky, P.E. (1986). Prevention of lethal murine graft versus host disease by treatment of donor cells with L-leucyl-L-leucine methyl ester. *J. Clin. Invest. 78*(5), 1415–1420.

Cirman, T., Orešić, K., Mazovec, G.D., Turk, V., Reed, J.C., Myers, R.M., Salvesen, G.S., and Turk, B. (2004). Selective disruption of lysosomes in HeLa cells triggers apoptosis mediated by cleavage of bid by multiple papain-like lysosomal cathepsins. *J. Biol. Chem. 279*(5), 3578–3587.

Conus, S., Pop, C., Snipas, S.J., Salvesen, G.S., and Simon, H.U. (2012). Cathepsin D primes caspase-8 activation by multiple intra-chain proteolysis. *J. Biol. Chem.* 287(25), 21142–21151.

Droga-Mazovec, G., Bojič, L., Petelin, A., Ivanova, S., Romih, R., Repnik, U., Salvesen, G.S., Stoka, V., Turk, V., and Turk, B. (2008). Cysteine cathepsins trigger caspase-dependent cell death through cleavage of bid and antiapoptotic Bcl-2 homologues. *J. Biol. Chem.* 283(27), 19140–19150.

de Duve, C. (1983). Lysosomes revisited. *Eur. J. Biochem.* 137(3), 391–397.

Ellegaard, A.M., Dehlendorff, C., Vind, A.C., Anand, A., Cederkvist, L., Petersen, N.H.T., Nylandsted, J., Stenvang, J., Mellemgaard, A., Østerlind, K., et al. (2016). Repurposing cationic amphiphilic antihistamines for cancer treatment. *EBioMedicine 9*, 130–139.

Ellegaard, A.M., Groth-Pedersen, L., Oorschot, V., Klumperman, J., Kirkegaard, T., Nylandsted, J., and Jäättelä, M. (2013). Sunitinib and SU11652 inhibit acid sphingomyelinase, destabilize lysosomes, and inhibit multidrug resistance. *Mol. Cancer Ther.* 12(10), 2018–2030.

Fehrenbacher, N., Gyrd-Hansen, M., Poulsen, B., Felbor, U., Kallunki, T., Boes, M., Weber, E., Leist, M., and Jäättelä, M. (2004). Sensitization to the lysosomal cell death pathway upon immortalization and transformation. *Cancer Res.* 64(15), 5301–5310.

Feldstein, A.E., Werneburg, N.W., Li, Z., Bronk, S.F., and Gores, G.J. (2006). Bax inhibition protects against free fatty acid-induced lysosomal permeabilization. *Am. J. Physiol. Gastrointest. Liver Physiol.* 290(6), G1339–G1346.

Firestone, R.A., Pisano, J.M., and Bonney, R.J. (1979). Lysosomotropic agents. 1. Synthesis and cytotoxic action of lysosomotropic detergents. *J. Med. Chem.* 22(9), 1130–1133.

Foghsgaard, L., Wissing, D., Mauch, D., Lademann, U., Bastholm, L., Boes, M., Elling, F., Leist, M., and Jäättelä, M. (2001). Cathepsin B acts as a dominant execution protease in tumor cell apoptosis induced by tumor necrosis factor. *J. Cell Biol.* 153(5), 999–1009.

Galluzzi, L., Vitale, I., Aaronson, S.A., Abrams, J.M., Adam, D., Agostinis, P., Alnemri, E.S., Altucci, L., Amelio, I., Andrews, D.W., et al. (2018). Molecular mechanisms of cell death: Recommendations of the Nomenclature Committee on Cell Death 2018. *Cell Death Differ.* 25(3), 486–541.

Geelen, M.J.H. (2005). The use of digitonin-permeabilized mammalian cells for measuring enzyme activities in the course of studies on lipid metabolism. *Anal. Biochem.* 347(1), 1–9.

Gómez-Sintes, R., Ledesma, M.D., and Boya, P. (2016). Lysosomal cell death mechanisms in aging. *Ageing Res. Rev. 32*, 150–168.

Groth-Pedersen, L., Aits, S., Corcelle-Termeau, E., Petersen, N.H.T., Nylandsted, J., and Jäättelä, M. (2012). Identification of cytoskeleton-associated proteins essential for lysosomal stability and survival of human cancer cells. *PLoS One 7*(10), e45381.

Guan, J.J., Zhang, X.D., Sun, W., Qi, L., Wu, J.C., and Qin, Z.H. (2015). DRAM1 regulates apoptosis through increasing protein levels and lysosomal localization of BAX. *Cell Death Dis. 6*, e1624.

Guicciardi, M.E., Deussing, J., Miyoshi, H., Bronk, S.F., Svingen, P.A., Peters, C., Kaufmann, S.H., and Gores, G.J. (2000). Cathepsin B contributes to TNF-α-mediated hepatocyte apoptosis by promoting mitochondrial release of cytochrome c. *J. Clin. Invest.* 106(9), 1127–1137.

Gyrd-Hansen, M., Farkas, T., Fehrenbacher, N., Bastholm, L., Hoyer-Hansen, M., Elling, F., Wallach, D., Flavell, R., Kroemer, G., Nylandsted, J., and Jäättelä, M. (2006). Apoptosome-independent activation of the lysosomal cell death pathway by caspase-9. *Mol. Cell. Biol.* 26(21), 7880–7891.

Hafner Česen, M., Pegan, K., Špes, A., and Turk, B. (2012). Lysosomal pathways to cell death and their therapeutic applications. *Exp. Cell Res.* 318(11), 1245–1251.

Hung, Y.H., Chen, L.M.W., Yang, J.Y., and Yuan Yang, W. (2013). Spatiotemporally controlled induction of autophagy-mediated lysosome turnover. *Nat. Commun. 4*, 2111.

Jahchan, N.S., Dudley, J.T., Mazur, P.K., Flores, N., Yang, D., Palmerton, A., Zmoos, A.F., Vaka, D., Tran, K.Q.T., Zhou, M., et al. (2013). A drug repositioning approach identifies tricyclic antidepressants as inhibitors of small cell lung cancer and other neuroendocrine tumors. *Cancer Discov. 3*(12), 1364–1377.

Johansson, A.C., Appelqvist, H., Nilsson, C., Kågedal, K., Roberg, K., and Öllinger, K. (2010). Regulation of apoptosis-associated lysosomal membrane permeabilization. *Apoptosis 15*(5), 527–540.

Kågedal, K., Zhao, M., Svensson, I., and Brunk, U.T. (2001). Sphingosine-induced apoptosis is dependent on lysosomal proteases. *Biochem. J. 359*(2), 335–343.

Karch, J., Schips, T.G., Maliken, B.D., Brody, M.J., Sargent, M.A., Kanisciak, O., and Molkentin, J.D. (2017). Autophagic cell death is dependent on lysosomal membrane permeability through bax and bak. *eLife 6*, e30543.

Kirkegaard, T., and Jäättelä, M. (2009). Lysosomal involvement in cell death and cancer. *Biochim. Biophys. Acta Mol. Cell Res. 1793*(4), 746–754.

Kirkegaard, T., Roth, A.G., Petersen, N.H.T., Mahalka, A.K., Olsen, O.D., Moilanen, I., Zylicz, A., Knudsen, J., Sandhoff, K., Arenz, C., et al. (2010). Hsp70 stabilizes lysosomes and reverts Niemann-Pick disease-associated lysosomal pathology. *Nature 463*(7280), 549–553.

Kornhuber, J., Tripal, P., Reichel, M., Mühle, C., Rhein, C., Muehlbacher, M., Groemer, T.W., and Gulbins, E. (2010). Functional inhibitors of acid sphingomyelinase (FIASMAS): A novel pharmacological group of drugs with broad clinical applications. *Cell. Physiol. Biochem. 26*(1), 9–20.

Kreuzaler, P., and Watson, C.J. (2012). Killing a cancer: What are the alternatives? *Nat. Rev. Cancer 12*(6), 411–424.

Kurz, T., Terman, A., Gustafsson, B., and Brunk, U.T. (2008). Lysosomes and oxidative stress in aging and apoptosis. *Biochim. Biophys. Acta Gen. Subj. 1780*(11), 1291–1303.

Li, N., Zheng, Y., Chen, W., Wang, C., Liu, X., He, W., Xu, H., and Cao, X. (2007). Adaptor protein LAPF recruits phosphorylated p53 to lysosomes and triggers lysosomal destabilization in apoptosis. *Cancer Res. 67*(23), 11176–11185.

Loison, F., Zhu, H., Karatepe, K., Kasorn, A., Liu, P., Ye, K., Zhou, J., Cao, S., Gong, H., Jenne, D.E., et al. (2014). Proteinase 3-dependent caspase-3 cleavage modulates neutrophil death and inflammation. *J. Clin. Invest. 124*(10), 4445–4458.

Petersen, N.H.T., Kirkegaard, T., Olsen, O.D., and Jäättelä, M. (2010). Connecting Hsp70, sphingolipid metabolism and lysosomal stability. *Cell Cycle 9*(12), 2305–2309.

Petersen, N.H.T., Olsen, O.D., Groth-Pedersen, L., Ellegaard, A.M., Bilgin, M., Redmer, S., Ostenfeld, M.S., Ulanet, D., Dovmark, T.H., Lønborg, A., et al. (2013). Transformation-associated changes in sphingolipid metabolism sensitize cells to lysosomal cell death induced by inhibitors of acid sphingomyelinase. *Cancer Cell 24*(3), 379–393.

Prudova, A., Gocheva, V., auf dem Keller, U., Eckhard, U., Olson, O.C., Akkari, L., Butler, G.S., Fortelny, N., Lange, P.F., Mark, J.C., et al. (2016). TAILS N-Terminomics and proteomics show protein degradation dominates over proteolytic processing by cathepsins in pancreatic tumors. *Cell Rep. 16*, 1762–1773.

Repnik, U., Distefano, M.B., Speth, M.T., Wui Ng, M.Y., Progida, C., Hoflack, B., Gruenberg, J., and Griffiths, G. (2017). L-leucyl-L-leucine methyl ester does not release cysteine cathepsins to the cytosol but inactivates them in transiently permeabilized lysosomes. *J. Cell Sci. 130*(18), 3124–3140.

Roberg, K., Kågedal, K., and Öllinger, K. (2002). Microinjection of cathepsin D induces caspase-dependent apoptosis in fibroblasts. *Am. J. Pathol. 161*(1), 89–96.

Shchors, K., Massaras, A., and Hanahan, D. (2015). Dual targeting of the autophagic regulatory circuitry in gliomas with repurposed drugs elicits cell-lethal autophagy and therapeutic benefit. *Cancer Cell 28*(4), 456–471.

Sukhai, M.A., Prabha, S., Hurren, R., Rutledge, A.C., Lee, A.Y., Sriskanthadevan, S., Sun, H., Wang, X., Skrtic, M., Seneviratne, A., et al. (2013). Lysosomal disruption preferentially targets acute myeloid leukemia cells and progenitors. *J. Clin. Invest. 123*(1), 315–328.

Taha, T.A., Kitatani, K., Bielawski, J., Cho, W., Hannun, Y.A., and Obeid, L.M. (2005). Tumor necrosis factor induces the loss of sphingosine kinase-1 by a cathepsin B-dependent mechanism. *J. Biol. Chem. 280*(17), 17196–17202.

Turk, V., Stoka, V., Vasiljeva, O., Renko, M., Sun, T., Turk, B., and Turk, D. (2012). Cysteine cathepsins: From structure, function and regulation to new frontiers. *Biochim. Biophys. Acta Proteins Proteom. 1824*(1), 68–88.

Vanden Berghe, T., Vanlangenakker, N., Parthoens, E., Deckers, W., Devos, M., Festjens, N., Guerin, C.J., Brunk, U.T., Declercq, W., and Vandenabeele, P. (2010). Necroptosis, necrosis and secondary necrosis converge on similar cellular disintegration features. *Cell Death Differ. 17*(6), 922–930.

Uchimoto, T., Nohara, H., Kamehara, R., Iwamura, M., Watanabe, N., and Kobayashi, Y. (1999). Mechanism of apoptosis induced by a lysosomotropic agent, L-leucyl-L- leucine methyl ester. *Apoptosis 4*(5), 357–362.

Xu, H., and Ren, D. (2015). Lysosomal physiology. *Annu. Rev. Physiol. 77*, 57–80.

Yamashima, T., and Oikawa, S. (2009). The role of lysosomal rupture in neuronal death. *Prog. Neurobiol. 89*(4), 343–358.

# 9 Rapid Isolation of Lysosomes from Cultured Cells Using a Twin Strep Tag

*Jian Xiong, Jingquan He, Michael X. Zhu, and Guangwei Du*

## CONTENTS

## 9.1 INTRODUCTION

Lysosomes are the major degradation compartments of the cells. These acidic organelles rely on hundreds of proteins that reside in them to carry out the degradation function (Xiong and Zhu, 2016). Besides proteins, lipid homeostasis in the lysosome also plays key roles in lysosomal functions. For example, defects in lysosomal cholesterol trafficking or phosphatidylinositol 3,5-bisphosphate [$PI(3,5)P_2$] production result in enlarged and defective lysosomes (Li et al., 2013; Liao et al., 2007). Impairments in the lysosomal function often cause accumulation of incompletely digested materials inside the organelles, leading to diseases which are referred to as lysosomal storage disorders or LSDs (Xiong and Zhu, 2016). Studies in recent years have also revealed that lysosomes function as not only degradation compartments but also as signalling hubs in response to cellular metabolic needs. For example, the activity of mechanistic target of rapamycin complex 1 (mTORC1) depends on the abundance of lysosomal luminal amino acids, which promotes the tethering of the protein complex to the lysosome to support anabolic activity when nutrient is sufficient (Castellano et al., 2017; Zoncu et al., 2011). Therefore, proteins, lipids and metabolites associated with the lysosome concurrently play critical roles in supporting lysosomal functions and cell signalling.

Because of the growing appreciation of the regulatory functions of lysosomes, there is a great need to understand how contents of both macromolecules and small metabolites are changed in response to alterations in the extracellular environment and intracellular activities, and how these changes regulate downstream signalling pathways and cellular functions. Recent advances in mass spectrometry-based large-scale analysis techniques have provided powerful means to analyze the global levels of proteins, lipids and small molecule metabolites for the understanding of lysosomal functions (Abu-Remaileh et al., 2017; Chapel et al., 2013; Evers et al., 2017; Markmann et al., 2017; Tharkeshwar et al., 2017). For example, several studies have attempted to reveal the metabolomics and proteomics of lysosomes under different growth conditions by isolating lysosomes and utilizing mass spectrometry with ever-increasing sensitivity to detect the abundance of proteins or metabolites within the organelles (Abu-Remaileh et al., 2017; Chapel et al., 2013). However, due to the highly dynamic nature of the lysosomes, it is extremely critical to rapidly enrich a relatively large quantity of lysosomes without contamination of other intracellular organelles.

The traditional method of lysosome purification utilizes density-gradient-based subcellular fractionation (de Araujo and Huber, 2007; Graham, 2001). However, most subcellular fractionation approaches bear inevitable disadvantages. For example, the lysosomes are often contaminated with other organelles. In addition, the entire process requires the use of ultracentrifugation that lasts for a long period of time (typically hours), making the procedure prone to alterations or further metabolism of some molecules, especially signalling molecules associated with the cytoplasmic leaflet of lysosomal membranes and small molecule metabolites commonly transported across the lysosomal membranes. Besides these methods, iron oxide-conjugated dextrans have also been used to load lysosomes through endocytosis and then the labelled lysosomes can be collected by magnets (Rofe and Pryor, 2016). However, dextrans can be enriched in different degrees in various endosome populations and lysosomes at different times of loading and chasing (Humphries et al., 2011). Moreover, accumulation of non-degradable dextrans over the long term may alter lysosomal contents and hence their functions (Kurz et al., 2008). Recently, lysosome isolation through immunoprecipitating an epitope-tagged lysosomal resident protein has been shown to potentially overcome these drawbacks of the traditional approaches (Abu-Remaileh et al., 2017; Zoncu et al., 2011). However, constitutive expression of a particular marker protein posts a risk of "spilling over" the marker to other organelles during its trafficking among different subcellular compartments, therefore introducing contamination as well (Chen et al., 2017). Here, we describe a twin Strep-tagged LAMP1 construct (Lyso-2Strep) under the control of an inducible promoter (Xiong et al., 2019). With this new tool, we are able to purify ~70% lysosomes with high purity from the post-nuclear supernatants (PNS) of cell lysates within 3 minutes (Figure 9.1). An advantage of this rapid purification procedure is demonstrated by differential association of mTORC1 with lysosomes purified from cells cultured in fed and nutrient-starved conditions (Xiong et al., 2019). In this chapter, we describe a detailed

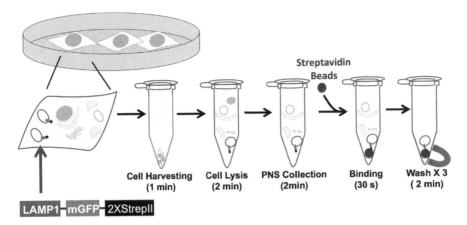

**FIGURE 9.1** Workflow of lysosome purification and time of each step using Lyso-2Strep. Cells expressing Lyso-2Strep are collected (1 minute), mechanically lysed (2 minutes) and centrifuged (2 minutes) to prepare post-nuclear fraction (PNS). Streptavidin magnetic beads are then incubated with PNS (30 seconds), and washed three times (2 minutes) to remove unbound materials.

protocol of lysosome isolation using this new method. Examples of experimental results can be found in the referenced publication (Xiong et al., 2019).

## 9.2  MATERIALS

1. Lyso-2Strep lentiviral construct (Figure 9.1).
2. Lentiviral packaging vectors pCMV-delta R8.2 (Addgene # 12263) and pMD2.g (Addgene # 12259).
3. HEK293T cells (ATCC).
4. Lipofectamine 3000 and Lipofectamine Plus reagent (Thermo Fisher # L3000015).
5. DMEM high glucose culture medium (Sigma # 5796).
6. Opti-MEM medium (Thermo Fisher # 51985034).
7. Fetal bovine serum (FBS) (GenDepot # F0901).
8. Polybrene (8 mg/ml).
9. Puromycin (10 mg/ml, InvivoGen).
10. Potassium-based phosphate-buffered saline (KPBS): 136 mM KCl, 10 mM $KH_2PO_4$, pH 7.4.
11. Phosphate-buffered saline (PBS): 137 mM NaCl, 8 mM $Na_2HPO_4$, 2.7 mM KCl, 1.47 mM $KH_2PO_4$, pH 7.4.
12. LysoTracker™ Red (1 mM in DMSO, Thermo # L7528).
13. VWR PTFE tissue grinders (VWR # 89026-398, VWR # 89026-386).
14. Magnetic streptavidin beads (Thermo Fisher # 88817).
15. Magnet stand (Thermo Fisher # 12321D).
16. 0.45-μm sterile low protein binding surfactant free cellulose acetate (SFCA) syringe filter (Thermo Fisher # 723-9945).

17. Antibodies: Antibodies for S6K (1:1000), SDHA (1:1000), Golgi-97 (1:1000) and Catalase (1:1000) were from Cell Signaling Technology (Danvers, MA). Antibody for α-tubulin (1:5000) was from Sigma-Aldrich (St. Louis, MO), for β-actin from Santa Cruz (Dallas, TX) and for LAMP1 and LAMP2 from the Developmental Studies Hybridoma Bank (Iowa City, IA). Goat anti-mouse and anti-rabbit IgGs conjugated with Dylight 800 and Dylight 680 (1:5000) were from Thermo Scientific (Waltham, MA).

## 9.3   METHODS

HEK293T and HeLa cells are cultured in DMEM high glucose medium supplemented with 10% FBS at 37°C and 5% $CO_2$, unless otherwise instructed. If the lysosomes are prepared for metabolite analysis, all organic solvents should be LC/MS grade and all chemicals should be of high purity. Microcentrifuge tubes used for this purpose should be pre-sterilized by radiation if necessary. Autoclaving should be avoided since vapour from autoclaving might introduce contaminants from water and compromise the purity of metabolite extraction.

### 9.3.1   GENERATION OF HELA CELLS STABLY INFECTED
### WITH THE LYSO-2STREP CONSTRUCT

(1) Seed HEK293T cells onto 6-well culture plates at ~60% confluence and incubate overnight.

   *Note*: HEK293T cells should be either split every other day or avoid over-confluence. We noticed a dramatically decreased virus titre once the HEK293T cells were in confluence for more than one day; however, passage numbers of HEK293T cells do not seem to affect virus packaging.

(2) Next day, at the time of transfection, cell density should reach ~80%.

(3) Dilute 1 μg Lyso-2Strep together with 1 μg pCMV-delta R8.2, 0.2 μg pMD2.g and 4 μl of Lipofectamine Plus reagent in 250 μl Opti-MEM in a microcentrifuge tube. In another microcentrifuge tube, dilute 8 μl of Lipofectamine 3000 in 250 μl Opti-MEM and add the mixture to the DNA tube. Briefly vortex and incubate at room temperature for 15 minutes.

   *Note*: The amount of DNA used in transfection and transfection procedure may vary with different transfection reagents.

(4) Remove culture medium from the HEK293T cells, leaving 1 ml in the well. Gently add the DNA-Lipofectamine mixture to cells drop-by-drop.

   *Note*: take care not to disturb the cells. Gently agitate the plate to allow even distribution.

(5) Incubate the plate for 6 hours at 37°C, 5% $CO_2$.

(6) At 6 hours after transfection, remove medium from the well and then add 2 ml prewarmed Opti-MEM supplemented with 5% FBS.

   *Note*: the removed medium contains a small amount of virus and therefore needs to be treated with bleach before disposal.

(7) At 24 hours post transfection, collect the 2 ml cell culture medium without the cells from the plate and store it in a 15 ml conical tube at 4°C. Add

another 2 ml prewarmed Opti-MEM supplemented with 5% FBS and return the plate to 37°C, 5% $CO_2$.

(8) At 52 hours post transfection, collect the 2 ml cell culture medium without the cells and pool it with the first collection for a total of 4 ml.

*Note*: the leftover cells should be treated with 10% bleach to eradicate all viruses.

(9) Centrifuge the pooled supernatant at 1000 g for 10 minutes at 4°C to remove cell debris, or pass them through a 0.45-μm sterile low protein binding SFCA syringe filter. Collect and transfer the supernatant and discard cell pellet. Aliquot the supernatant in new microcentrifuge tubes at 1 ml per tube and store them in a −80°C freezer.

(10) Seed HeLa cells in a 35-mm culture dish at ~30–50% confluence and incubate them overnight at 37°C, 5% $CO_2$.

(11) Next day, remove the medium from the HeLa cells and add 1 ml of prewarmed lentiviral supernatant from step 9, followed by the addition of polybrene to reach a final concentration of 8 μg/ml (1:1000 dilution of the stock).

(12) Next day, trypsinize and collect all the HeLa cells from the well. Incubate them in a 100-mm culture dish at 37°C, 5% $CO_2$.

(13) At 2 days after lentiviral transduction, replace the culture medium and add 2 μg/ml puromycin.

*Note*: the sensitivity of the target cells to puromycin should be tested by performing a puromycin dose-cell viability assay. The concentration of puromycin used should be the lowest dose that kills all non-transduced cells within 48 hours.

(14) Two or three days after puromycin selection, split the cells into several 100-mm dishes for cryopreservation.

## 9.3.2  PURIFICATION OF LYSOSOMES FROM HELA CELLS STABLY EXPRESSING LYSO-2STREP

(1) Two or three days before lysosome isolation, plate HeLa cells stably expressing Lyso-2Strep in DMEM containing 10% FBS at 50–70% confluency. Supply doxycycline at the final concentration of 1 μg/ml to induce the expression of the fusion protein.

(2) One day before lysosome isolation, re-plate cells on a 15-cm cell culture dish in DMEM containing 10% FBS without doxycycline and culture them overnight. Cell density should reach 90% the next day (~20 million cells in total).

*Note*: One 15-cm dish contains about 20 million HeLa cells; however, if cells are flat and big, more cells may be needed for some applications.

Lysosomal proteins traffic through the endoplasmic reticulum and Golgi apparatus before they reach lysosomes. We routinely remove doxycycline by reseeding cells in order to minimize the presence of newly synthesized Lyso-2Strep proteins on non-lysosomal compartments. This step may be skipped.

(3) On the day of lysosomal isolation, pre-chill centrifuge, all buffers and tubes to 4°C.

(4) Treat cells with appropriate stimuli as needed. For amino acid starvation, one plate of cells grown in normal culture medium is used as a control; one plate of cells is starved in amino acid-free medium for 1 hour; and another plate of cells is first amino acid starved for 1 hour and then followed by refeeding with the normal culture medium.

(5) At the end of the treatment, remove the medium and immediately add ~20 ml of pre-chilled PBS to wash off the residual medium and then remove the wash buffer as much as possible.

(6) Repeat wash in step 5.

(7) Add 1 ml of pre-chilled KPBS to the plates and detach the cells with a cell lifter. Collect all the cells into a microcentrifuge tube and centrifuge at 1000 g for 30 seconds.

(8) Remove the supernatant, resuspend the cells with 1 ml of KPBS, then transfer the cell suspension to a Dounce homogenizer.

(9) Stroke the plunger 25–30 times to break the cells.

*Note*: The space between the plunger and vessel varies even among the same batch of homogenizers. We strongly recommend adding water to the homogenizer to test the tightness of the homogenizer before use. Homogenizers of similar tightness should be used in order to accomplish similar yields when several lysosome samples are compared in biochemical assays.

Cells may be also mechanically disrupted by nitrogen decompression using Parr 4639 cell disruption vessels (Cat #4639, Parr Instrument Company), which offers a very fast and consistent cell lysis. However, for cells with small sizes, this method may not be very efficient.

(10) Transfer the homogenate to a new microcentrifuge tube and centrifuge at 1000 g for 2 minutes to remove nuclei.

(11) While waiting for centrifugation, mix streptavidin magnetic beads thoroughly and transfer 200 µl beads to a microcentrifuge tube.

*Note*: The yield of lysosomes may be further increased by using more beads. The size of the magnetic beads is very critical. Among 50 nm, 1 µm, 5 µm and 25 µm beads we have tested, the beads with 1 µm diameter showed the most recovery of the lysosomes (Xiong et al., 2019). Among the few manufacturers we have tested, magnetic streptavidin beads from Thermo Fisher worked the best. If a faster recovery is needed, we suggest further testing the isolation using beads between 0.2 µm and 2 µm (in diameter).

(12) Wash the beads twice with KPBS and resuspend them with 800 µl of PNS from step 10 by gently pipetting up and down until no more visible pellets of the beads are present in the tube.

*Note*: Make sure that the cell pellet is not disturbed when taking out PNS.

(13) Incubate the bead-PNS mixture in a rotator for 0.5–2 minutes at 4°C.

*Note*: Due to the high affinity between the twin Strep tag and streptavidin, the binding between lysosomes and beads is faster than the typical antibody-based methods. In our hands, the maximal lysosome capture efficiency is achieved in 0.5–1 minute, and a longer incubation time does not seem to increase the recovery of the lysosomes (Xiong et al., 2019). We recommend checking the recovery efficiency at different time points of incubation if the speed of isolation is critical.

(14) Briefly centrifuge the samples for ~2 seconds in a microcentrifuge to collect all the mixtures from the lid and body of the tube and then place the tubes against the magnetic stand to allow the beads to be attracted to the magnet.

(15) Remove the supernatants and resuspend the beads in 1 ml KPBS, transferring the mixture to a new tube to avoid potential non-specific binding to the wall of the microcentrifuge tube.

(16) Wash the beads twice by resuspending with 1 ml KPBS and collect beads with magnet.

*Note*: For lysosome integrity evaluation, spare 50 μl for LysoTracker staining (step 18). For metabolite analysis in lysosomes, after suspending beads with KPBS during the last wash, spare 100 μl for immunoblot analysis (step 17).

(17) For immunoblot analysis, elute the beads with 200 μl 1× SDS sampling buffer containing 2%-mercaptoethanol, vortex for 10 seconds and briefly centrifuge. Incubate the mixture for 10 minutes in a 37°C water bath or boil the sample for 5 minutes.

*Note*: If the proteins of interest are multi-transmembrane proteins, the sample should not be boiled. Multi-transmembrane proteins might aggregate and fail to properly migrate in SDS-PAGE. The purity of isolated lysosomes can be determined by immunoblotting using antibodies against lysosomal proteins, such as LAMP1 and LAMP2, as well as other intracellular organelles, such as HSPA9 (mitochondria), calnexin (endoplasmic reticulum), EEA1 (early endosomes), catalase (peroxisomes) and tubulin (cytoskeleton) (Xiong et al., 2019). Only the lysosomal proteins should be detected by immunoblotting in a successful lysosome purification. To assess the changes of signalling molecules associated with lysosomes upon amino acid treatments, we measured the level of mTORC1 by immunoblotting as well, and observed decreased levels of mTOR, raptor and phosphor-mTOR (S2448) in lysosome preparations isolated from amino acid-starved cells (Xiong et al., 2019).

(18) To assess the integrity of the extracted lysosomes, add 1 μl LysoTracker Red to 50 μl beads suspension and incubate for 5 minutes. Wash once with 200 μl KPBS and subject the sample to fluorescence imaging.

*Note*: Staining of purified lysosomes by LysoTracker indicates their intactness and a low pH in their lumen, as LysoTracker only labels acidic compartments.

(19) For amino acid extraction, add 60 μl of 50% methanol (v/v in $H_2O$) to the beads and vortex for 10 seconds. Collect the mixture by a brief centrifugation and vortex for another 10 seconds. Leave the mixture on ice for 5 minutes, then collect beads with the magnetic stand. Transfer the supernatant to a clean glass sample bottle and keep the sample at −20°C or −80°C for storage.

(20) Lysosomes may also be eluted from the beads by KPBS containing 20 mM biotin.

### 9.3.3 AMINO ACID ANALYSIS BY LC-MS

(1) Spike 5 μl of isotopic labelled amino acid standard mix into each sample.
(2) Set the parameters of HPLC and MS as follows: Gas temperature, 250°C; Gas flow, 14 l/min; Nebulizer gas pressure, 20 psi; Sheath gas temperature, 350°C; Sheath gas flow, 12 l/min; Capillary voltage, 3000 V positive and 3000 V negative; Nozzle voltage, 1500 V positive and 1500 V negative.

*Note*: approximately 8–11 data points are acquired for each of the detected amino acids.
(3) Include three runs for each sample by loading 20 μl of the same sample three times.

*Note*: because amino acids are small molecules, we used 30 minutes as the interval between each loading. For the analysis of larger metabolites, longer intervals may be required.
(4) Amino acid metabolites are identified by using 0.1% formic acid as buffer (A) and 0.1% formic acid in acetonitrile as buffer (B) using Zorbax eclipse XDB C-18 Chromatography column (Agilent Technologies). The samples can be analyzed on 6490 triple quadrupole mass spectrometer coupled with 1290 series HPLC system equipped with a degasser, binary pump, thermostatted autosampler and column oven (Agilent Technologies, Santa Clara, CA).
(5) LC-MS analysis is performed in MRM mode. Data analysis is carried out by using Agilent Mass Hunter workstation software. All the identified amino acids may be normalized against the spiked isotopic labelled standard.

## 9.4 CONCLUSION AND PERSPECTIVES

A rapid and efficient lysosomal purification method is critical to the characterization of the proteins, lipids and metabolites in the lysosomes, thus helping us understand lysosomal functions. The method described in this chapter allows rapid isolation of ~70% of total lysosomes from the PNS, which are free of detectable contamination from other organelles (Xiong et al., 2019). The lysosomes purified with this method are intact, they preserve the activity of the signalling molecules on the organellar membrane (e.g. mTORC1) and they can be used for metabolomic analysis (Xiong et al., 2019). The same procedure described in this chapter can also be applied to purify other organelles such as mitochondria and peroxisomes in cells expressing the twin Strep tag fused to the mitochondrial and peroxisomal targeting sequences (Mito-2Strep and Pero-2Strep), respectively (Xiong et al., 2019). This fast purification method will likely find its use in many applications where rapid isolation of subcellular compartments with high fidelity is required. We also anticipate that this method will be exploited for analyzing lysosome contents of various molecules and lysosomal organization under different conditions, revealing greater mechanistic details of the regulation of these organelles on cellular function.

## ACKNOWLEDGEMENTS

We thank Dr. Takanari Inoue (John Hopkins University) for the LAMP-CFP-FKBP plasmid. This study was supported in part by grants from American Heart

Association (19TPA34910051 to G.D.) and National Institutes of Health (AR075830 to G.D, and NS092377 to M.X.Z).

## REFERENCES

Abu-Remaileh, M., Wyant, G.A., Kim, C., Laqtom, N.N., Abbasi, M., Chan, S.H., Freinkman, E., and Sabatini, D.M. (2017). Lysosomal metabolomics reveals V-ATPase- and mTOR-dependent regulation of amino acid efflux from lysosomes. *Science 358*(6364), 807–813.

Castellano, B.M., Thelen, A.M., Moldavski, O., Feltes, M., van der Welle, R.E., Mydock-McGrane, L., Jiang, X., van Eijkeren, R.J., Davis, O.B., Louie, S.M., Perera, R.M., Covey, D.F., Nomura, D.K., Ory, D.S., and Zoncu, R. (2017). Lysosomal cholesterol activates mTORC1 via an SLC38A9-Niemann-Pick C1 signaling complex. *Science 355*(6331), 1306–1311.

Chapel, A., Kieffer-Jaquinod, S., Sagne, C., Verdon, Q., Ivaldi, C., Mellal, M., Thirion, J., Jadot, M., Bruley, C., Garin, J., Gasnier, B., and Journet, A. (2013). An extended proteome map of the lysosomal membrane reveals novel potential transporters. *Mol Cell Proteomics 12*(6), 1572–1588.

Chen, W.W., Freinkman, E., and Sabatini, D.M. (2017). Rapid immunopurification of mitochondria for metabolite profiling and absolute quantification of matrix metabolites. *Nat Protoc 12*(10), 2215–2231.

de Araujo, M.E., and Huber, L.A. (2007). Subcellular fractionation. *Methods Mol Biol 357*, 73–85.

Evers, B.M., Rodriguez-Navas, C., Tesla, R.J., Prange-Kiel, J., Wasser, C.R., Yoo, K.S., McDonald, J., Cenik, B., Ravenscroft, T.A., Plattner, F., Rademakers, R., Yu, G., White, C.L. 3rd, and Herz, J. (2017). Lipidomic and transcriptomic basis of lysosomal dysfunction in progranulin deficiency. *Cell Rep 20*(11), 2565–2574.

Graham, J.M. (2001). Isolation of lysosomes from tissues and cells by differential and density gradient centrifugation. *Curr Protoc Cell Biol*. Chapter 3, Unit 3.6.

Humphries, W.H.T., Szymanski, C.J., and Payne, C.K. (2011). Endo-lysosomal vesicles positive for Rab7 and LAMP1 are terminal vesicles for the transport of dextran. *PLoS One 6*(10), e26626.

Kurz, T., Terman, A., Gustafsson, B., and Brunk, U.T. (2008). Lysosomes in iron metabolism, ageing and apoptosis. *Histochem Cell Biol 129*(4), 389–406.

Li, X., Wang, X., Zhang, X., Zhao, M., Tsang, W.L., Zhang, Y., Yau, R.G., Weisman, L.S., and Xu, H. (2013). Genetically encoded fluorescent probe to visualize intracellular phosphatidylinositol 3,5-bisphosphate localization and dynamics. *Proc Natl Acad Sci USA 110*(52), 21165–21170.

Liao, G., Yao, Y., Liu, J., Yu, Z., Cheung, S., Xie, A., Liang, X., and Bi, X. (2007). Cholesterol accumulation is associated with lysosomal dysfunction and autophagic stress in Npc1$^{-/-}$ mouse brain. *Am J Pathol 171*(3), 962–975.

Markmann, S., Krambeck, S., Hughes, C.J., Mirzaian, M., Aerts, J.M., Saftig, P., Schweizer, M., Vissers, J.P., Braulke, T., and Damme, M. (2017). Quantitative proteome analysis of mouse liver lysosomes provides evidence for mannose 6-phosphate-independent targeting mechanisms of acid hydrolases in mucolipidosis II. *Mol Cell Proteomics 16*(3), 438–450.

Rofe, A.P., and Pryor, P.R. (2016). Purification of lysosomes using supraparamagnetic iron oxide nanoparticles (SPIONs). *Cold Spring Harb Protoc 2016*(4), pdb prot084822.

Tharkeshwar, A.K., Trekker, J., Vermeire, W., Pauwels, J., Sannerud, R., Priestman, D.A., Te Vruchte, D., Vints, K., Baatsen, P., Decuypere, J.P., Lu, H., Martin, S., Vangheluwe, P., Swinnen, J.V., Lagae, L., Impens, F., Platt, F.M., Gevaert, K., and Annaert, W. (2017). A novel approach to analyze lysosomal dysfunctions through subcellular proteomics and lipidomics: The case of NPC1 deficiency. *Sci Rep 7*, 41408.

Xiong, J., He, J., Xie, W.P., Hinojosa, E., Ambati, C.S.R., Putluri, N., Kim, H.E., Zhu, M.X., and Du, G. (2019). Rapid affinity purification of intracellular organelles using a twin strep tag. *J Cell Sci 132*(24). doi:10.1242/jcs.235390.

Xiong, J., and Zhu, M.X. (2016). Regulation of lysosomal ion homeostasis by channels and transporters. *Sci China Life Sci 59*(8), 777–791.

Zoncu, R., Bar-Peled, L., Efeyan, A., Wang, S., Sancak, Y., and Sabatini, D.M. (2011). mTORC1 senses lysosomal amino acids through an inside-out mechanism that requires the vacuolar $H^+$-ATPase. *Science 334*(6056), 678–683.

# 10 A Transcriptomic Analysis and shRNA Screen for Intracellular Ion Channels and Transporters Regulating Pigmentation

*Donald C. Koroma, Salwa Y. Hafez,*
*and Elena Oancea*

## CONTENTS

## 10.1   INTRODUCTION

We owe the colour of our skin, hair, and eyes to the pigment produced in melanocytes, specialized cells that synthesize and store melanin. Melanocytes in the skin,
hair, and eyes, as well as retinal pigmented epithelial cells, contain melanosomes,
unique organelles that provide the optimal environment for melanin synthesis and
storage (Marks and Seabra 2001, Hearing 2005) (Figure 10.1). Melanosomes are
lysosomal-related organelles derived from the endocytic pathway that share similarities to other lysosomal-related organelles like the platelet-dense and basophil granules (Raposo and Marks 2007). The endosome-derived organelles are involved in

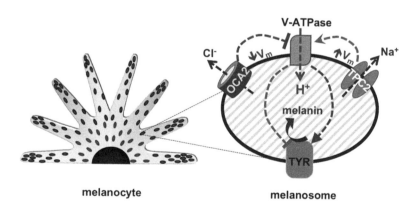

**FIGURE 10.1**   Melanosomal channels and transporters regulate luminal pH and tyrosinase
(TYR) activity in melanocytes. Melanocytes are pigment-producing cells that synthesize and
store melanin in specialized lysosomal-related organelles named melanosomes. Melanosomal
channels and transporters tightly regulate the ionic milieu by controlling the flow of ions and
melanogenic substrates into and out the melanosome lumen to influence pH and melanin
synthesis. Melanosome luminal pH regulates the activity of the main melanogenic enzyme,
TYR, and determines the rate of melanin synthesis. Vacuolar ATPases (V-ATPases) transport
protons ($H^+$) into the melanosome lumen to acidify it and inhibit TYR activity and melanin
synthesis. OCA2, encoded by the gene mutated in oculocutaneous albinism type II, is an
anion channel that conducts $Cl^-$, decreasing the driving force on the electrogenic V-ATPase
when $Cl^-$ is taken out of the melanosome. In contrast, two-pore channel 2 (TPC2) is a melanosomal cation channel that conducts $Na^+$ out of the lumen, increasing the driving force on
the V-ATPase, which, in turn, will acidify the melanosome.

different cellular functions: degradation of proteins, immune responses, and, in the case of melanosomes, pigmentation of the eyes, hair, and skin (Lin and Fisher 2007). Their specialized functions are achieved, in part, due to the activities of transporters, ion channels, and receptors localized to their limiting membranes (Bellono et al. 2014, Bellono, Escobar, and Oancea 2016, Bellono and Oancea 2014). The activity of these transmembrane proteins is required for establishing and regulating the unique luminal milieu necessary for the function of these organelles (Schiaffino and Tacchetti 2005, Bellono, Escobar, and Oancea 2016, Bellono et al. 2014). The luminal pH, in particular, is critical for the organellar function, and each organelle has its unique pH that appears to be tightly regulated (Faundez and Hartzell 2004). For example, the acidic pH of lysosomes (pH 4–5) is critical for optimal activity of their degradative enzymes, while melanosomes require a near-neutral pH for the activity of the main melanogenic enzyme, tyrosinase (TYR), necessary for melanin synthesis (Brilliant and Gardner 2001, Halaban et al. 2002).

Defects in melanosomal function result in albinism, characterized by total or partial lack of pigment in the skin, hair, and eyes. Albinism occurs at a frequency of ~1:20,000 in the US, with significantly higher incidence (>1:1,400) in Africa (Luande, Henschke, and Mohammed 1985). The lack of pigment in albinism causes severe visual impairment and elevated susceptibility to skin cancers. Of the seven types of oculocutaneous albinism identified so far, OCA1–7 (Montoliu et al. 2014), five types (OCA1–4 and OCA6) are caused by mutations in genes encoding putative melanosomal transmembrane proteins. Three of these five transmembrane proteins (OCA2, 4, and 6) have the topology of an ion channel or transporter (predicted by UniProtKB, www.uniprot.org) with unknown function, while the protein encoded by the gene mutated in OCA5 is yet to be identified (Kausar et al. 2013). In addition to mutations in melanocyte-specific genes that lead to albinism, there are other identified mutations that cause diseases associated with hypopigmentation or hyperpigmentation (Chow et al. 2007, Bowman et al. 2019, Wang et al. 2015), suggesting that proteins that are not melanocyte-specific can also regulate pigmentation.

Melanosomal transporters and ion channels localized to the delimiting membrane control the movement of ions and other melanogenic substrates between the cytosol and melanosomal lumen (Bellono and Oancea 2014, Bellono, Escobar, and Oancea 2016, Bellono et al. 2014). They work to influence the melanosome ionic milieu, including pH, which, in turn, controls melanin synthesis (Bellono et al. 2014, Bellono, Escobar, and Oancea 2016, Brilliant and Gardner 2001). The melanosomal pH is primarily controlled by vesicular ATPases (V-ATPases), multi-subunit proton pumps that acidify endocytic vesicles (Mindell 2012). Importantly, because V-ATPases are electrogenic (Stauber and Jentsch 2013, Jentsch 2015), the rate of $H^+$ transport depends on the organellar membrane potential ($V_m$) (Faundez and Hartzell 2004) (Figure 10.1). In melanosomes, V-ATPase mediated transport of $H^+$ acidifies the lumen, thus decreasing TYR activity and melanin synthesis (Wang and Hebert 2006, Ancans et al. 2001, Olivares and Solano 2009). Because melanosomes have almost neutral pH for optimal TYR activity, additional regulatory mechanisms must be involved in their luminal pH regulation.

Recently, we have uncovered two melanosomal ion channels that indirectly regulate luminal pH: the anion channel OCA2, encoded by the gene mutated in oculocutaneous albinism type 2 (Bellono et al. 2014), and the cation channel two-pore channel type 2 (TPC2) (Bellono, Escobar, and Oancea 2016, Ambrosio et al. 2016). OCA2 conducts Cl⁻ from the lumen into the cytosol, thus leaving an excess of positive charges in the lumen, which decrease the driving force of the V-ATPase, resulting in higher luminal pH, increased TYR activity, and augmented melanin synthesis (Bellono et al. 2014) (Figure 10.1). In contrast, TPC2 transports Na⁺ out of the melanosomal lumen to decrease the melanosomal pH and negatively regulate melanin synthesis (Bellono, Escobar, and Oancea 2016) (Figure 10.1). Despite our recent progress in understanding melanosomal physiology, OCA2 and TPC2 do not tell the whole story. The regulation of the melanosomal milieu employs complex mechanisms that remain to be elucidated. These mechanisms not only maintain the luminal ionic balance and regulate the pH, but are also responsible for importing the amino acid tyrosine (Bar-Peled and Sabatini 2014) (Milkereit et al. 2015), the primary melanin substrate, the copper cofactor necessary for TYR function (Setty et al. 2008), as well as other critical factors and co-factors necessary for optimal melanosomal function. Transport of amino acids and other substrates often occurs in conjunction with cations like Na⁺ or with other amino acids, transported in the same or opposite directions (DeFelice and Goswami 2007). In addition, for the OCA2 channel to conduct Cl⁻ from the lumen to the cytosol, a Cl⁻ gradient must be maintained, perhaps supported by a Cl⁻ transporter.

To gain more insight into how intracellular ion channels and transporters modulate the function of melanosomes, we analyzed transcriptomic data of primary human epidermal melanocytes obtained by our lab and others (Haltaufderhyde and Oancea 2014, Reemann et al. 2014) to identify candidate intracellular ion channels and transporters that might regulate melanosomal function. We then established shRNA-based high-throughput assays to test and validate the ability of the candidates to modulate melanocyte pigmentation. Here we describe the transcriptomic analyses employed to select the candidates (Figure 10.2A) and the optimized protocol used for the shRNA-mediated changes in pigmentation (Figure 10.3). As a proof of concept and to develop proper controls for the shRNA screen, we used the protocols described here to test three known regulators of pigmentation: the melanogenic enzyme TYR, mutated in OCA1 (Montoliu et al. 2014), OCA2, and TPC2. While TYR and OCA2 are known to be positive regulators of pigmentations (loss of function mutations in these genes lead to albinism), TPC2 is a negative regulator, as reduced TPC2 expression leads to hyperpigmentation of melanocytes (Bellono, Escobar, and Oancea 2016, Ambrosio et al. 2016). The transcripts encoding these three proteins satisfied all the criteria used for our transcriptomic analyses (Figure 10.2B). Moreover, the 96-well plate-based shRNA screen correctly identified TYR and OCA2 as positive regulators and TPC2 as a negative regulator of pigmentation (Figure 10.4A). These results and the effect of the shRNA on reducing the expression of respective transcripts were validated using the 6-well plate protocol (Figure 10.4B). We also tested our co-localization marker and found that all three proteins were localized to melanosomes when expressed in MNT-1 cells (Figure 10.5). The proof of concept results obtained for the positive and negative controls for our screen predict identification of novel pigmentation modulators and regulatory mechanisms for melanosomes.

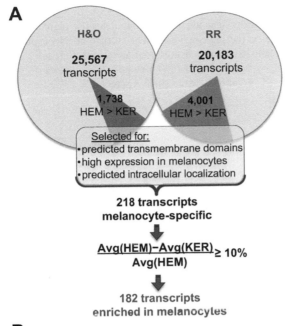

| Gene Symbol | H&O | | | RR | | |
|---|---|---|---|---|---|---|
| | HEM expression (FPKM) | % enriched in HEM vs. KER | | HEM expression (RPKM) | % enriched in HEM vs.KER | |
| TYR | 1517.2 ± 65.0 | 99.9 | | 381.6 ± 62.6 | 97.1 | |
| SLC45A2 | 91.8 ± 40.2 | 100 | | 83.8 ± 22.2 | 98.2 | |
| OCA2 | 241.4 ± 61.6 | 99.9 | | 51.5 ± 14.6 | 95.9 | |
| TPCN2 | 52.1 ± 7.2 | 88.6 | | 21.1 ± 2.1 | 92.5 | |
| MC1R | 13.4 ± 4.9 | 94.4 | | 2.9 ± 0.4 | 91.5 | |

**FIGURE 10.2** Identification of candidate ion channels and transporters that regulate pigmentation based on transcriptomic analyses. (A) We used two independent sets of RNASeq data (H&O and RR, Haltaufderhyde and Oancea 2014, Reemann et al. 2014) from human epidermal melanocytes (HEM) and human epidermal keratinocytes (KER) to identify transcript that were expressed in melanocytes at higher levels than the MC1R gene that encodes the HEM-specific melanogenic G-protein coupled receptor, and that had higher expression in melanocytes than keratinocytes (HEM – KER >0). The abundance of the transcripts was measured in fragments per kilobase million (FPKM) in H&O data set and in reads per kilobase of transcript, per million mapped reads (RPKM) in RR data set. We identified 1,738 and 4,001, respectively, highly and differentially expressed transcripts in HEM vs KER. Further selection of the transcripts from both data sets for encoded proteins, with >1 predicted transmembrane domain and predicted intracellular localization (based on UniProtKB, NCBI, The Human Protein Atlas, and GeneCards databases), resulted in 218 candidates. We further selected for transcripts that were enriched in HEM by calculating percentage enrichment and obtained 182 candidates with average mRNA levels enriched by ≥10% in HEM vs KER.

**FIGURE 10.2 (CONTINUED)**

(B) Representative transcripts encoding known regulators of pigmentation fulfil the selection criteria used to select the 182 candidates. The average mRNA expression of these genes encoding known melanogenic and melanosomal proteins are greater than MC1R's average transcript expression by at least threefold. These known regulators of pigmentation will be further tested and used as controls for the shRNA screen.

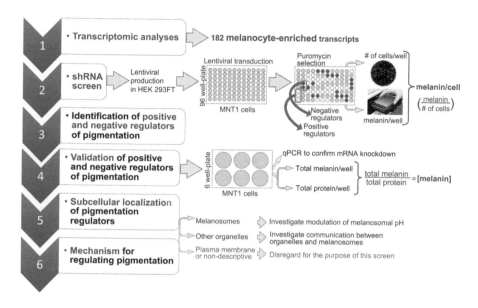

**FIGURE 10.3**   Workflow for identifying putative intracellular ion channels and transporters that regulate melanosomal function.

## 10.2   96-WELL PLATE SHRNA SCREEN FOR PIGMENTATION REGULATORS

### 10.2.1   Transcriptomic Analyses of HEM-Specific Transcripts

**Rationale:** Melanosomes are organelles unique to pigment cells, including epidermal melanocytes. We reasoned that proteins critical for the ability of melanosomes to produce melanin can be encoded by either (i) genes that are unique to pigment cells, similar to those mutated in different types of OCA, or (ii) genes that serve different roles in other cells and in melanocytes are localized to and repurposed to function in melanosomes, similar to TPC2, a lysosomal channel in other cells. Because melanocytes contain a large number of melanosomes, melanosomal proteins will presumably be expressed at high levels in melanocytes, but not in other cells.

We and others have obtained transcriptomic (RNAseq) data from primary human epidermal melanocytes (HEM) and also from human primary epidermal keratinocytes (KER) (Haltaufderhyde and Oancea 2014, Reemann et al. 2014), the cells that surround the epidermal melanocytes and form the outer most layer of our skin. We used the data sets from our lab (H&O) (Haltaufderhyde and

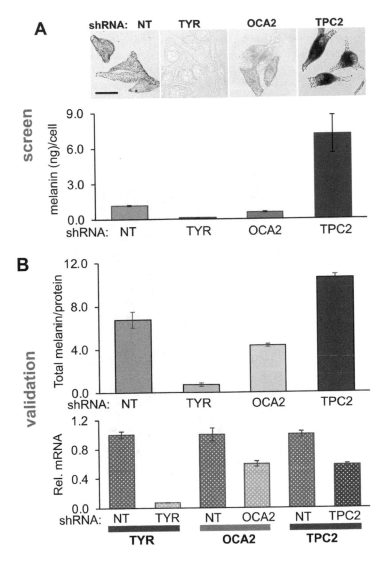

**FIGURE 10.4** TYR, OCA2, and TPC2 are appropriate controls for the shRNA screen as positive (TYR and OCA2) and negative (TPC2) regulators of pigmentation. (A) Using the described protocol for the 96-well plate shRNA screen and targeting TYR, OCA2, or TPC2 resulted in significant changes in MNT1 cells pigmentation. MNT1 cells expressing shRNA targeting TYR or OCA2 appeared depigmented (top: bright field images, scale bar: 20 μm) and had significantly less melanin/cell compared to non-targeting (NT) shRNA control. In contrast, MNT1 cells expressing shRNA targeting TPC2 were highly pigmented (top: bright field image) and had significantly higher melanin/cell values compared to NT shRNA control. Bars represent averages ± SEM of 3–6 independent experiments, $p < 0.0001$ for TYR and OCA2 and $p = 0.0097$ for TPC2. (B) The results obtained in (A) for TYR, OCA2, and TPC2 using the 96-well plate protocol were validated using the 6-well plate validation protocol. Results of classic melanin per protein assays show a significant decrease in total melanin for MNT1 cells expressing shRNA targeting TYR or OCA2, in contrast to TPC2, which

**FIGURE 10.4 (CONTINUED)**

exhibits a significant increase in total melanin, thus validating the initial results obtained in (A). Bar graphs represent averages ± SEM from 3 independent experiments, $p < 0.01$ for all conditions. Quantitative PCR using cDNA obtained from MNT1 cells expressing shRNA targeting TYR, OCA2, or TPC2 showed significantly decreased mRNA levels of the targeted transcripts compared to NT control. Bars represent averages ± SEM from 3 independent experiments, $p < 0.001$ for all conditions.

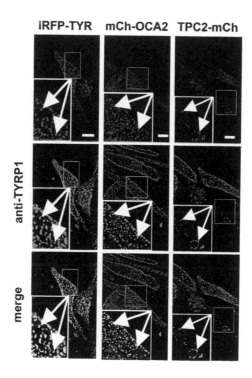

**FIGURE 10.5** Melanosomal localization of fluorescently tagged TYR (iRFP-TYR), OCA2 (mCherry-OCA2), and TPC2 (TPC2-mCherry) in MNT1 pigmented cells. MNT1 cells expressing iRFP-TYR, mCherry-OCA2, or TPC2-mCherry were fixed and immunostained with an antibody against tyrosinase-related protein 1 (TYRP1), shown in green, used as a melanosomal marker. All three proteins showed significant co-localization with the anti-TYRP1 antibody (bottom row). Arrows in enlarged images of the outlined fields indicate co-location (yellow) of TYR, OCA2, or TPC2 with TYRP1 (scale bar: 10 μm).

Oancea 2014) in conjunction with NCBI KER data and also data (H&O) from Reeman et al. (RR) (Reemann et al. 2014) to first identify transcripts that are highly expressed in HEM but not in KER (Figure 10.2A). Differentially expressed transcripts were identified by calculating the average expression of each transcript in keratinocytes [KER (FPKM)] and subtracting it from the corresponding value in melanocytes [HEM(FPKM)]. As a cutoff for expression level of HEM transcripts, we used the average transcript level of the melanocyte-specific G-protein-coupled receptor melanocortin 1 receptor (MC1R) (Figure 10.2B), a master regulator of pigmentation at the plasma membrane (Schioth et al. 1999, Wolf Horrell, Boulanger, and D'Orazio 2016). We reasoned that, unlike melanosomal proteins that need to be expressed in each melanosome or in a sub-set of melanosomes, plasma membrane receptors do not require high expression due to downstream amplification of their activities by second messenger. We found that 1,738 of the 25,267 transcripts in H&O data set and 4,001 of the 20,183 transcripts in the RR data set had higher average expression in HEM than KER and were higher in HEM than the value obtained for MC1R (Figure 10.2B).

An inherent characteristic of transcripts encoding melanosomal transporters, ion channels, and receptors is the presence of transmembrane domains. From the two sets of differentially expressed transcripts, we selected only those predicted to have >1 transmembrane domain based on UniProtKB database (www.uniprot.org). The Human Protein Atlas and GeneCards were then used to further select transcripts encoding proteins with predicted intracellular localization based on Compartments (compartments.jensenlab.org). We obtained 218 such transcripts common to both data sets, RR and H&O. We further selected these transcripts by calculating their fractional representation in HEMs compared to KERs, as shown in Figure 10.2A and setting the threshold to >10% enrichment in HEMs. The enrichment scores allowed for comparison of individual transcripts across both H&O and RR data-sets and the scores for all the identified transcripts were positively correlated. In total, we obtained 182 transcripts that fulfilled all our selection criteria, not including known genes encoding melanosomal proteins. As expected, transcripts encoding known melanosomal proteins with a role in pigmentation, like OCA2, TPCN2, and SLC45A2 (the gene mutated in OCA4), fulfilled all the selection criteria, exhibiting a >80% enrichment in melanocytes (Figure 10.2B). A large majority of the 182 selected transcripts encode proteins with unknown function, in addition to other transcripts for which a function in melanocytes has not been characterized.

## 10.2.2 96-WELL-BASED LENTIVIRAL SHRNA PRODUCTION

**Rationale:** To test which of the identified 182 candidates have a role in melanocyte pigmentation, we developed a protocol for a shRNA screen based on the collection available from the Broad Institute. This collection contains 3–6 shRNAs targeting each transcript (978 shRNAs total for the 182 candidates), with individual shRNAs cloned in the pLKO.1 lentiviral vector containing the puromycin resistance gene. To screen multiple transcripts simultaneously, we adapted and optimized the Broad Institute protocol for viral particle production in 96-well plates (Figure 10.3). The preparation steps for viral production were crucial for optimal efficiency of the screen.

Cells: Lentiviral particles were generated in low passage HEK293FT cells. Upon thawing cells from cryopreservation, HEK293FT cells must be passaged at least two times before seeding for lentiviral production. HEK293FT cells were not cultured for more than 10 passages.

Vectors: To produce lentiviral particles, each shRNA in pLKO.1 was transfected together with the packaging plasmid pCMV-dR8.91 and pVSV-G envelope plasmid. The DNA concentration of all three plasmids, shRNA/pLKO.1, pCMV-dR8.91, and pVSV-G was normalized to 50 ng/μl.

Protocol: The HEK293FT cells were seeded in antibiotic-free media at 40–50% confluence (~22,000 cells per well of 96-well plate) one day before transfection and grown to 70–80% the day of the transfection. To make sure that the cells were evenly seeded to form a monolayer, the cell suspensions were thoroughly mixed to avoid clumping. Post seeding, the 96-well plate was immediately placed on a flat surface and incubated at 37°C for 24 h.

Prior to transfecting the HEK293FT cells, the following transfection reagents and master mixes were prepared:

**VC** master mix: for each well, 2 μl pCMV-dR8.91 and 0.2 μl of pVSV-G were added to 10 μl of OPTI-MEM medium to obtain 100 ng pCMV-dR8.91 and 10 ng pVSV-G, respectively. The mix can be scaled to any number of shRNAs.

**MR** master mix: concurrently, a master mix of the transfection agent was prepared in a separate tube by adding 0.6 μl of TransIT-LT1 to 10 μl OPTI-MEM medium per well.

Using a multi-channel pipette (or a robotic arm), 10 μl of the **MR** master mix was transferred to each well of a deep and round bottom 96-well plate.

On a separate round bottom 96-well plate, to each well were added 10 μl of **VC** master mix plus 2 μl of the desired **shRNA/pLKO.1** (to get 100 ng), which were mixed thoroughly by pipetting. The resulting solution was incubated at room temperature for 10 min. The **VC/shRNA** mix was then transferred to each well of the 96-well plate containing the **MR** master mix and dispensed by pipetting rigorously to produce bubbles, which were required for optimal transfection efficiency. The **MR/VC/shRNA** mix was incubated at room temperature for 25–30 min for optimal results. The **MR/VC/shRNA** mix was carefully transferred (to prevent the cells from detaching) to 70–80% density HEK293FT cells seeded the previous day.

To visually determine transfection efficiency, a control well was transfected with cDNA encoding GFP in the same pLKO.1 vector backbone as the shRNAs. The percentage of HEK293FT cells displaying green fluorescence revealed the transfection efficiency, indicative of the virus titre.

The cells and transfection mixtures were incubated for 6–10 h, before the cell media was replaced with 100 μl viral harvesting – high BSA – media. The first round of virus was collected 48 h post transfection by removing 100 μl of the media and replacing it with 100 μl fresh, high BSA media, without disturbing the remaining HEK293FT cells. The collected virus was stored in deep 96-well plates at 4°C until the next harvest. The second round of virus was collected 48 h after the first collection (96 h after transfection) and pooled with the first virus collection. The pooled virus was stored at −80°C for at least 24 h prior to viral transduction to get rid of any lingering HEK293FT cells (which died in the process of freezing and thawing the virus).

### 10.2.3 Lentiviral Transduction of MNT1 Cells

We used MNT1 pigmented melanoma cells to test the effect of shRNAs on pigmentation. Although these cells are highly pigmented, we were able to measure both shRNA-mediated increases and decreases in pigmentation for our control transcripts (Figure 10.4A).

MNT1 cells were seeded at 25,000 cells/well in a 96-well plate, ~24 h prior to transduction. On the day of transduction, the old media was removed, and the cells were washed with PBS. Then, 200 µl of the pooled virus plus polybrene to a final concentration of 8 µg/ml (i.e. 1.3 µl of 600 µg/ml polybrene per 100 µl of virus) were added to each well.

After 24 h of incubation with viral particles, the cells were washed with PBS, and the viral media was replaced with a cell-type-specific medium with 1 µg/ml puromycin to select the cells that were successfully transduced with lentivirus and thus expressing shRNA.

For improved viral transduction efficiency, especially when viral titre was low, the antibiotic selection could start 48 h post viral transduction. Cell media was changed every 2–3 days with fresh media containing 1 µg/ml puromycin. The cells were kept under puromycin selection even after the cells that were not transduced were eliminated. This method allows for the successful selection of the MNT1 cells within 5–6 days post viral transduction.

Since MNT1 cells are highly pigmented, we passaged the cells once or twice post selection, to eliminate residual melanin. This step is particularly important for measuring the effects of shRNAs that cause decreased pigmentation.

Alternatively, to avoid the potential effects of high pigmentation, MNT1 cells can be treated with the tyrosinase inhibitor propylthiouracil (PTU, 300 µM) to block melanin synthesis prior to viral transduction. Ten days of PTU-treatment resulted in completely depigmented MNT1 cells. These cells can then be transduced with shRNA-containing lentiviral particles and released from PTU inhibition on the day of transduction. The effect of shRNAs that causes an increase in pigmentation will be more evident in the depigmented cells in the first few days after PTU is removed and before the MNT1 cells fully restore their normal pigmentation levels (3–4 days).

## 10.2.4 HIGH-CONTRAST BRIGHT FIELD IMAGING TO DETERMINE CELL NUMBER

The size of a 96-well limits the number of cells that can be cultured in it, making it difficult to measure melanin and protein contents for each well using the standard protocol (Ozdeslik et al. 2019). The standard protocol requires cells to be lysed, transferred to a tube, and centrifuged in order to separate the soluble protein from the melanin-containing pellet, a procedure that would be very inefficient for 96-well plates and unsuitable for high-throughput analysis. In addition, the small number of cells in each well represents a major challenge for measuring total melanin and total protein. To circumvent this problem, we used a plate imager to quantify the number of cells in each well of the 96-well plate, to which melanin content can then be normalized.

To determine the number of cells that were successfully selected in each well, the 96-well plates were placed into the incubator chamber of the Opera Phenix (PerkinElmer) cell counter at 37°C and 5% $CO_2$. Using a 10x lens and the default phase contrast programme on the Opera Phenix, the number of cells in each well was determined by taking high-contrast bright field images of multiple quadrants of each well. The Opera Phenix analysis software was used to stitch together the images from each quadrant to produce a single image of all the cells in the well, which was then used to determine the number of cells in each well. As a control, the total number of objects in a blank control well was subtracted from the number of objects in each well.

### 10.2.5  MELANIN MEASUREMENT

After obtaining the cell count for each well of the 96-well plate, the same cells were washed with 100 µl of PBS, before 100 µl of 1 N NaOH was added to release and dissolve their melanin content. The cells in NaOH were incubated overnight at room temperature on a circular shaker. The next day, cell homogenates were incubated at 85°C for 30 min. After the incubation, the homogenates were mixed thoroughly by pipetting up and down with a multi-channel pipette. A plate reader was used to measure the absorbance of each well at 405 nm.

A melanin standard curve was obtained by measuring the absorbance at 405 nm of 100 µl of synthetic melanin with concentrations between 0 µg/ml and 200 µg/ml in individual wells of a 96-well plate. The absorbance values were plotted as a function of synthetic melanin concentration to generate a standard curve. The standard curve was used to determine the melanin concentration in each experimental well. Cellular melanin concentration was calculated as melanin (in ng) per total number of cells in each well.

Similar to the results obtained for our known regulators of pigmentation controls (Figure 10.4A), we expect that shRNAs targeting some of our candidates will lead to either a decrease in pigmentation (positive regulators) or an increase in pigmentation (negative regulators). It is important to evaluate the effect on pigmentation of all the shRNAs targeting a particular transcript, compare the effects with the positive and negative controls, and only then proceed to validation if at least half of the shRNAs targeting the same candidate exhibit a similar trend and cause a significant change in pigmentation compared to non-targeting shRNA or GFP transduced cells.

## 10.3  VALIDATION OF SHRNA EFFECTS ON PIGMENTATION

The validation step will be used for the shRNAs that have a significant effect on MNT1 pigmentation (increase or decrease) measured as described above in Sections 10.2.4 and 10.2.5. The validation step will scale up the number of cells for a small number of candidates and employs the standard techniques for measuring melanin concentration. In addition, we will validate that the effect of each shRNA on pigmentation is due to decreased mRNA levels of the targeting transcript. We expect the effect of individual shRNAs on pigmentation to correlate with the effect on the mRNA levels of the targeted candidate (Figure 10.4B).

### 10.3.1  DETERMINE TOTAL MELANIN PER PROTEIN

MNT1 stably expressing various targeted and scrambled shRNA were grown in 6-well plates to 50–80% confluence. The cells were lysed with 100 µl of lysis buffer and collected with a cell scraper in 1.5 ml tubes, homogenized and spun down at 14,000 rpm for 30 min to separate the soluble protein from the melanin-containing pellet. The volume of the soluble protein fraction (supernatant) was measured before transferring it to a new tube. The protein content of each sample was determined using a BCA protein assay kit and the total protein for each sample was obtained by multiplying the protein content by its corresponding volume.

The melanin pellet was then resuspended in 100 μl of 1 N NaOH and incubated at 85°C for 1 h with intermittent vortexing to completely dissolve the melanin. The precise volume of the solubilized melanin in each tube was recorded and the melanin concentration was determined by measuring absorbance at 405 nm with a Nanodrop and using a calibration curve of synthetic melanin (as described in Section 10.2.5, but measuring the absorbance of each sample by Nanodrop). Samples that were highly pigmented and had absorbance values above the maximum detectable range were further diluted in 1 N NaOH. The total melanin content was obtained by multiplying the melanin concentration determined from the standard curve by the volume of the solubilized melanin for each sample, taking the dilution factor into consideration for the highly pigmented samples. The melanin concentration in each well was calculated as total melanin per total protein (Bellono, Escobar, and Oancea 2016, Bellono et al. 2014, Wicks et al. 2011).

## 10.3.2 QUANTITATIVE POLYMERASE CHAIN REACTION (qPCR)

Another well of the 6-well plate containing the same MNT1 cells used for melanin assays was used to extract RNA with RNeasy Plus Kit (Qiagen). The extracted RNA was reverse transcribed using iScriptTM Reverse Transcription Supermix (Bio-Rad) and the resulting cDNA used for qPCR. The reactions were set up according to the manufacturer's recommended protocol using iTaqTM Universal SYBR Green Master MiX (Bio-Rad) and VIIA-7 Real-Time PCR System (Applied Biosystems). The mRNA level of each targeted gene was determined relative to β-actin mRNA level in controls (Haltaufderhyde and Oancea 2014). The primer pairs used for the transcripts shown in Figure 10.4B (TYR, OCA2, and TPC2) are included in Appendix I.

## 10.4 POSSIBLE MECHANISMS MEDIATING THE CHANGES IN PIGMENTATION

### 10.4.1 IMMUNOSTAINING AND FLUORESCENCE IMAGING

**Rationale:** Our goal is to identify novel intracellular ion channels and transporters regulating pigmentation. Most such proteins known so far are localized to the melanosomal membrane. We will therefore test which of the candidates identified are localized to melanosomes, using co-localization studies with TYR-related protein 1 (TYRP1) immunostained with the monoclonal TA-99 antibody, an established melanosomal marker. Since the majority of our candidates are proteins with unknown functions, it is highly unlikely that we will find validated antibodies available to immunostain the endogenously expressed proteins. As an alternative, we will clone the cDNA for the respective candidates from HEMs as fusion proteins with HA or mCherry tags at either N- or C-termini and express the constructs in MNT1 cells. The localization of the expressed proteins to melanosomes will then be quantified using co-localization with TYRP1 immunostained with the TA-99 antibody. If no melanosomal localization is detected, then co-localization with other known organellar markers (lysosomes, endosomes, recycling endosomes, etc.) will be investigated.

As a proof of concept and control for changes in localization due to overexpression of tagged proteins, we showed that the three pigmentation regulators that we chose as controls (TYR, OCA2, and TPC2) tagged with mCherry or iRFP localized to melanosomes when expressed in MNT1 cells (Figure 10.5). MNT1 cells were seeded on coverslips coated with Poly-L-Lysine (Sigma) at 40–50% density and transfected the following day with 1 µg of the iRFP- or mCherry-tagged candidate cDNA and 1 µl of PolyMag Neo (OZ BIOSCIENCES) transfection reagent and magnet. At 24–48 h after transfection, the cells were fixed with 4% paraformaldehyde and permeabilized with 0.2% (w/v) saponin in 0.1% (w/v) BSA. The melanosomes were immunostained using mouse anti-TYRP1 antibody TA-99 (1:50 dilution, Biolegend) that was detected by goat anti-mouse secondary antibody conjugated to Alexa 488 (Invitrogen) (Bellono et al. 2014, Bellono, Escobar, and Oancea 2016). The cells were imaged using a laser-scanning confocal microscope (Olympus FV3000) with a 63× objective. The images were deconvoluted using the default settings of the built-in cellSens FV3000 software. Co-localization of the melanosomal proteins with TYRP1 can be quantified using Image J software.

## 10.5   RESULTS AND DISCUSSION

Our transcriptomic analyses revealed that many uncharacterized genes encoding putative transporters and ion channels are highly and differentially expressed in HEM, compared to KER. Although transcript levels do not always correlate with the amount of protein synthesized, transcripts encoding known melanogenic proteins (Figure 10.2B) that localize to melanosomes (Figure 10.4) are highly expressed in HEM, compared to the plasma membrane melanogenic receptor MC1R (Figure 10.2B). The transcriptomic analyses and shRNA screen presented here could effectively identify melanosomal regulators of pigmentation. In addition, our transcriptome analyses and shRNA screen could be adapted and used to identify uncharacterized proteins with functional relevance to other organelles.

Our transcriptomic analysis is inherently biased towards transcripts encoding proteins with transmembrane domain and excludes transcripts that encode novel soluble proteins, which may also be involved in regulating melanosomal function. Additionally, the comparative analyses of transcriptomic data of HEM from our lab with a KER dataset from NCBI could introduce experimental biases because these RNA-sequencing experiments were done by two distinct groups using cell samples from different individuals. Therefore, we included the RNA-sequencing data from Reemann et al. (2014), that analyzed HEM and KER from the same individuals and analyzed all their samples under identical experimental conditions to minimize experimental variation. Nevertheless, the high number of overlapping candidates between the two sets of data is reassuring. The arbitrary cutoff of 10% enrichment applied during the last selection step could exclude some putative candidates that are repurposed for melanosome function in melanocytes and are not expressed at significantly higher levels.

The use of the Opera Phenix high content cell imager to count the cells in each well was essential for comparing the relative melanin concentration across wells and conditions. However, the number of cells that the Opera Phenix imager can accurately detect plateaus around 12,000 cells per well. Therefore, additional steps of standardizing the number of cells in each well were taken to enable comparison of the relative melanin concentration across wells and conditions. To circumvent these issues, we identified wells that were overly confluent and in which individual cells could not be easily distinguished by the software and reduced the number of cells in those wells by reseeding the cells at 50–80% of their initial confluency. In addition, only wells that were 50–80% confluent were selected for counting post selection with puromycin. The cells in all the selected wells were resuspended, thoroughly mixed, and evenly reseeded 24–48 h prior to counting with the Opera Phenix imager.

Furthermore, for wild type MNT1 cells, the melanin concentration per cell increased with the cell density, which led us to conclude that the relative change in melanin per cell across conditions is only comparable for an equal number of cells per well. Therefore, to account for the increasing melanin concentration per cell across conditions, the proportional melanin per cell for each condition was calculated and graphed. This was made possible given that the rate of change of melanin per cell was linear for 4,000–12,000 cells, implying that the rate of change of melanin per cell is directly proportional to the number of cells and their melanin content.

We designed our shRNA screen to target transcripts encoding predicted transmembrane proteins highly expressed and enriched in epidermal melanocytes, as compared to keratinocytes. The selected transcripts encode putative intracellular channels or transporters that might function in pigmentation. The transcriptomic analysis and shRNA screen described here could be adapted to screening for different organellar functions that have a measurable cellular readout, similar to how melanosomal function affects cellular pigmentation. The number of candidates encoding poorly characterized proteins as well as channels and transporters with unknown function in melanocytes hold the promise of finding novel regulators of pigmentation and uncovering new cellular and molecular mechanisms.

## ACKNOWLEDGEMENTS

We thank members of the E.O. lab for stimulating discussions and suggestions and Joshaya Trotman for valuable technical support during the optimization of the protocol. We especially thank Dr. Mickey Marks (University of Pennsylvania) who provided us with the shRNA library. This work was supported by National Institute of Arthritis and Musculoskeletal and Skin Diseases Grant R01AR071382 to E.O., R01AR071382-02S1 to D.K. and by a scholarship to S.Y.H. from King Saud bin Abdulaziz University for Health Sciences, College of Medicine-Jeddah.

## OVERVIEW OF PROTOCOL FOR SHRNA SCREEN FOR MELANOCYTES PIGMENTATION GENES

### SCREEN FOR CANDIDATE PIGMENTATION GENES – 96-WELL PLATE

1. Lentiviral production of shRNA in 96-well plate
2. Lentiviral transduction of MNT1 cells in 96-well plate
3. Puromycin selection of MNT1 cells expressing shRNA
4. Determination of pigmentation of MNT1 cells expressing shRNA
   (a) Count cells/well using high-throughput bright field imaging
   (b) Measure solubilized melanin/well using plate reader
   (c) Calculate melanin/cell for each well

### VALIDATION OF IDENTIFIED CANDIDATES – 6-WELL PLATE

For transcripts that show a significant change in MNT1 pigmentation for more than one targeting shRNA, repeat steps 1–3 above in 2 individual wells of a 6-well plate.

- 1st well: **Determine melanin concentration (total melanin/total protein) of MNT1 cells expressing shRNA**
  - Lyse cells with lysis buffer:
    → supernatant → BCA assay → calculate total protein
    → pellet → solubilize in 1 N NaOH at 85°C → measure absorption at 405 nm → calculate total melanin
    [melanin] = total melanin/total protein
- 2nd well: **Determine mRNA levels of transcripts targeted by shRNA using qPCR**
  - Extract RNA → RT reaction to obtain cDNA → qPCR with transcript-specific primers and actin primers as control → determine transcript of interest for CTRL vs shRNA targeting the transcript of interest, relative to actin levels.

Represent as bar graphs for each transcript of interest: [melanin] and mRNA levels (relative to actin) for control and each of the shRNAs tested. Transcripts that show a change in pigmentation in the same direction for more than 50% of the shRNAs tested are further investigated.

## PROTOCOL FOR SHRNA SCREEN FOR MELANOCYTES PIGMENTATION GENES

### I.  96-WELL-BASED LENTIVIRAL SHRNA PRODUCTION IN HEK293FT CELLS

HEK293FT cells – freshly thawed and passaged at least two times before seeding – could not be used for more than 10 passages.

**DAY 1:**
Seed HEK293FT at 40–50% confluence (~22,000 cells per well of 96-well plate) in antibiotic-free media.

- Mix thoroughly the cell suspensions to avoid clumping
- Seed cells evenly to form a monolayer
- Place a 96-well plate immediately on a flat surface at 37°C and 5% $CO_2$ for 24 h

Cell will be 70–80% on the day of transfection (next day)

**DAY 2:**

Normalize the concentrations of shRNA/pLKO.1, pCMVdR, and pVSV-G plasmids to 50 ng/μl

Prepare the following transfection reagents and master mixes:

*VC master mix:*

Add per well of 96-well plate:

- 2 μl pCMV-dR8.91 at 50 ng/μl → 100 ng/well
- 0.2 μl pVSV-G at 50 ng/μl → 10 ng/well
- 10 μl of OPTI-MEM

→ Scale up to the number of wells corresponding to the number of shRNAs to be tested.

Transfer to a round bottom 96-well plate:

- 10 μl of **VC** master mix
- 2 μl of **shRNA**/pLKO.1 at 50 ng/μl → 100 ng shRNA/well

Mix thoroughly by pipetting → incubate for 10 min

*MR master mix:*

Add per well of 96-well plate:

- 0.6 μl of TransIT-LT1
- 10 μl OPTI-MEM

→ Scale up to the number of wells/shRNAs to be tested

Transfer to each well of a deep and round bottom 96-well plate:

- All 10.6 μl of the **MR** master mix
- All 12 μl of the **VC + shRNA**, added by pipetting vigorously to produce bubbles
  → Incubate at room temperature for 25–30 min (max 30 min for best results).
  → Transfer mix slowly and carefully to the HEK293FT cells seeded the previous day.

Incubate the cells with the transfection mix for 6–10 h, then replace it with 100 μl media with high BSA (viral harvesting media).

**Control for transfection efficiency:** transfect cells with GFP in the same vector as the shRNA plasmids → visualize GFP expression, which reflects transfection efficiency.

**DAY 4:**

- Collect the *first round of virus* (~48 h post transfection) by removing 100 μl of the media containing the viral particles
- Replace the collected media with 100 μl of fresh high BSA media added very slowly not to disturb the remaining HEK293FT cells
- Store the collected virus in deep 96-well plates at 4°C until the next harvest

**DAY 6:**

- Collect the *second round of virus* (~48 h after the first collection) and pool with the first round of virus
- Store pooled virus at −80°C for 24–48 h prior to viral transduction to get rid of any lingering HEK293FT cells

## II.   LENTIVIRAL TRANSDUCTION OF MNT1 CELLS

**DAY 1:**

Seed MNT1 pigmented melanoma cells 25,000/well of a 96-well plate

**DAY 2:**

MNT1 cells should be ~60–70% confluent
Remove media and wash cells with 1× PBS

To each well add:

- 200 μl of the pooled virus
- Polybrene – 2.66 μl of 600 μg/ml → final polybrene concentration = 8 μg/ml
  *polybrene concentration needs to be adjusted for each cell type
  → incubate for 24 h

**DAY 3:**

- Wash cells with 1× PBS
- Replace viral media with MNT1-specific media with 1 μg/ml puromycin for selecting cells expressing shRNA
- Change cell media every 2–3 days with fresh media containing 1 μg/ml puromycin
- This method allows for the successful selection of the MNT1 cells within 5–6 days post viral transduction
    Maintain MNT1 cells in puromycin after selection.
    Optional: For improved viral transduction efficiency, start the antibiotic selection 48 h post viral transduction, especially if viral titre appears not to be high based on the number of GFP-expressing cells.
    Option for positive regulators of pigmentation:

- Treat MNT1 cells with the tyrosinase inhibitor propylthiouracil (PTU, 300 μM in cell media) for 10 days (passage cells twice during this time) to block melanin synthesis → cells will become depigmented
- Transduce MNT1 cells with shRNA-containing lentivirus and remove PTU from the media the day of transduction
- Measure melanin/cell (as described below) 5 days after starting puromycin selection.

## III.  High-Contrast Bright Field Imaging to Determine Cell Number

- Image individual wells of a 96-well plate at 37°C and 5% $CO_2$ using a high-content screening system (Opera Phenix High-Content Screening System)
- Use the 10× lens and the default phase contrast programme on the Opera Phenix
- Determine the number of cells in each well by acquiring high-contrast bright field images of multiple quadrants of each well
- Use the analysis software on the Opera Phenix to stitch together the images and generate a single image of all the cells in each well
- Use the stitched image to determine the total number of cells in each well using the Opera Phenix analysis software
- Control: count the total number of objects in a blank well control and subtract it from the total number of cells in each well

## IV.  MNT1 Melanin Quantification Using Plate Reader

Generate a standard melanin curve:

- Varying concentrations (0.00, 3.13, 6.25, 12.50, 25.00, 50.00, 100.00, and 200.00 μg/ml) of synthetic melanin are made in 1 N NaOH
- The absorbance of each standard solution is measured in a plate reader at 405 nm, by adding 100 μl of each standard solution to a clean well of the same 96-well plate used to culture the MNT1 cells
- The absorbance values obtained from the synthetic melanin measurements are plotted to generate a standard curve
  - Use the same 96-well plate used for counting cells/well to quantify melanin/well
  - Wash each well with 100 μl of 1× PBS
  - Add 100 μl of 1 N NaOH solution to each well to release and dissolve the melanin from the MNT1 cells
  - Shake the 96-well plate overnight in a circular motion at room temperature
  - Next day, incubate 96-well plate at 85°C for 30 min
  - Mix the homogenate in each well thoroughly by pipetting up and down
  - Measure the absorbance of each well at 405 nm using a plate reader

- Calculate the melanin concentration in each well using the calibration curve determined above
- Calculate cellular melanin concentration by dividing the [melanin] to the total number of cells in each well

## V.  VALIDATION OF IDENTIFIED CANDIDATES

### V.A.  Determine melanin concentration (total melanin/ total protein) of MNT1 cells expressing shRNA

- Plate MNT1 cells (pre-treated with PTU) in 6-well plates and allow them to grow to 50–80% confluence
- Generate lentiviral particles in HEK293FT cells (as described above) encoding shRNAs targeting transcripts identified as positive or negative regulators of pigmentation in the screen
- Transduce MNT1 cells with lentiviral particles and select with puromycin for 5 days
- Split each well of selected MNT1 cells into two wells
- Lyse cells in one of the two wells with Lysis Buffer and transfer to 1.5 ml tubes
- Centrifuge the lysate at 14,000 rpm for 30 minutes to separate the melanin from the soluble fraction (supernatant)
- Transfer the supernatant to a new 1.5 ml tube and measure its volume by pipetting, as precisely as possible
- Determine the protein content of each sample using a BCA protein assay kit
- Calculate the total protein for each sample by multiplying the protein concentration by its volume
- Add 100 µl of 1 N NaOH to the pellet containing melanin and incubate at 85°C for 1 h with intermittent vortexing to completely dissolve the melanin
- Measure the volume of the solubilized melanin by pipetting, as precisely as possible
- Determine the melanin concentration of the pellet by measuring absorbance at 405 nm with a spectrophotometer and using a calibration curve of synthetic melanin also obtained with a spectrophotometer (as in IV)
- Calculate total melanin content of each sample by multiplying the volume of the solubilized melanin by the melanin concentration
- Calculate melanin concentration for each sample by dividing the amount of total melanin by total protein, as calculated above

### V.B.  Determine mRNA levels of transcripts targeted by shRNA using qPCR

- Use the second well of selected MNT1 cells to extract RNA using the RNeasy Plus Kit (Qiagen)
- Reverse transcribe the extracted RNA using iScriptTM Reverse Transcription Supermix (Bio-Rad) and use the resulting cDNA for qPCR

- Set up qPCR reactions using an iTaqTM Universal SYBR Green Master MiX (Bio-Rad) and a VIIA-7 Real-Time PCR System (Applied Biosystems), according to the manufacturers' protocols
- The mRNA level of each targeted gene was determined relative to β-actin mRNA level in controls

## APPENDIX I – REAGENTS, VECTORS, AND PRIMERS

Reagents:

- TransIT-LT1: (Mirus, MIR 2300)
- Synthetic Melanin: (SIGMA, M0418-100MG)
- Polybrene: (SIGMA, H9268)
- N-Phenylthiourea/Propylthiouracil (PTU): (SIGMA, P7629)
- BCA protein assay kit: (PierceTM, ThermoFisher Scientific, 23227)
- Qiagen RNeasy Plus Kit: (Qiagen, 74134)
- iScriptTM Reverse Transcription Supermix: (Bio-Rad, 1708841)
- iTaqTM Universal SYBR Green Master MiX: (Bio-Rad, 1725121)
- VIIA-7 Real-Time PCR System: (Applied Biosystems System)
- Puromycin: (Invivo-Gen, ant-pr-1)
- 96-Well Clear Round Bottom: (Corning®, 3795)

Vectors:

- pLKO.1
- pCMVdeltaR8.9 (GenScript, lot: U9580CK130S-1/G193486)
- pVSV-G (GenScript, lot: U5824CI190S-1/G178153)
- GFP in pLKO.1 pRosetta: (Addgene #59700, pLKO.1 vector backbone)
- Non-target shRNA/PLKO.1(sh NT): (SIGMA, SHC002)
- Tyrosinase shRNA (sh TYR): (SIGMA, TRCN0000373833)
- mCherry-OCA2: pcDNA4TO vector backbone
- TPC2-mCherry/EGFP-N3: peGFP-C3 vector backbone
- piRFP-N3-Tyrosinase: (Addgene #80152, piRFP682 vector backbone)

qPCR Primers:

- TYR (NM_000372.5)
  - Forward: TGTCCCAGGTACAGGGATCT
  - Reverse: CTTCTTGAAGAGGACGGTGC
- OCA2 (NM_000275.3)
  - Forward: ATGTCCAGCTCCAGGTCTA
  - Reverse: TGAACTCTGGATGGTAAACAGG
- TPC2 (NM_139075.4)
  - Forward: CTGTGCCTCTTCACCATGT
  - Reverse: GCAGGTTCTGGAAGTAGGTC

- β-actin (NM_001101.5)
  - Forward: GGCATCCTCACCCTGAAGTA
  - Reverse: AGCACTGTGTTGGCGTACAG

## APPENDIX II – SOLUTIONS AND CELL MEDIA

MNT1 Media:

- 360 ml DMEM-GlutaMAX (ThermoFisher SCIENTIFIC, 10569044)
- 50 ml AIM (ThermoFisher SCIENTIFIC, 12055091)
- 90 ml Fetal Bovine Serum
- 5 ml Penicillin-Streptomycin (5,000 U/mL, ThermoFisher SCIENTIC, 15070063)

HEK293FT Media:

- 500 ml DMEM-GlutaMAX (ThermoFisher SCIENTIFIC, 10569044)
- 50 ml Fetal Bovine Serum
- 5 ml Penicillin-Streptomycin (5,000 U/mL, ThermoFisher SCIENTIFIC, 15070063)

HEK293FT High BSA Viral Harvesting Media:

- 500 ml DMEM-GlutaMAX (ThermoFisher SCIENTIFIC, 10569044)
- 50 ml Fetal Bovine Serum
- 5 ml Penicillin-Streptomycin (5,000 U/mL, ThermoFisher SCIENTIFIC, 15070063)
- 6.16 g BSA (FsherScientific, SH30574.02)

Lysis Buffer: 1% TRITON X-100 in 1× PBS, pH 7.4
Opti-MEM: (ThermoFisher SCIENTIFIC, 31985062)

## REFERENCES

"Broad institute protocols." https://portals.broadinstitute.org/gpp/public/resources/protocols.
"GeneCards." https://www.genecards.org/Guide/GeneCard.
"Genetics home refrence." https://ghr.nlm.nih.gov/condition/oculocutaneous-albinism.
"Homo sapiens; RNA-Seq - SRA - NCBI." https://www.ncbi.nlm.nih.gov/sra?term=SRX118281.
"The human protein atlas", https://www.proteinatlas.org/.
Ambrosio, A. L., J. A. Boyle, A. E. Aradi, K. A. Christian, and S. M. Di Pietro. 2016. "TPC2 controls pigmentation by regulating melanosome pH and size." *Proc Natl Acad Sci U S A* 113(20):5622–7. doi:10.1073/pnas.1600108113.
Ancans, J., D. J. Tobin, M. J. Hoogduijn, N. P. Smit, K. Wakamatsu, and A. J. Thody. 2001. "Melanosomal pH controls rate of melanogenesis, eumelanin/phaeomelanin ratio and melanosome maturation in melanocytes and melanoma cells." *Exp Cell Res* 268(1):26–35. doi:10.1006/excr.2001.5251.

Bar-Peled, L., and D. M. Sabatini. 2014. "Regulation of mTORC1 by amino acids." *Trends Cell Biol* 24(7):400–6. doi:10.1016/j.tcb.2014.03.003.

Bellono, N. W., I. E. Escobar, A. J. Lefkovith, M. S. Marks, and E. Oancea. 2014. "An intracellular anion channel critical for pigmentation." *eLife* 3:e04543. doi:10.7554/eLife.04543.

Bellono, N. W., I. E. Escobar, and E. Oancea. 2016. "A melanosomal two-pore sodium channel regulates pigmentation." *Sci Rep* 6:26570. doi:10.1038/srep26570.

Bellono, N. W., and E. V. Oancea. 2014. "Ion transport in pigmentation." *Arch Biochem Biophys* 563:35–41. doi:10.1016/j.abb.2014.06.020.

Bowman, S. L., J. Bi-Karchin, L. Le, and M. S. Marks. 2019. "The road to LROs: Insights into lysosome-related organelles from Hermansky-Pudlak syndrome and other rare diseases." *Traffic.* doi:10.1111/tra.12646.

Brilliant, M., and J. Gardner. 2001. "Melanosomal pH, pink locus protein and their roles in melanogenesis." *J Invest Dermatol* 117(2):386–7. doi:10.1046/j.0022-202x.2001.01462.x.

Chow, C. Y., Y. Zhang, J. J. Dowling, N. Jin, M. Adamska, K. Shiga, K. Szigeti, M. E. Shy, J. Li, X. Zhang, J. R. Lupski, L. S. Weisman, and M. H. Meisler. 2007. "Mutation of FIG4 causes neurodegeneration in the pale tremor mouse and patients with CMT4J." *Nature* 448(7149):68–72. doi:10.1038/nature05876.

DeFelice, L. J., and T. Goswami. 2007. "Transporters as channels." *Annu Rev Physiol* 69:87–112. doi:10.1146/annurev.physiol.69.031905.164816.

Faundez, V., and H. C. Hartzell. 2004. "Intracellular chloride channels: Determinants of function in the endosomal pathway." *Sci STKE* 2004(233):re8. doi:10.1126/stke.2332004re8.

Halaban, R., R. S. Patton, E. Cheng, S. Svedine, E. S. Trombetta, M. L. Wahl, S. Ariyan, and D. N. Hebert. 2002. "Abnormal acidification of melanoma cells induces tyrosinase retention in the early secretory pathway." *J Biol Chem* 277(17):14821–8. doi:10.1074/jbc.M111497200.

Haltaufderhyde, K. D., and E. Oancea. 2014. "Genome-wide transcriptome analysis of human epidermal melanocytes." *Genomics* 104(6):482–9. doi:10.1016/j.ygeno.2014.09.010.

Hearing, V. J. 2005. "Biogenesis of pigment granules: A sensitive way to regulate melanocyte function." *J Dermatol Sci* 37(1):3–14. doi:10.1016/j.jdermsci.2004.08.014.

Jentsch, Thomas J. 2015. "Discovery of CLC transport proteins: Cloning, structure, function and pathophysiology." *J Physiol* 593(18):4091–109. doi:10.1113/jp270043.

Kausar, T., M. A. Bhatti, M. Ali, R. S. Shaikh, and Z. M. Ahmed. 2013. "OCA5, a novel locus for non-syndromic oculocutaneous albinism, maps to chromosome 4q24." *Clin Genet* 84(1):91–3. doi:10.1111/cge.12019.

Lin, J. Y., and D. E. Fisher. 2007. "Melanocyte biology and skin pigmentation." *Nature* 445(7130):843–50. doi:10.1038/nature05660.

Luande, J., C. I. Henschke, and N. Mohammed. 1985. "The Tanzanian human albino skin. Natural history." *Cancer* 55(8):1823–8.

Marks, M. S., and M. C. Seabra. 2001. "The melanosome: Membrane dynamics in black and white." *Nat Rev Mol Cell Biol* 2(10):738–48. doi:10.1038/35096009.

Milkereit, R., A. Persaud, L. Vanoaica, A. Guetg, F. Verrey, and D. Rotin. 2015. "LAPTM4b recruits the LAT1-4F2hc Leu transporter to lysosomes and promotes mTORC1 activation." *Nat Commun* 6:7250. doi:10.1038/ncomms8250.

Mindell, J. A. 2012. "Lysosomal acidification mechanisms." *Annu Rev Physiol* 74:69–86. doi:10.1146/annurev-physiol-012110-142317.

Montoliu, L., K. Gronskov, A. H. Wei, M. Martinez-Garcia, A. Fernandez, B. Arveiler, F. Morice-Picard, S. Riazuddin, T. Suzuki, Z. M. Ahmed, T. Rosenberg, and W. Li. 2014. "Increasing the complexity: New genes and new types of albinism." *Pigment Cell Melanoma Res* 27(1):11–8. doi:10.1111/pcmr.12167.

Olivares, C., and F. Solano. 2009. "New insights into the active site structure and cata-lytic mechanism of tyrosinase and its related proteins." *Pigment Cell Melanoma Res* 22(6):750–60. doi:10.1111/j.1755-148X.2009.00636.x.

Ozdeslik, R. N., L. E. Olinski, M. Trieu, D. Oprian,and E. Oancea. 2019. "The human nonvi-sual opsin 3 regulates pigmentation of epidermal melanocytes through functional inter-action with melanocortin 1 receptor." *PNAS 2019* 116(23):11508–11517. doi: 10.1073/pnas.1902825116.

Raposo, G., and M. S. Marks. 2007. "Melanosomes--Dark organelles enlighten endosomal membrane transport." *Nat Rev Mol Cell Biol* 8(10):786–97. doi:10.1038/nrm2258.

Reemann, P., E. Reimann, S. Ilmjarv, O. Porosaar, H. Silm, V. Jaks, E. Vasar, K. Kingo, and S. Koks. 2014. "Melanocytes in the skin--Comparative whole transcriptome analysis of main skin cell types." *PLoS one* 9(12):e115717. doi:10.1371/journal.pone.0115717.

Schiaffino, M. V., and C. Tacchetti. 2005. "The ocular albinism type 1 (OA1) protein and the evidence for an intracellular signal transduction system involved in melanosome bio-genesis." *Pigment Cell Res* 18(4):227–33. doi:10.1111/j.1600-0749.2005.00240.x.

Schioth, H. B., S. R. Phillips, R. Rudzish, M. A. Birch-Machin, J. E. Wikberg, and J. L. Rees. 1999. "Loss of function mutations of the human melanocortin 1 receptor are com-mon and are associated with red hair." *Biochem Biophys Res Commun* 260(2):488–91. doi:10.1006/bbrc.1999.0935.

Setty, S. R., D. Tenza, E. V. Sviderskaya, D. C. Bennett, G. Raposo, and M. S. Marks. 2008. "Cell-specific ATP7A transport sustains copper-dependent tyrosinase activity in mela-nosomes." *Nature* 454(7208):1142–6. doi:10.1038/nature07163.

Stauber, T., and T. J. Jentsch. 2013. "Chloride in vesicular trafficking and function." *Annu Rev Physiol* 75:453–77. doi:10.1146/annurev-physiol-030212-183702.

Wang, N., and D. N. Hebert. 2006. "Tyrosinase maturation through the mamma-lian secretory pathway: Bringing color to life." *Pigment Cell Res* 19(1):3–18. doi:10.1111/j.1600-0749.2005.00288.x.

Wang, S., Z. Y. Tsun, R. L. Wolfson, K. Shen, G. A. Wyant, M. E. Plovanich, E. D. Yuan, T. D. Jones, L. Chantranupong, W. Comb, T. Wang, L. Bar-Peled, R. Zoncu, C. Straub, C. Kim, J. Park, B. L. Sabatini, and D. M. Sabatini. 2015. "Metabolism. Lysosomal amino acid transporter SLC38A9 signals arginine sufficiency to mTORC1." *Science* 347(6218):188–94. doi:10.1126/science.1257132.

Wicks, N. L., J. W. Chan, J. A. Najera, J. M. Ciriello, and E. Oancea. 2011. "UVA phototrans-duction drives early melanin synthesis in human melanocytes." *Curr Biol* 21(22):1906–11. doi:10.1016/j.cub.2011.09.047.

Wolf Horrell, E. M., M. C. Boulanger, and J. A. D'Orazio. 2016. "Melanocortin 1 receptor: Structure, function, and regulation." *Front Genet* 7:95. doi:10.3389/fgene.2016.00095.

# Index

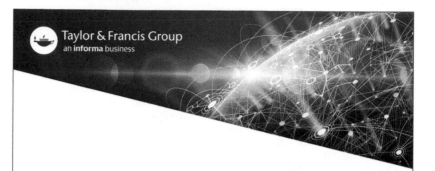